Beyond Infertility

THE NEW PATHS TO PARENTHOOD

Susan Lewis Cooper
Ellen Sarasohn Glazer

LEXINGTON BOOKS
An Imprint of Macmillan, Inc.
NEW YORK

Maxwell Macmillan Canada
TORONTO

Maxwell Macmillan International
NEW YORK   OXFORD   SINGAPORE   SYDNEY

April, 1994

Library of Congress Cataloging-in-Publication Data

Cooper, Susan
　　Beyond infertility : the new paths to parenthood /
Susan Lewis Cooper, Ellen Sarasohn Glazer.
　　　　p. cm.
　　Includes bibliographical references and index.
　　ISBN 0-02-911813-1
　　1. Human reproductive technology—Popular works. 2. Infertility—
Psychological aspects
I. Glazer, Ellen Sarasohn. II. Title.
RG133.5.C67　1994
616.6'9206–dc20　　　　　　　　　　　　　　　　　93-50684
　　　　　　　　　　　　　　　　　　　　　　　　　　CIP

Copyright © 1994 by Lexington Books
An Imprint of Macmillan, Inc.

Lexington Books
An Imprint of Macmillan, Inc.
866 Third Avenue, New York, N. Y. 10022

Maxwell Macmillan Canada, Inc.
1200 Eglinton Avenue East
Suite 200
Don Mills, Ontario M3C 3N1

Macmillan, Inc. is part of the Maxwell Communication
Group of Companies.

Printed in the United States of America
printing number

1 2 3 4 5 6 7 8 9 10

*For the women and men who have included us
in their journey through infertility: their struggles
and their resilience enabled us to write this book.*

Contents

Acknowledgments

Although we are solely responsible for the content of this book, we are well aware that it is the product of the wisdom and experience of many people, without whom it could never have been written. First and foremost, we thank our patients, to whom this book is dedicated. They have informed our work over the years and challenged us in immeasurable ways. The case examples and the quotations throughout the book come directly from them; indirectly their teachings and their presence are a part of every page. Most important, as we said in our dedication, their determination, struggle, and resilience have taught us that people can indeed move beyond infertility.

We are fortunate to have access to the finest physicians and medical personnel, who are not only skilled practitioners but compassionate human beings. Peter Martin, M.D., reviewed chapters 1 and 9. He also suggested that we put together a glossary and helped us with it. Patricia McShane, M.D., reviewed chapters 5 and 6. Natalie Schultz, M.D., reviewed chapter 8 and helped with chapter 3. Steven Bayer, M.D., helped with chapter 3. In addition, Shari Litch, Ph.D., helped with chapters 5 and 9, and Anne Danforth, R.N., provided careful explanations about many of the protocols involved in ART treatment. We thank them all.

There were many professionals throughout the country who willingly offered their expertise and patiently responded to our telephone calls for information or explanations. In particular, we thank Andrea Braverman, Ph.D., for her help with the chapters on gestational care and ovum donation. Her insight and wisdom, as well as discussions about terminology, guided us at many points along the way. We thank Ali Domar, Ph.D., for discussing her research with us on the Mind/Body Program and for sending us her articles, and Elaine Gordon, Ph.D., for her insights about ovum donation and embryo adoption.

Susan Crockin also helped us immeasurably. Her knowledge of reproductive law and her familiarity with litigation in the field assured us that we were receiving the most accurate information. Our legal knowledge, and we hope the reader's, benefited greatly from her expertise.

We thank Nancy Hughes, Ph.D., of Hagar Associates in Topeka, Kansas, for her help with chapters 7 and 8. We also thank William Handel, Ralph Fagan, and Hilary Hanafin, Ph.D., at the Center for Surrogate Parenting, for sharing their expertise and experience with surrogacy and for welcoming Ellen at their center. Without their help, chapters 7 and 8 could not have been written. In particular, Hilary Hanafin offered immeasurable help. With graciousness and clarity, she communicated her depth of understanding of surrogacy. In addition, Shirley Zager of the Organization for Parenting Through Surrogacy, and Fay Johnson, director of its national headquarters, contributed immensely to our knowledge of surrogacy. We appreciate having been able to hook up with Fay in New Hampshire over lunch.

Jean Kollantai of the Center for Loss in Multiple Birth was also a great help in our chapter on pregnancy loss. She went out of her way to educate us about the many dimensions of loss in multiple gestation.

Barbara Raboy of the Sperm Bank of California, Ronda Wilkin of California Cryobank, and Lisa Aymat of Xytex patiently answered countless questions about their policies and procedures. We were impressed with how all of these banks, though very different, are grappling with many of the psychosocial and ethical issues discussed in chapter 5.

Judith Ribbler, M.L.S. information specialist extraordinaire, as well as Susan's friend and running partner, was always available, and always willing, to do yet another search—always late at night because she insisted on saving us money. We appreciate her diligence and support.

Margaret Zusky, our editor, believed in this book from day one. More important, she believed that we could write it together. Her faith that our different styles would enhance the book rather than detract from it kept us going when we were feeling most doubtful.

A number of other individuals graciously responded to our requests for contact and information, and each, in her own way, has added to our book: Marie Campo, Debbie Howell, Booker Heppenstall, Stacy Lee, Cristy Montgomery, and Candace Turner.

We are fortunate to belong to the Psychological Special Interest Group of the American Fertility Society. This group consists of professionals from across the country who are interested in the psychological aspects of infertility. Over the past four years, through this organization, we have met a number of highly skilled, perceptive clinicians who have added to our knowledge and have helped to shape our thinking. Although space does not permit us to list the countless names of members, we want to acknowledge this important organization.

We are privileged to live in an area where there are not only many skilled physicians but also many skilled therapists and counselors as well. We have had the benefit and opportunity of meeting monthly with nine other colleagues—all professionals from various mental health disciplines—in what has come to be a peer support and supervision group, which we affectionately refer to as the Friday Group. During our meetings we discuss and debate current issues in infertility, as well as psychological and ethical dilemmas. We also discuss difficult cases and offer help to one another when it is requested. In a field that unfortunately all too often breeds competition, our Friday Group is refreshingly collaborative in nature. The mutual enrichment the group offers is indeed special, and our thinking (as well as our clinical judgment) has been influenced by each group member. Because each person contributes a unique perspective to the group and has enriched our experience in her own way, we thank each person individually: Judith Bernstein, R.N.C., M.S.N.; Alma Berson, Ph.D.; Mara Brill, M.D.; Geri Ferber, Ph.D.; Adele Kauffman, Ph.D.; Susan Levin, LICSW; Deborah Silverstein, LICSW; Jeane Springer; LICSW; Sharon Steinberg; R.N., M.S. In particular, we thank Susan Levin, Jeane Springer, and Sharon Steinberg for working with us on the ovum donation chapter. Their contributions enriched the material.

No book on infertility would be complete without mentioning RESOLVE Inc. It was through RESOLVE that we first met and through RESOLVE that we found an outlet for both our personal and professional interest in infertility. RESOLVE, founded by Barbara Eck Menning, serves as an anchor for infertile people, as it once was an anchor for us.

S.L.C., E. S. G.

There have been many moments over the past eighteen months, particularly in the last few, when I had a difficult time reconciling how I could be writing a book for people who desperately wanted to become parents while at the same time ignoring my own children. I had to trust that the strength of family bonds would result in their forgiveness. I am well aware, however, that this chapter in all of our lives will be remembered as a time when Mom was almost always irritable and their reasonable requests were too often denied. Though now sixteen and twelve, my children, Seth and Amanda, are the real reason I wrote this book. If I had not had to struggle to get them, I would never have known the torment of infertility, and in all likelihood my career would have taken another direction. I want to thank Seth and Amanda for their interest in and support of my work, and for their pride in me, which I know is always there, even when I am barely being civil. I thank my husband, Marc, who was also ignored for most of the past eighteen months. Without his (almost) unqualified support of my writing endeavor, I doubt that I could have written this book. His confidence in me gave me a needed boost when my spirits were low.

I thank my parents, Doris and Allen Lewis, for being proud and devoted parents and grandparents and for being understanding when they too were being ignored.

I thank my college roommate, Marjorie Saltzberg, CSW, for reading an early draft of chapter 1, for her feedback and perceptions, and for always being there. Deborah Silverstein, LICSW, friend and colleague at Focus Counseling and Consultation, Inc. also read an early draft of chapter 1 and substituted for me at IVF America-Boston this past summer, so I could write this book. Deborah has been an important influence in shaping the way I have come to understand adoption, including the adoption of gametes. Her clear perceptions and insights have helped clarify my own views. I wish also to thank my friend and colleague, Cathy Heenan, Ed.D., for her wise counsel; I have come to rely on it. Although she has not read parts of the book, she has been part of my process.

In considering those factors that helped keep me sane this year, I think about Focus, a home for the past fifteen years. Focus has always been a stable force in my life—another place to grow professionally, to keep me balanced, and to remind me that working in an infertility setting, though immeasurably challenging and fulfilling, is not the only clinical work I enjoy.

Finally, I thank everyone at IVF America Program-Boston who has been a source of support, learning, and inspiration over the past four and a half years. I came to IVFA 'accidentally,' but it has been one of the most gratifying 'accidents' I have ever had. Working there has provided me with many opportunities for which I am extremely grateful: to be involved in a clinic that is doing state-of-the-art medicine—and doing it with utmost skill and integrity; to work with some of the finest and most compassionate physicians I have ever encountered; and to work as part of a team that puts patients' needs first. Although the staff is too large for me to thank everyone, a few people have been extremely helpful to me, especially this past year while working on this book. Patricia McShane, M.D., medical director of IVF America, who helped with this book, is an outstanding, caring physician. Her sound medical judgment and keen understanding of the emotional and psychosocial impact of infertility is something I have come to count on. Peter Martin, M.D., who also helped with this book, is another person I have come to rely on for similar reasons. He puts patients first; the only times I have ever heard him complain or get upset are when some inefficiency in the system has, or might, cause hardship or inconvenience to a patient. Lee Hoffman, executive director, is a wonderful and supportive boss, and I thank her for trusting and valuing me. I thank Anne Danforth, R.N., manager of patient services, who mysteriously manages to keep track of everything that is happening in the program—and to solve problems as well. She has been an important source of help and support at work. Finally, I thank my colleague, partner, and friend, Adele Kauffman, Ph.D. She has offered me the benefit of her careful judgment, provided needed support, and been a sounding board when I needed one.

S.L.C.

First and foremost, I thank my daughters, Elizabeth and Mollie Glazer. Without their patience and acceptance, I would never have been able to prepare this manuscript. They allowed me to hog the computer, to edit on family vacations, and to spend time in New Hampshire with Susan. Beyond tolerating the preparation of this manuscript, they were each immensely helpful to me as I grappled with questions involving the best interests or children. I greatly appreciated their candid reactions to each of the third party parenting options and feel proud of the depth of understanding that they have about assisted reproduction. Now, as in times past, they are the reason I write about parenthood.

There are several people in my personal and professional lives without whose help I could not have completed this project. Each was there with what I needed, when I needed it.

My running buddy, Natalie Schultz, M.D., was there each day at 5:30 A.M.—come rain, snow, sleet, or hail. In addition to her companionship, which I treasure, she provided me with medical information and consultation. I respect and admire the good judgment and compassion that she brings to the practice of reproductive medicine.

Steve Bayer, M.D., my colleague and friend, was gracious and responsive when I went to him with medical questions. I continue to appreciate the support that he offers to my clinical practice as well as my writing.

Larry Selter, M.D., helped me remain emotionally grounded while writing this book. He enabled me to see that the project could—and should—unfold in unexpected ways and to appreciate the rewards that could come from the process as well as the product.

Roanne Weisman, my friend and neighbor, willingly provided a home away from home for my chapters. She offered me the peace of mind of knowing that if my house burned down, or if robbers decided to come and steal the manuscript, all would not be lost.

Finally, I thank my friend and colleague, Sylvia Freed, LICSW. For this project, as for earlier ones, she offered a sense of humor, a willing distraction, and a shoulder to lean on.

There are several people who, although they did not have direct involvement in this book, have informed my thinking and shaped my career. Without their wisdom and guidance, I would not have been able to write this book.

I am especially indebted to the staff at the Fertility Center at New England Memorial Hospital in Stoneham, Massachusetts. At a time when many are questioning the quality and ethics of medical care, it is indeed a pleasure and a privilege to be part of such a responsible and compassionate medical team. Although I am unable to list the entire staff—which numbers over fifty individuals—I do want to acknowledge the contributions of certain of my colleagues.

In addition to Steve Bayer, M.D., whom I mentioned earlier, I thank Rob McInnes, M.D., Nancy Harrington, R.N., and Paula Ayers, R.N. I feel respect and gratitude, also, to the program's former medical director, Vito Cardone, M.D. and its former biologist, Michael Lee, M.A. Both are outstanding professionals who taught me a great deal.

Joan Jack of Serono Symposia, USA, has offered me a range of professional opportunities over the past few years. Many of these have enabled me to develop comfort and experience in public speaking.

Michael Hubner, LICSW, has shared her expertise in cancer and infertility. By introducing me to the medical, emotional, social and ethical issues involved in this dual diagnosis, she enabled me to do some of the most satisfying work of my career.

Margarete Sandelowski, Phd., Betty Harris, Phd., and Diane Holditch-Davis, Phd., have written several wise and insightful papers which have been immeasurably helpful to me. Although I have never spoken with any of them directly, their cogent observations of infertility have helped shape my thinking.

A special thanks to my parents, Ira Sarasohn and Shirlee Sarasohn, and my step-mother, Helen Sarasohn. They taught me, long ago, that loving families can be formed in "nontraditional" ways. I feel extraordinarily fortunate to have all of them there for me.

Finally, I thank the Cooper family: Marc, for loaning me Susan for eighteen months (and always maintaining a sense of humor about it!); Seth, for attempting (unsuccessfully) to tackle my computer phobia; and Amanda, for caring for my dog, J.P, when I was too busy and too frazzled to tend to him.

E.S.G.

Introduction

Beyond Infertility began as a second edition of our first book, *Without Child*. Published in 1988, *Without Child* was our attempt to present, mainly through the writings of others, a comprehensive look at the experience of infertility. As it went to press, however, we realized that although it captured the timeless emotions of infertility, dramatic changes in the field of reproductive medicine—in particular, the rapid proliferation of advanced reproductive technology—would soon make parts of the book outdated.

In 1990 we decided that the time had come to update *Without Child*. We thought it would be a simple project. With the addition of some medical facts here and there, a chapter on ovum donation, and some new essays, we would have an infertility book for the 1990s. Slowly and hesitantly we began to work on revising our book. With the passage of another year, however, we realized that we had not made much progress. As we explored the reasons and attempted to develop a plan, we realized that neither of us was excited about revising that book. By then, it had become clear to us how dramatically the world of reproductive medicine had changed and how much we had learned. We had to begin again.

And so *Beyond Infertility* was conceived. It has had a lengthy gestation, and the process of writing it has been complex and challenging for both of us in a number of ways. *Beyond Infertility* has forced each of us individually, and the two of us as coauthors, to confront the depth of emotions involved in infertility. They are emotions that we thought we knew well, both as former infertility patients and as long-time mental health clinicians in the field. What we did not realize, however, was the degree to which the expansion of reproductive options has intensified the feelings that people have about infertility, as well as their determination to fight it.

Writing *Beyond Infertility* has also forced us to take a careful look at the medical advances in reproductive medicine and to examine what they mean. In our practices, we see countless couples going through the various assisted reproductive procedures. We also see people setting out on new frontiers such as microinsemination. What we did not fully appreciate, however, until half way through this book, were the ways in which in vitro fertilization (IVF) revolutionized and redefined reproduction. Its arrival in 1978 opened doors to an array of new reproductive options, and those options brought on their heels many new dilemmas and decisions.

We had many memorable and enjoyable moments together. *Beyond Infertility* was written not only on our individual computers but also on long runs or walks around the Brookline reservoir. It was debated on airplanes, edited in a canoe, expanded at the New Orleans zoo, and often conceptualized over ice cream or sushi.

Writing *Beyond Infertility* has also taken us on difficult personal journeys. We set out as close friends and colleagues who rarely disagreed with each other. It never occurred to us that writing a book together (which we had done before) could push our relationship to the limit and that there would be moments when we each felt like resigning from the project. Some of our difficulties, we realized, had to do with the weight of the material; we were struggling with social, psychological, emotional, and ethical questions that had no simple answers—or any answers at all. Other difficulties stemmed from the fact that two strong-willed people—each of whom is always right—were trying to collaborate. Thankfully, our friendship has endured, and even flourished, in our struggles. We hope that the book that has emerged out of this process, although different from one we would each have written alone, reflects the best of us. We hope it combines our differences in a way that illuminates the material, makes it easily readable, and does justice to the profound nature of the subject matter.

Over the past fifteen years we have borne witness to revolutionary changes in reproductive medicine. Vast numbers of couples who were once considered sterile become parents through the assisted reproductive technologies. At the same time, increasing numbers of people, faced with an irreparable reproductive loss, have turned to third-party parenting options such as ovum or sperm donation, surrogacy, and gestational care. In sitting with couples, hearing their stories and listening to their pain, we have learned a great deal about the experience of infertility. In having the privilege of working with exceptional physicians, embryologists, and nurses, we have also had the opportunity to expand our medical knowledge greatly. *Beyond Infertility* is our attempt to pass our understanding and knowledge on to others.

We have come to understand from our patients—and from searching our own souls as well—that people have intense and often very different feelings about genetic continuity. There are those for whom continuing bloodlines or lineage is essential, others for whom passing on traits means a great deal, and still others for whom genetics is unimportant but for whom the biological experience of pregnancy and childbirth is a major longing. The significance people attach to these various aspects of reproduction and parenting in large measure determines the decisions they make and the paths they take.

The new reproductive possibilities indeed create profound dilemmas, choices, and decisions. In *Beyond Infertility* we look at the ways in which couples confront these choices. Although certain patterns emerge, the journey through infertility varies considerably from one couple to another. Some of these differences have to do with diagnosis, cost, availability of treatment, and geography; others have to do with temperament and stamina and the feelings people have, as individuals and as a couple, about the nature of parenthood. We hope that it will be clear throughout this book that the decisions that are right for one couple are not necessarily right for another.

Beyond Infertility is about the remarkable advances in reproductive medicine, the decisions facing infertile people as a result of those advances, and the intense emotions that accompany them throughout their experience. Although these emotions are timeless, there are several ethical dilemmas that have arisen only in recent years. We see throughout the book that the new reproductive options involve complex, and often disturbing, questions about what is in the best interest of children. For instance: Is it in the best interest of any child to be the product of third-party reproduction? Is it in the best interest of a child to know the truth about his or her origins, if knowledge of that truth may potentially give rise to conflict about one's identity? Is it in the best interest for adults to create new children through donor gametes when there are vast numbers of existing children without parents? Believing that reproductive decisions should be guided by a respect for the rights of unborn children, yet empathizing with the pain of infertile people, we see, throughout much of this book, that profound conflicts arise between the longings of adults to reproduce and the needs of both existing and unborn children.

Our readers need an explanation about what is missing in this book. Although it is written for everyone who is infertile, it is written in language directed toward heterosexual couples. Our intention is not to exclude single people or lesbian couples, because we know well that both groups suffer the pain of infertility—pain that is intensified by the fact that their sorrow is less often appreciated and understood and by the fact that their access to treatment may be more limited. Rather, for the sake of simplicity and because most people currently pursuing treatment are heterosexual couples, it was impossible, in the space we had, to do justice to the infertility experiences of single women and lesbian couples. We hope, however, that most of what is included will be of relevance and help to each of these groups.

Our readers will notice that we make virtually no mention of secondary infertility (infertility that occurs after a couple has had a biological child), despite the fact that as many as one-third of the couples we see already have a child. With divorce and second marriages, there are also increasing numbers of couples in which one or both partners has a child(ren) from another marriage. Again, we do not address these groups directly because of space limitations. We believe, however, that much of what we say pertains to couples with secondary infertility.

Another group, which we mention only briefly in one chapter, are grandparents. We are keenly aware of the pain felt by the parents of infertile couples and, though to a lesser extent, the pain of many parents of gamete donors and surrogates. *Beyond Infertility* is largely about loss, and thus it is important to acknowledge that "infertile grandparents" also suffer loss: the actual or threatened loss of their grandchildren and the loss of time. Although many of their children will become parents, one way or another, the years of struggle with infertility will rob everyone of precious grandparenting time.

Readers will notice also that we have not included chapters on two important options for resolving infertility. One is traditional adoption, a time-honored alternative path to parenthood. It is a very large topic, and there are many excellent and current books on this subject; furthermore, the process does not involve reproductive medicine. The second option not included is child-free living, as it too is unrelated to reproductive medicine.

We have divided *Beyond Infertility* into two parts. The first half of the book focuses on the pursuit—and specifically, the high-tech pursuit—of biogenetic children. We begin with a general discussion of the emotional experience of infertile couples in the 1990s and then follow them through their experiences with assisted reproductive technology (ART). We also discuss the excruciatingly difficult experience of those couples who achieve pregnancy through the ARTs, only to go on to suffer pregnancy loss. The first part of the book ends with an examination of the process of moving on. There we look at how a couple decides that they are ready to let go of the hope they will conceive and bear a child together. Chapter 4 is about letting go and moving on.

The second half of the book focuses on alternative paths to parenthood: third-party reproduction. Ironically, two of these alternatives, donor insemination and surrogacy, do not rely on advances in reproductive medicine. They have existed for a long time; according to some historians, they date back to the Bible. However, it has been primarily in the last decade that both ethicists and mental health professionals have taken an in-depth look at whether, due to psychosocial issues generated by third-party reproduction, these options are in the best interest of children.

One of the biggest challenges we faced in writing this book—the magnitude and complexity of which we had not anticipated—involved language. More specifically, our problem involved arriving at the language that best expresses how we conceptualize some of the reproductive options (and processes) described in this book. In our efforts to find and use language that was both descriptive and respectful, we encountered some perplexing dilemmas. The one that was most troubling was what to call the process by which one woman gestates a baby for another couple. This process, commonly referred to as *gestational surrogacy* or *gestational carrier* programs is an option that has ties to two distinct areas: surrogacy and in vitro fertilization Because we understand and respect both sides of the debate, we wanted to find language that captured most accurately our understanding of this option, without offending those who are involved with it daily. We eventually decided to call the process *gestational care*, and the woman who gestates the baby the gestational carrier (or carrier).

Another language dilemma we encountered was what to call a child who is born from and genetically connected to both parents. Although the terms *biological child* and *genetic child* are used interchangeably by most people, we decided to refer to the offspring just described as *biogenetic children*, a term we feel captures the connections they have to their parents through both pregnancy and genes. In chapter 6 we refer to the woman who gestates and births her child as a result of ovum donation as the *biological mother*, because she has a biological connection to her child through the process of gestation and birth, although she does not have a genetic connection to him/her. In chapter 8 we refer to the woman who provides an egg, used to create an embryo/fetus that is gestated by another woman, as the *genetic mother*.

A third language question arose each time we referred to the mental health professionals working in infertility centers. Since psychiatrists, psychologists, clinical social workers and psychiatric nurses all work with infertility patients, we wanted to emphasize this point. Thus rather than select a generic term, such as program counselor, we decided to make reference to each of these disciplines at various points throughout the book. When case material is presented we use the title of the clinician familiar with the case.

As *Beyond Infertility* goes to press, we find ourselves reflecting back on why we wrote this book. We would be dishonest if we do not say it had something to do with helping our personal careers as well as our self-esteem as professionals. Such motivations are always true for professionals who write. But primarily we wrote this book because it was a way to challenge us in our work, because we feel profoundly connected to the struggles of infertile people, and because it was inside us crying to be born. Although we know that in this rapidly progressing field of reproductive technology, (even as we write this news is breaking about the cloning of embryos) it may be outdated almost as soon as it is published, we hope that our readers will find *Beyond Infertility* a valuable resource—at least throughout the nineties.

PART 1

The Pursuit of High Technological Treatment

1

The Emotional Experience
of Infertility

The book of Samuel in the Old Testament tells the story of Elkanah, a pious man who has two wives, Hannah and Peninnah. Peninnah has many children, but Hannah, his more beloved wife, is barren. Peninnah taunts Hannah that the Lord has shut up her womb. Hannah weeps and cannot eat. Elkanah asks, "Hannah, why weepest thou? And why eatest thou not? And why is thy heart grieved? Am not I better to thee than ten sons?" Later Hannah prays to the Lord and weeps again, vowing that if the Lord gives her a son, then she "will give him unto the Lord all the days of his life, and there shall be no razor come upon his head." As Hannah is praying, Eli, the priest, watches her lips moving, though no sound emerges from her. He assumes that she is drunk and asks her to put away her wine. Hannah speaks intensely: "I am a woman of a sorrowful spirit; I have drunk neither wine nor strong drink, but I poured out my soul before the Lord." Eli responds by reassuring her that the Lord will answer her prayers. As promised, Hannah conceives, bearing a son, Samuel.

Although the Old Testament is replete with references to infertility, the story of Hannah is especially important because it illustrates the timelessness of the emotions that surround infertility. We see in this short passage the pain of an infertile woman, overcome with despair. She is so saddened by her condition that she is unable to eat, and she cries frequently. Furthermore, she is pained and jealous by the fecundity of her rival, who appears insensitive to her condition. Her husband, Elkanah, feeling helpless and desperate to make her happier, attempts to use logic to help her feel better. Like many of today's husbands, he cannot understand why his love of her, and the special attention he gives her, is not enough to make her happy.

Hannah, like many of today's infertile women, looks outside her marriage for support and understanding. She turns to Eli, the high priest, hoping that he will understand her feelings, but he too fails to understand her pain and mistakes her grief for intoxication. Finally, Hannah, resorts to bargaining with God—practically giving up her very soul—in her desperation to conceive.

Thousands of years later, infertility remains a common and intensely painful experience, afflicting approximately one in six couples of reproductive age. Although the medical picture has changed drastically from when prayer was the only "cure," all the emotions expressed in Hannah's story—depression, jealousy, helplessness, despair, misunderstanding, and insensitivity—are, to greater or lesser degrees, a part of every infertile couple's experience.

As recently as a generation ago, many people believed the emotions that infertile women felt were their own doing, that infertility was "in a woman's head." Women were told (and still are told) to relax, take a vacation, stop trying so hard, or adopt—and they would become pregnant. The common belief among psychiatrists and psychologists was that underlying psychopathology was the root of infertility. Studies about the psychological aspects of infertility were aimed at proving this point. The pathology attributed to infertile women included unconscious hostility toward their mothers and toward the female role, unresolved oedipal issues, and other demeaning psychological interpretations. In other words, underlying psychopathology and unresolved emotional conflicts were thought to be a primary cause of infertility. Much more is understood today about the medical causes of infertility, and it is well recognized among physicians, as well as mental health professionals who treat infertile couples, that psychological stress is a by-product of infertility rather than a primary cause of it.

There are many people outside the field of reproductive technology who believe that the new technologies are a shot in the dark and that infertile couples who go to great lengths to achieve pregnancy are more psychologically disturbed than those who end treatment before subjecting themselves to its rigors. They see these couples as being lost in endless, blind pursuit of pregnancy, unable or unwilling to accept reality. Although there are occasionally infertile couples who are unbalanced, mental health professionals have not come to this conclusion, through either clinical work or research. Mazure and Greenfeld, a psychologist and clinical social worker as well as researchers in the field of infertility, also concluded that infertile women are not more disturbed than their fertile counterparts. After reviewing dozens of research articles about psychological issues related to in vitro fertilization (IVF) treatment, they summarized their conclusions in the following way:

> Probably the single most important finding has been that, in general, IVF/ET [embryo transfer] participants score within normal limits on measurements of preexisting psychopathology. Furthermore, the data do not support the notion of an increased incidence of psychiatric diagnoses or psychosexual disorders in IVF/ET participants. In fact, the data suggest that these couples often present with considerable psychological determination and some may have developed ways of managing stress without becoming overtly anxious.[1]

Estimates are that between 30 and 40 percent of infertility problems reside exclusively in the woman, 30 to 40 percent exclusively in the man, and approximately 30 to 40 percent are shared between husband and wife. Because of the remarkable achievements in the field of reproductive medicine, more than half of all couples who are treated for infertility eventually give birth to biological children. Those who do are eternally grateful, though the emotional experience of infertility is not erased by the birth of a healthy child, as the birth often comes only after prolonged suffering.

The assisted reproductive technologies (commonly referred to as the ARTs) have revolutionized the field of reproductive medicine. Couples once considered sterile have gone on to have successful pregnancies and healthy babies. Although the new technologies are remarkable, they involve enormous physical and emotional energy, a large financial investment (except for those couples who have insurance coverage), and medical risk. Those who decide to undergo one or more cycles of assisted reproductive technology usually do so only after extensive treatment has resulted in repeated failure. Couples therefore approach the new technologies feeling much like

Hannah did when she approached Eli, the priest: helpless, hopeless, depressed, jealous, and despairing.

Beyond Infertility focuses on the new reproductive technologies and on third-party medical alternatives to biogenetic parenting. However, in order to understand what faces a couple about to embark in the world of ART, it is necessary to understand where they have been—socially, emotionally, and psychologically. Thus we begin our book by focusing on the couple's emotional experience of infertility prior to undergoing ART.

Emotional Effects of Infertility on Women

From the time they are young girls and become aware of pregnancy, most women learn (and believe) that their biological destiny is to bear children. Although times have changed dramatically and men's and women's roles are no longer so rigid, most women today were raised to expect that they will be the primary caretakers of their children. No matter to what extent a woman has developed a career or a professional identity, the image of herself as a mother tends to be the psychological backdrop from which she operates. When a woman decides to have children but discovers she is infertile, her self-image is assaulted.

If much of her personal identity is tied to being a mother, an infertile woman is likely to feel that her life has no purpose. She may feel she is no longer sexually desirable. She may suffer feelings of inadequacy, fearing she is unlovable and unable to nurture. Like Hannah, women who strongly desire children may become despondent, feeling helpless and out of control. In general, the longer that infertility continues, the more helpless they feel, and the more helpless they feel, the more depressed they become.

In an effort to cope with their infertility, many women search for an explanation for their affliction. They examine their lives and may conclude they are being punished for an unforgivable past sin. Often they become plagued by guilt remembering acts of pride or vanity or focusing on imagined moral failings. If the woman has been sexually active in the past, she may decide that she is being punished for sexual transgressions—that her pelvic inflammatory disease or adhesions are a message from God that she went astray. Similarly, women who had prior abortions or gave birth out of wedlock are particularly prone to feelings of guilt about past actions or decisions. Indeed it is difficult to avoid having such feelings when one has experienced the agony of an abortion or the feelings of emptiness after having made an adoption plan for one's birthchild.

The Meaning of Pregnancy. The loss of the pregnancy and childbirth experience is immensely significant for almost all women. Since their bodies are designed to house babies, a belief reinforced throughout their lives, the inability to bear a child and give birth can create profound grief that reaches into the core of the self.

For many women a pregnant belly is the ultimate sign of femininity, its absence may be interpreted as meaning they are not real women. For those who have looked forward to pregnancy for much of their lives, the loss can feel enormous. Many believe that the process of gestation creates magical feelings of emotional and physical connection to their child and fear that motherhood without it would be inauthentic. Furthermore, because pregnancy, and subsequent parenthood, involves the creation of an extraordinarily intimate bond with another person—vastly different than is experienced between lovers yet compelling in its urgency—the inability to bear a child can create feelings of emptiness and sadness unlike any other experience in her life. Infertility can create feelings so intense that a women may fear she will never again feel happy or fulfilled unless she can give birth.

Diagnosis and Treatment. Unlike ancient times when the causes of infertility were unknown, today we have a sophisticated understanding of many medical conditions that contribute to or cause infertility. We also have an array of treatment options ranging from pharmacology, to surgery, to the new reproductive technologies. Each of these options offers hope, yet each comes with its own physical, emotional, and financial price tag. And while treatment often "corrects" the problem—endometriosis or adhesions can be removed, tubes can be unblocked, hormones can induce ovulation—pregnancy does not always follow.

Although a woman's partner may share some of her anguish, many of the costs are hers alone, as she bears the physical burden of infertility almost exclusively. It is she who must take her temperature each morning before rising and check her urine to determine whether and when she is ovulating. And it is she who must undergo painful, invasive, expensive, and time-consuming diagnostic procedures. Furthermore, treatment, even for male infertility, almost exclusively involves the woman and is but one of the unfair ironies of infertility.

The Mind-Body Connection

Women experiencing infertility are told over and over again that they should "relax," "take a vacation," "stop working so hard," or worse, "stop trying so hard to get pregnant." Although advice givers are trying to help, they do reflect popular beliefs that stress may be a cause of infertility. What they are forgetting is that the stress infertile women experience is, more than anything else, a by-product of infertility, probably not the cause (at least not the prevailing cause). Although it is rarely helpful to tell an infertile woman (or man) to relax, or not try so hard, and she will get pregnant (that just makes her feel more stressed), it is also true that reducing stress can help a person's overall well-being, and whether pregnancy occurs or not, the burden of infertility may be somewhat relieved.

For many years scientists insisted that the mind and the body were separate entities, neither affecting nor being affected by the other. However, research has shown that the mind and body are in fact connected; hormones released by the brain when people are stressed may contribute, over time, to physical dysfunction. Although the prevailing view is that infertility is not the result of stress but that the converse is true, it is important to acknowledge the way in which the mind-body connection may play a role, if only a small one, in some aspects of infertility.

M. Seibel and J. McCarthy, reproductive endocrinologists who have written about stress and conception, describe the role of the hypothalamus and pituitary gland in ovulation. Chemical signals released by the brain and hypothalamus stimulate the ovaries to produce luteinizing hormone (LH) and follicle-stimulating hormone (FSH), which then cause ovulation to occur. When people experience stress, their body produces hormones in response to stress, which can then cause a disruption in the sequence of events necessary for ovulation. Nerve fibers located throughout the spinal cord link the brain to the ovaries, uterus, and fallopian tubes. Seibel and McCarthy speculate that emotional stress may also interfere with pregnancy by disrupting the activity of the fallopian tubes.[2]

Boston's New England Deaconess Hospital offers the Mind/Body Program for Infertility Patients through its Department of Behavioral Medicine. The program is based on the understanding that infertility frequently leads to stress, causing anger, anxiety, and depression—emotions that are unpleasant in themselves and may also aggravate conditions that can cause infertility. The main thrust of the program is on teaching participants to elicit the relaxation response, a behavioral technique aimed at reducing stress and tension. The program emphasizes self-empathy and includes yoga, exercise, and nutrition counseling.

Two studies researching the effects of the Mind/Body Program (the aim of the second study was to replicate the results of the first) produced noteworthy results. Based on pre and post measures of depression, anxiety, and anger, results indicated that the women who participated (fifty-four in the first study, fifty-two in the second) demonstrated statistically significant decreases in depression, anxiety, and fatigue and increases in vigor. (The first study also indicated significantly decreased anger on one of the measures, and the second study showed a trend toward decreased anger on the same measure, but it was not considered statistically significant.) Interestingly, 34 percent of the women in the first study got pregnant within six months of completing the program, and 32 percent of the women in the second study got pregnant within six months of completing the program. The researchers concluded: "Although it is tempting to suggest that the behavioral treatment led to an increased chance of conception, the conception rate may be within the normal range for women who aggressively seek treatment from experienced infertility specialists who offer a wide modality of technologically sophisticated treatments."[3]

These studies are important because women about to embark on the new reproductive technologies frequently ask their caregivers whether reducing stress will help them become pregnant. They wonder if they should take a leave of absence from work or plan a vacation on a remote island just prior to beginning treatment. Both authors, as well as other clinicians with whom we have conferred (including Domar, the primary researcher in the studies just mentioned), have seen pregnancies in severely anxious patients. One woman was so anxious throughout her cycle that three nurses had to hold her arm down when she was having blood drawn. Another patient was so upset that a psychologist had to accompany her to *the retrieval* in order to help her relax. She was equally shaken during her embryo transfer and reported being very anxious during the following two weeks. Both women experienced uneventful though highly anxious pregnancies and gave birth to healthy children.

It is still too early to know whether stress reduction programs do, in fact, improve conception rates. It is important to recognize, however, that whether or not the stress felt as a result of infertility makes conception more difficult, it does interfere with the well-being of infertile women. Programs aimed at teaching relaxation techniques in order to reduce stress have been well received. Those who have participated frequently comment that regardless of whether conception occurs, they feel their experience in the program will help them throughout life.

Women and Relationships

One of the reasons that infertility is so painful to women is that it affects their interpersonal relationships, which they value and nurture. Women, who are used to turning to others for comfort, find that these relationships often cause pain. Since most people form friendships with those who are at approximately their age and stage of life, infertile couples often find that while their friends and relatives are having babies, they are undergoing invasive diagnostic tests and treatments.

Women can feel inferior to fertile friends who conceive and give birth with ease. As friends move on in life—having children, buying houses, progressing in their careers—infertile women may feel left behind. Their lives, which in all probability are on hold, appear stagnant in contrast. It is painful for them to visit friends whose lives are consumed with the demands of young children—demands of which infertile women are envious.

Relationships with family members may be even more stressed. When siblings, especially younger ones, have children, infertile women may experience a multitude of mixed feelings—on the one hand, they are glad to have a new niece or nephew, on the other hand, they are sad being reminded of their own longings and how they feel deficient. Not only are they not providing cousins for their nieces and nephews, but, more important, they are not bearing grandchildren to carry on the family legacy. Relationships with relatives may be especially trying during holidays or other life cycles events, many of which focus on children. They are reminders that time is passing them by and that what they want most in life seems to be eluding them.

The issue of privacy can be difficult for infertile women. Despite the fact that they tend to be more open than men and to seek out others for support in times of crisis, infertile women still struggle with questions about how much of their experience they want to share. Although some are extremely open and discuss their treatment in detail, others view infertility as personal business and do not feel comfortable discussing it with anyone. Many others decide to be selectively open, revealing their problem only to close friends or relatives.

Whether one has chosen to be open or private, it is impossible to avoid painful encounters with others. The fertile world often has no idea how to react to infertility. With the best of intentions, many quote "experts" they saw on television or articles they read in the newspaper. Sometimes they pass on stories—of their neighbor who adopted and shortly after got pregnant, or of their second cousin who was successfully treated by a specialist a thousand miles away.

Infertility and Career

In recent years work has taken on new meaning in women's lives. While it was unusual a generation ago for a woman to place importance on a career—and even more unusual for her to return to a job after the birth of a child—the past twenty years have heralded a revolution in the world of work. The women's movement has created new career opportunities for women, and these opportunities, together with economic necessity, have prompted most women, including mothers, to work outside the home. Yet even women who have been highly successful in their careers, who believe they have shed the chains of their past conditioning, feel a tremendous gap in their lives when they decide to have a child and discover they are infertile. The emotional pain they feel may be a surprise, particularly if their career has previously been an important source of pleasure and self-esteem. Shops specializing in maternity clothes for career women seem to proliferate, causing more pain to infertile women by the implicit message that they can have it all.

Women find that their infertility affects their career in a variety of ways. They may be unhappy in their jobs, desiring a change or a return to school to further their education. Many are afraid to shift gears, fearful that a new employer would not be supportive of their infertility treatment—or a pregnancy—should it occur. Other women remain stuck in their jobs because they need to maintain their company's medical insurance in order to continue treatment; otherwise they might have to change physicians or endure a waiting period for a preexisting condition.

Some women struggle with whether to resign from their jobs altogether or to work part time in order to pursue treatment. They wonder whether reducing their work load will alleviate much of the stress they feel and hope that relief from stress might increase their chances of becoming pregnant. Not many working women have this option, but those who do and avail themselves of it frequently report a greater sense of well-being (though not necessarily a higher pregnancy rate).

Other women take a very different approach. Aware that infertility has assaulted their self-esteem, they hold fast to their careers as a vital source of fulfillment. However, for some of these women, career satisfaction breeds additional conflict; they fear that their infertility may be punishment for their successful career—that they may have gotten their priorities wrong. This message is sometimes reinforced, especially to older career women. It is not unusual to hear comments such as, "you should have had children before you went to graduate school."

Ancient women who were infertile did not have a career to fall back on. Their lives were geared toward raising a family, and their desperation was probably obvious to everyone when children were not forthcoming. The modern infertile career woman may direct a company and appear to be busy, competent, and in control of her life. Inwardly, however, she may be suffering, feeling just as bereft as Hannah when she poured out her anguish to God.

Emotional Effects on Men

In biblical times it was assumed that the woman bore the responsibility for a barren marriage. Despite our modern sophisticated understanding of reproduction and the fact that approximately 30 to 40 percent of infertility problems are male related, this presumption persists. Stigma surrounding male infertility, together with limited advances in treating this problem, have perpetuated a public view that "real" men are strong, virile, and fertile. The encouraging news is that in the past few years enormous advances have been made in treating male problems through the technique of in vitro fertilization and microassisted fertilization. The latter procedure (made possible by the development of IVF), still in its infancy, promises to be a turning point in the treatment of male infertility.

Identity

Many men spent a fair amount of their adolescence and young adulthood avoiding pregnancy. Equating sexual performance with fertility, they assumed that if they were able to reach orgasm, they must have plenty of sperm. Most learned to be responsible, remembering that it "just takes one sperm" to fertilize an egg. Years later, as infertility patients, they learn that their information was incomplete; even though it only takes one, that sperm needs to be accompanied by another 20 million. This news can be confusing, as well as surprising, especially to those who were once the unwitting partner in an accidental pregnancy. They never imaginined that when they were finally ready for parenthood their sperm would be inadequate. Because we live in a society in which fertility, virility, and masculinity are equated, even those young men who fear the consequences of "getting their girlfriend pregnant" may feel a strange mixture of pride and regret when an accident happens. The unwanted pregnancy is viewed as proof of their manhood.

This notion of proving manhood through conception remains subconscious in many men. Thus, when conception seems impossible, men commonly feel damaged and defective. Even those who are enlightened or liberated from the constraints of sex roles—those who understand that masculinity is not tied to fertility—may experience shame and humiliation. A few become impotent. Others, more successful at preserving sexual performance, feel helpless and ineffectual in other areas of their lives.

Historically physicians have colluded in protecting infertile men from their condition. Rather than acknowledging male infertility for what it is—an unfortunate medical condition with profound emotional ramifications—they have unintentionally perpetuated the shame that surrounds it by attempting to camouflage the problem. Couples have reported being ushered into their physician's office, being told the "bad news," and immediately presented with a "solution"—donor sperm. Their physicians assured them that donor insemination is the best "treatment" for male infertility, that it is superior to adoption because no one ever has to know about the husband's infertility, and that there is no need ever to reveal the truth to anyone, including the child. The unspoken but powerful message is that their condition is so humiliating that it has to be hidden. (These assumptions will be discussed in detail in chapter 5.)

Diagnosis and Treatment

Every test attempting to diagnose problems with sperm—with the exception of blood tests that determine the presence of either antibodies or sexually transmittable diseases—requires the man to produce a sperm sample. Since the most accurate results come from fresh samples, physicians prefer that men produce their sample via masturbation, on the premises. Unlike tests for the woman, producing a sperm sample is neither physically painful nor time-consuming; it is just humiliating. Although men who must produce regularly as part of a treatment plan may become accustomed to the process, most are initially horrified at the idea that staff, and possibly other patients, will know that they are masturbating. Some programs try to reduce men's embarrassment by situating collection rooms away from the traffic flow, yet the experience always feels uncomfortable.

Although most infertility treatment primarily involves the woman, infertile men may also undergo pharmacological treatment or surgical procedures to correct their problem. These procedures include the use of medications to improve sperm count or motility, and the use of surgery to treat a blockage of the reproductive tract, to repair a varicocele in the testicle, or to reverse a vasectomy. Although most men tolerate medications or surgery fairly well, some men have a rough time. One man who was unprepared for having to miss five days of work after a varicocelectomy, commented that he felt like he had "been kicked in the scrotum." Another man with low motility who was prescribed Clomid (a fertility drug commonly given to women but also used to treat male infertility) said he feared that he would wake up one morning and discover he had grown breasts.

When pharmacological or surgical treatment fails to improve the sperm quality or quantity, in vitro fertilization may be the only way to achieve pregnancy. For these couples, IVF is not only recommended as a treatment, but it is also recommended as a diagnostic intervention to see if fertilization can occur. (see Chapter 5, DONOR INSEMINATION). Infertile men feel guilty watching their wives undergo high-tech treatment—being injected with powerful medications, having blood drawn daily, enduring an invasive surgical procedure, as well as depression and mood swings—because of their problem.

Thus, many couples weary, after years of testing and treatment, having assumed that eventually a sperm would find its way to an egg and that pregnancy would occur, find themselves on the doorstep of an IVF program. Although IVF is an ordeal, (see chapter 2), many couples with male problems do have success. This outcome goes a long way toward restoring a man's sense of self-esteem. However, those for whom IVF fails—especially those for whom fertilization did not occur—feel all the more assaulted and helpless.

Relationships with Family and Friends

Men have a more difficult time than women talking about their problems. They tend to isolate themselves when they are upset or depressed. Men also have different coping mechanisms; they are better at compartmentalizing their feelings—pushing them aside until they are ready to face them. Thus, infertility—although it may be more painful for women because their identity feels at stake—is probably more isolating for men, because they do not readily share their problems.

Society unfortunately has perpetuated a sense that male infertility is shameful, and many men fear that their manhood will be called into question if they discuss their problem with others. Often it is. For example, one man decided to mention his problem to a friend. He revealed that he and his wife would probably adopt because he had an infertility problem. The friend replied, "I'm sorry. You would have made a great father." Other men have had the unpleasant experience, after confiding to a friend, of the latter boastingly offering to "solve the problem for them." These experiences are in contrast to the experience of many women who readily seek help by confiding in others and who, more often than not, are offered compassion rather than insult.

Many men feel extremely vulnerable talking to their families about infertility. Because over the years lineage has been more emphasized for men (even when a woman retains her surname after marriage, most often their children are given the husband's surname), men are likely to feel they will let down their parents and grandparents if they cannot reproduce. The brother of an infertile man commented, after learning his sibling was adopting a baby, "I guess I'll just have to carry on the family name." Those who do tell parents about their infertility often hear responses that convey disbelief or shock about their problem. Since much of the world assumes that infertility is a condition that belongs solely to women, families of infertile men sometimes react in a way that indicates they cannot accept this news. It is common for parents to react defensively when their son mentions his infertility—protesting that it could not have been anything they did that caused it.

Career

Although most men's identities are primarily shaped by their work, most also look forward to being husbands and fathers. In fact, some of the emphasis they place on career involves preparation for the role as breadwinner or family provider. A man who encounters infertility may feel that his other accomplishments are superfluous, since he will not have to provide for any children.

Infertility affects the career decisions of men differently than it does women. It is the rare man who finds himself in a stopgap job, waiting to have a child, intending to leave or work part time in order to provide child care for his infant. Men also do not have to contend with thinking about how a pregnancy would affect their work performance, should any complications arise. Consequently, it is unusual for a man who wants to make a career move to think about whether such a move would be unfair to his employer.

Insurance coverage is a factor in the decisions infertile men make regarding their work. Some stay in jobs because they offer excellent health benefits, including infertility coverage. Sometimes a particular insurance company pays for IVF when other plans do not, even though there is not a state mandate. (For couples who think IVF is the next step, coverage may be crucial.) A few insurance companies are also beginning to offer adoption benefits, and couples who are considering adoption may be reluctant to lose that benefit as well.

Because timing is key to infertility treatment, a man's job may be affected by his mate's biological calendar. For example, if a couple is involved in intrauterine inseminations, the man must be available when his wife is ovulating because inseminations must be timed precisely; a twenty-four-hour delay means a missed opportunity. Men who travel must adjust their schedule to their wife's calendar, which can roughly, but not accurately, be determined in advance.

Infertility as a Marital Crisis

Marriage rarely has a predictable course. Couples encounter many unexpected twists and turns along the way, including detours and roadblocks that challenge their individual and collective strength. The journey begins with courtship, connection, and sexual attraction. When couples enter into marriage they do so because they are in love and because they believe they share common goals, interests, and values. For many couples, having children is central among these goals. When they decide to pursue parenthood, they anticipate that their sexual union, which has always brought them pleasure, will bring them children.

For some couples, infertility is the first roadblock they face. Although they may have expected adversity at various points in their marriage, this first one comes much sooner than expected. Infertility is a major life crisis—for some the worst crisis that a couple will endure in their lifetime. Infertility involves profound feelings of loss and despair, and prior to resolution, it affects practically every important decision or event in their lives. Furthermore, the duration of infertility is uncertain, making it almost impossible to believe the crisis will ever be over.

One of the first steps in a couple's journey through infertility is to see a physician. The difficulty of this step cannot be minimized: they are taking a very private part of their lives out of their bedroom and into a medical office. For many, it is a bewildering and humiliating experience: couples are asked to discuss certain aspects of their sexual relationship, and they are told when to have sexual relations and when to abstain.

Once they have entered the medical world, couples face a series of questions and decisions involving time, money, jobs, relationships, moves, and quality of life. They must make decisions that affect them physically and that have potential consequences for their future health. All of these deliberations happen in the midst of profound emotional pain and in an array of complicated and conflicting pieces of information. In addition, their journey is not always in tandem; their timing may be very different, both emotionally and practically. For example, one spouse may be ready to move on to IVF, while the other wants to continue inseminations. Thus, couples may find that their previously happy marriage is coming unhinged: tension, resentment, and distance may have replaced the mutual support, spontaneity, and joy they once treasured.

The journey through infertility in the nineties is often longer and more uncertain than it was previously because there are so many treatment options and alternative routes to parenthood. Complicating the journey, but no different from other aspects of marriage, is that the experience of infertility involves both an individual process and a couple process.

An Emotional Endurance Test

Infertility has frequently been described as a roller coaster ride—an endless process in which couples are filled with hope one day, only to come crashing down the next. Another way to describe the experience is as an emotional endurance test. Powerful and often overwhelming feelings—anger, depression, jealousy, helplessness, despair, and loss—engulf men and women, testing their strength as individuals and as a couple.

Although the journey through infertility involves learning a vast amount of information and making rational decisions about treatment, it is, more than anything else, a tumultuous emotional experience. This experience, as Barbara Eck Menning, founder of RESOLVE, Inc. (a national, non profit organization for infertile people) first pointed out, can be described by Elisabeth Kübler-Ross's five stages of grieving: denial, anger, bargaining, depression, and acceptance.[4] These stages are not experienced in a linear fashion, as they may be by someone who is dying or losing a loved one. The nature of the infertility roller coaster—with its ups and downs of hope and despair—precludes a smooth journey toward resolution. Rather, couples move in and out of the various stages depending on the time of the month, test results, new treatments being tried, or how many of their friends recently announced a pregnancy.

Because people move so easily in and out of the different stages, it can be difficult to make decisions, and even more difficult to accept one's ever-changing feelings. A woman who feels she has overcome her feelings of anger and jealousy may be surprised to find herself shredding a baby announcement she just received. A man who has recently agreed to adopt may be shocked when he finds himself bargaining with God to make his wife pregnant. Eventually, however, the intensity of the infertility crisis begins to subside, whether or not couples are pursuing ART, and they work their way to the stage of acceptance and resolution.

The Major Losses of Infertility

The intense feelings that engulf couples on their journey through infertility are the result of the many losses that confront them. The nature of these losses, as well as the significance of each, varies from person to person. We have categorized them into primary and secondary losses.

Primary losses refer to the experiences that are a direct outgrowth of reproduction, without which many people believe they will never feel whole: the loss of the pregnancy-childbirth experience; the loss of genetic continuity, and the loss of parenting. Although couples live with the fear of facing all three losses, many find, as they make their way through treatment, that only the first two come to pass.

The loss of the pregnancy-childbirth experience is a major loss for women. Many infertile women report having longed for the experience of pregnancy for years, regarding it as fulfillment of their biological destiny. This loss is one that belongs solely to them. Although a man may regret not being able to watch his wife's belly expand or to feel his child moving in her womb, his identity is not threatened in the way a woman's is by the inability to experience pregnancy.

The loss of genetic continuity is another major loss that infertile couples must face. For a man, whose only connection to his unborn child is a genetic one, this loss may be central. There are two parts to genetic continuity: genetics (the transmission of traits or similarities) and genealogy (the continuation of one's bloodline).

Although the exact formula of the nature/nurture debate has not been—and will probably never be—settled, it is increasingly understood that genes play a major role in who we are. They are responsible not only for physical traits and talents, but they are also a large determinant of personality and temperament as well. And although it is common for parents to produce biological children who are very different from them, it is more likely that their children will possess some familiar traits. Couples facing infertility realize they may not be able to look at their offspring and see parts of themselves reflected back—or parts of their grandparents or great-grandparents.

The inability to have genetic children means the loss of genealogical continuity. For some people, especially those who come from families that emphasized bloodlines or family trees, this loss is profound. Those whose families were rooted in strong ethnic or religious traditions may also feel the loss of genealogical continuity. Many facing infertility say that although there is no one trait or group of traits they feel a need to pass on, they do feel compelled to continue the bloodline that began generations ago.

Another primary loss is the loss of the parenting experience. It is true that adoption, while not curing infertility, does cure childlessness. Yet infertile couples, accustomed to loss, disappointment, and feelings of unworthiness and unaccustomed to success, fear that should they choose adoption, no agency or birthparent would chose them. Furthermore, many couples experiencing infertility do not know if they will adopt, should their efforts to conceive fail.

Secondary losses affect the way in which infertile people view themselves and the world around them. These losses, which affect infertile people to greater or lesser degrees, include the loss of self-esteem, the loss of control over one's life and the loss of sexual intimacy and pleasure. Due to the nature of the infertility journey, including the disappointments and disillusionments that appear every step along the way, these losses are not easily repaired, even when a biological child appears at the end of the road.

As men and women travel the rocky terrain of infertility, facing one hurdle after another, their self-esteem plummets, threatening to be the most enduring loss of all. Since infertility affects sexual identity, self-image, and self-worth—all parts of self-esteem—couples experience the inability to bear a biological child, or to bear one only after enormous effort, as a blow to the self. Years after the crisis has ended, it is common for both men and women to report that although they are happy and fulfilled, infertility had an unfortunate and lasting effect on them.

The loss of control over one's life, or more aptly, the illusion of control, is one of the painful lessons of infertility, especially for couples who have been able to accomplish their other goals through hard work and concentration. The doctoral dissertation by one of the authors studied thirty infertile women over several months. Results indicated that the passage of time negatively affected their overall feeling of being in control of their life. The longer the period of infertility, the more likely a woman was to feel that luck or chance determines her fate.[5] Thus, infertility teaches that life is not always fair—that those who play by the rules and try hard are not necessarily rewarded for their efforts. This loss of control sometimes makes couples wonder why they keep pursuing what feels like an elusive dream.

The loss of sexual pleasure is another painful loss—for some the most painful one—that affects infertile couples. Years of sex on demand wreck havoc on their sexual relationship. The longer the infertility continues, the worse it becomes. Although the ability to separate sexual intimacy from reproduction helps some couples to preserve their sexual relationship, unless they are being treated with intrauterine insemination (IUI) or ART, it is virtually impossible to do so.

Because coitus is a precondition for reproduction, at least prior to undergoing high-tech procedures, the issue of sexuality is constantly in the foreground of a couple's relationship. Lovemaking, once a warm, intimate, and pleasurable experience, becomes a dreaded chore—a means to an end. The thought of sexual intercourse can fill previously passionate couples with dread. Although there are many reasons that a couple's sexual relationship is adversely affected by infertility, because sex is rarely discussed—even with physicians, counselors, or other infertile people—couples may feel that they are alone in experiencing this problem.

Prior to being treated with IUI or one of the assisted reproductive technologies, most couples spend months or years having sexual relations according to the calendar. Couples soon discover that infertility takes the spontaneity out of sex. Attempting to conceive means having sex regularly around the time of ovulation. The man must be able to maintain an erection and reach orgasm; the woman only has to be a receptacle for his sperm. Often couples are given advice about having intercourse in certain positions—advice that is designed to facilitate conception (and probably does not) but that inevitably reduces spontaneity.

Because infertility takes the privacy out of sexuality, a couple's bedroom becomes associated with the infertility clinic, and this association usually decreases desire. Despite the sexual revolution, men and women rarely discuss their sex lives with anyone other than their partner, and infrequently even with him or her. The infertility workup by its very nature means that a couple's sex life, once private, is now scrutinized. Privacy is further compromised by certain diagnostic tests, such as the postcoital test in which a woman's cervical mucus is examined under a microscope subsequent to sexual intercourse. During sexual relations prior to this test, couples describe feeling as if they are being watched by their physician.

The anxiety and tension that surround infertility can build to such a degree that intercourse cannot take place. Husbands feel anxious about having to perform. Wives feel anxious that their husbands will not be able to perform. Men may begin to feel rejected, believing that their wives want a baby more than they want their husband. When men feel that the completion of the sexual act is their wife's first priority rather than a mutual exchange of pleasure, they tend to lose interest.

Infertile women frequently fear they are sexually undesirable, and a woman may interpret her mate's lack of interest in sex as confirmation of that fear, further contributing to her lack of desire. Similarly for men, because fertility and virility tend to be equated, infertile men may feel emasculated, particularly if there is a male infertility factor involved. Men with no prior history of sexual inadequacy or dysfunction can become impotent after they learn about their infertility problem. Women whose identities are closely tied to being a mother, and most are, feel the burden of infertility constantly.

Thus, sexual pleasure is another loss for many infertile couples who previously enjoyed that aspect of their relationship. Yet this loss is even greater, because sex not only provides loving couples with physical pleasure, but it also enhances emotional intimacy. At the time when couples most need to be close—in the midst of a major life crisis—they no longer have access to a path they once treasured together.

There are other losses as well, such as time, money, career advancement, and certain relationships, about which infertile couples have many regrets. Although these losses are important, they do not alter the couple's basic sense of themselves or of the world; they are usually outgrowths of putting life on hold. Time lost and money spent on treatment are gone forever. There is no way to make up for those years or those dollars. However, some of the other losses are more easily recoverable. Relationships can usually be mended, and careers can be furthered, though not necessarily on the original time line.

The Experience of Disconnection

When women and men suffer from prolonged infertility, the communication and understanding they previously shared often breaks down. Men, who are used to being in control and being able to use logic and reasoning to solve problems, may feel useless. Women may feel despondent, resentful of their pregnant friends and relatives, and they are rarely interested in socializing, especially with pregnant women or those with young children. In fact, they begin to lose much of their enthusiasm and motivation for all aspects of life. No matter what a man offers—reassurances, presents, flowers, dinners out—it makes no difference to a woman consumed with grief and despair. Men worry that infertility will cause their wife to have a mental breakdown or an emotional collapse. Because they feel so helpless and because helplessness is so intolerable, men may withdraw emotionally. When they do, women feel abandoned, alone in their crisis, fearing that their husbands do not understand how they feel and may not even desire a child at all. Instead of emotionally connecting, men and women slowly disconnect.

Another breakdown in communication occurs when women broach the subject of adoption or other alternatives to biogenetic children. Because men are generally more optimistic about an eventual pregnancy than women, at the point when women are ready to consider alternatives or begin to accept that they may never have a child, their partners may be unwilling to consider such a possibility. Women, whose bodies have been invaded on a regular basis, may believe unequivocally that their bodies will continue to fail them. Considering other options or alternatives may restore hope that they will become parents someday, giving them the fuel they need to remain in treatment for a while longer. It can be frightening, however, to discover they perceive this important matter so differently from their mate. Although they are part of a couple, they are also individuals, and their pacing may be very different. Though it can be frightening to feel so far apart from their mate, these perceived differences about moving on may actually reflect differences in timetables rather than differences about second choices.

What both mates feel in common, however, is sadness and loss, but the loss springs from different sources. The primary loss felt by the woman is the loss of a baby, creating feelings of emptiness inside her and fears that she will never feel fulfilled if she cannot give birth. The primary loss felt by the man, is the loss of his mate, coupled with the fear that she will never return emotionally to her previous self.

Dilemmas and Decision Making

Much of a couple's journey through infertility involves their emotions, yet they are also called upon to make countless decisions to which they must apply understanding, reason, and logic. These decisions are related to medical treatment, money, privacy, work, and, for some couples, alternatives to biological parenthood. Because these decisions are so challenging, the potential for conflict between them always exists.

As we shall see throughout this book, the medical aspects of infertility are extremely complicated, and there are no easy answers. Rather, there are difficult concepts to understand and many pieces of the puzzle to grasp before couples can evaluate their options. In the course of an infertility investigation and in the ensuing treatment, decisions must be made relative to diagnostic procedures, medications, surgery, inseminations, or the new reproductive technologies.

The ideal investigation involves close collaboration between physician and patients, yet it is ultimately up to each couple to decide what treatment to pursue. In general, the treatments that offer the highest probability of success are the most invasive and the most expensive and pose the greatest number of side effects. Couples must negotiate how, when, and what options they will pursue, as well as how long they will pursue them and when to change courses. These choices can be overwhelming, making the goal— overcoming infertility—appear insurmountable.

Sandelowski and associates refer to the process of deciding on a route to parenthood as "mazing," defined as the "tortuous process of negotiating the paths to parenthood." The formula that couples use—their "calculus of pursuit"—is based on the amount of money, time, and physical and psychic energy that are required for each particular treatment option, and that the couple have available and are willing to invest in the process. Sandelowski and associates describe six patterns of pursuit that couples may follow: sequential tracking (pursuing one avenue at a time), backtracking (returning to a former treatment regimen), getting stuck (continuing a particular treatment regimen over and over), paralleling (pursuing more than one option); taking a break (temporarily withdrawing from treatment), and drawing the line (deciding to end treatment). Most couples in pursuing parenthood follow various patterns at different points in their process.[6]

No matter how it is defined, the decision-making process for infertile couples is, as Sandelowski describes, "tortuous." The feelings that infertility evokes can be overpowering, making it even more difficult to apply logic and reasoning to the process. Although more than half of those who pursue treatment will ultimately give birth to a biogenetic child, the time they spend doing so may be far longer than they could have imagined. Some couples will leave no stone unturned in their efforts to reproduce, others opt out of treatment early on. And because spouses frequently disagree on timing, on treatments, and on alternatives, the potential for conflict is great.

Other decisions facing couples involve money. Treatment is very costly, and finances can be a key element in a couple's calculus of pursuit. In some states where insurance coverage for infertility is mandated, couples with health insurance have fewer decisions to make that are connected to their financial situation. Couples who live in states where coverage is not mandated may feel forced to choose the least expensive option even if it is not their first choice. Couples who do not have health insurance, an increasingly common situation, may be forced to remain childless because the treatment they need is out of their financial reach. Currently the health care system in this country is being completely revamped. It is unknown at this time whether infertility-or certain aspects of its treatment-will be routinely covered by health insurance in the future.

Couples with some financial resources are frequently forced to choose between the new reproductive technologies or another costly purchase, such as a down payment on a new house. Or they may feel pressed to choose between an IVF cycle and an alternative family-building method, such as adoption. Each option is expensive, and many couple's budgets cannot accommodate both, at least not at the same time.

Another decision couples must negotiate, and another factor in their calculus of pursuit, is how much time they will spend pursuing medical options. Because the emotional experience of infertility tends to be different for men and women and because the woman is usually the one who goes through the bulk of the diagnostic procedures and treatments, time is perceived differently by her than by her partner. A year or two of infertility treatments can feel like five years to a woman who has looked forward to motherhood for almost a lifetime. When she feels ready to consider alternative parenthood options, her partner, believing pregnancy will happen sooner or later, may feel that any option other than biological parenthood is unacceptable.

Couples need to determine as well how public to be about their infertility. Some people (usually women, for reasons that we have previously discussed) have a greater need to talk about infertility to others, to seek counseling, to join RESOLVE, or participate in support groups. Additional pressure is put on a relationship when one spouse desires privacy and the other needs to talk about the problem. Some couples who have different needs in this area actually agree to disagree, allowing one another the leeway each needs to feel comfortable.

Infertile couples face decisions about putting life on hold or moving on. Many couples who planned to purchase homes soon after the birth of their first child are frustrated in their small space yet unable to think about buying a house because they have no idea if they will ever need more than one bedroom. Changing careers, changing jobs, or returning to college or graduate school are other decisions that many infertile people postpone while their life is on hold. Some women feel it would be unfair to a new employer if they became pregnant and left or took a long maternity leave shortly after beginning a new job. Others choose to stay in an unfulfilling job because their boss and co-workers are understanding about infertility and because their work hours are flexible. Still others feel forced to stay in jobs because their health insurance benefits offer excellent coverage for infertility.

When infertility becomes prolonged, couples must consider alternatives to biogenetic parenting. This process can be excruciatingly painful; it forces couples to face the myriad losses they have already experienced and may continue to experience. Many who embark on the new reproductive technologies decide to postpone thinking about alternatives, knowing they are capable of pursuing only one avenue at a time. Others, who know they want to be parents, are not willing to pin all their hopes on advanced technology and have already decided on a second choice. The range of possibilities includes child-free living, adoption, donor sperm, donor ovum, gestational care, surrogacy, or embryo donation, depending on the diagnosis given to the couple.

Regardless of how it is resolved, the journey through infertility is emotionally charged from beginning to end. Yet, since infertility is not commonly understood to be a major life crisis, except by those who have faced it or who work in the field, few couples receive support and acknowledgment for this crisis. A study published in 1985 that involved 200 couples prior to their undergoing IVF treatment indicated that 49 percent of the women and 15 percent of the men considered infertility the most upsetting experience in their lives.[7] Another study, which surveyed ninety-four IVF patients, indicated that of those who had experienced divorce or the death of a family member, 63 percent claimed that infertility was equal to or worse than divorce and 58 percent claimed it was worse than the death of a loved one.[8] An even more recent study comparing the psychiatric symptoms of infertile women to those with other serious medical conditions, showed that infertile women were as depressed and anxious as those who had cardiac disease, cancer, hypertension, or who were HIV positive. Only women who experienced chronic pain had higher scores for depression and anxiety than did infertile women.[9]

Based on our years of experience working with infertile couples, we have come to similar conclusions. We are reminded of a woman interviewed with her husband just prior to undergoing an IVF cycle. The woman had been treated for breast cancer aproximately ten years before and had been battling infertility for four years. At one point she remarked that "infertility is much harder emotionally on me than having cancer." The woman explained that she always believed that she would survive cancer, despite the fact that her prognosis was unclear, but she was less sure that she would emotionally survive the inability to bear a child.

We have attempted to convey in this chapter a sense of the emotional experience of infertile couples prior to their embarking on their next journey—a journey through the world of assisted reproductive technology. Although the road has been difficult and may become even more so, infertile couples prove to be surprisingly resilient. The experiences they have had prior to ART, both physical and emotional, will guide their approach to the new technologies and will, in large measure, help shape the decisions they make from this point forth.

2

In Vitro Fertilization and the Assisted Reproductive Technologies

In vitro fertilization forms the cornerstone of the new reproductive technologies. When Louise Brown, the world's first IVF baby, was born in 1978, probably few people, if any, could foresee all the reproductive possibilities that would occur as the result of being able to harvest human eggs and fertilize them outside the body. Now, embryos can be frozen, stored, and implanted in the couple at a later date, or they can be donated to another infertile couple, who can then legally adopt them at the four-cell stage, enabling the latter to gestate as well as rear their child. As a result of IVF, a woman can carry another couple's genetic child, if the genetic/rearing mother is unable to do so for medical reasons. Finally, a woman can now donate eggs to an infertile woman who cannot produce viable eggs. These eggs can then be fertilized with the latter's husband's sperm and gestated in the uterus of the rearing mother.

Reproductive medicine has indeed come a long way, yet not everyone regards these technologies positively. Ardent feminists, for example, believe that the new technologies dehumanize and degrade women, and religious fundamentalists believe they are an affront to God. What is clear, however, is that these technologies are here to stay, and they bring with them new dilemmas and decisions about family building.

Couples who begin the process of ART frequently look back and wonder how they got there. If they had been asked early on in their treatment process whether they would ever try IVF, many would have readily said no. Yet months or years later, these same couples find themselves in a new world of high-tech terminology and treatment, investing large sums of money, facing medical risks, and embarking on an even steeper emotional roller coaster than the one from which they recently disembarked. It is important to point out, however, that part of the emotional difficulty of doing ART is that it feels like the end of the line—the last possible (and unlikely) chance of having a biological child. For a small group of couples, those with hopelessly blocked or absent tubes, IVF is their last resort. Yet for many other couples who are ART candidates, trying one or more of the new reproductive options does not mean that they cannot return to less invasive treatments.

In this chapter we will focus on those reproductive technologies in which only the couple's gametes (eggs or sperm) are used in order to be gestated by the woman and raised by the couple. We will use the term *assisted reproductive technology* (ART) for the high-tech procedures in which superovulation is usually, but not always, a part of the process. In this chapter, we briefly discuss the differences between technologies in which fertilization takes place outside the body and those in which fertilization occurs naturally inside the body though we will refer to all of them as ART, since much of the process is the same, both medically and emotionally.

Initial Considerations

Rarely do couples consider the new reproductive technologies from the start of their treatment, and many are surprised when their physician first mentions this possibility. Their reaction may indicate the level of denial under which they were operating— "That's only for couples who are really infertile. We just need a little help getting pregnant." Others, especially those who need to be anticipating the next step, may be the first to bring up the subject to their physician. Regardless of who initiates the discussion, couples generally give a great deal of consideration to this decision, finding that the medical, emotional, ethical, and financial issues are extremely complicated.

Ethical Issues

For some people, pursuing high-tech treatment for reproductive difficulties poses an ethical dilemma. For example, the Vatican has advised Catholics that IVF is morally unacceptable; rather, fertilization of egg and sperm must occur within the body, as God intended it. Gamete intrafallopian transfer (GIFT) is a more acceptable procedure to some prominent Catholic figures, since fertilization occurs within the fallopian tubes. Although sperm is almost always obtained through masturbation, that method of collection is not acceptable to the church, which requires couples to collect semen in a condom (that has tiny holes) while having sexual intercourse.

Practicing Catholics who are candidates for the ARTs find themselves torn between the teachings of their religion and the desires of their heart. Further, they may be confused by the church's teaching that married couples should procreate and that children are highly valued and desired. Some couples turn to priests for advice and guidance and frequently receive their support. Many, perhaps predominantly the younger clergy, tend to believe that the love between husband and wife, and their desire to have progeny, should be the central ingredient in the creation of their family. Catholic couples who seek and receive the blessing of a priest come to ART programs at greater peace with themselves and with their decision.

A different moral issue is the one raised by radical feminists: that IVF was developed not in order to help infertile couples but in order to give men greater control over women's bodies. They argue that the new reproductive technologies dehumanize women, that male physicians will use women's bodies to further their technological experiments, and that reproduction will become artificial. Elaine Baruch writes,

> It is a common belief among feminists now that the new technology with its *in vitro* fertilization and embryo transfer was designed less to help the infertile than to appease men's envy of women's re-

productive power . . . It is no small surprise to find that on the issue of reproductive technology, some radical feminists sound more like the women of the New Right than anyone else. They too fear men's intrusion into motherhood, the *sanctum sanctorum*.[1]

Elizabeth Bartholet, author of *Family Bonds*, is another critic. She believes that ART clinics intentionally mislead infertile couples, who feel that the only meaningful resolution to infertility is to bear a biogenetic child. She feels that political and social conditioning have helped shaped these attitudes and that proper counseling can help infertile couples change their perspective. Bartholet also believes that adoption is both unaffordable and unreachable for many people and that it is touted as a last resort—an unappealing alternative that ranks only slightly above childlessness. Having gone through years of infertility herself, including several failed IVF cycles when she was in her forties, she resolved her infertility by adopting two children from Peru. Bartholet, delighted, in love with, and awed by her family, has truly been converted—a goal that we would hope for all couples who eventually embark on a second- (or third-) choice route to parenthood.[2]

Although some clinics performing ART services are not reputable and do take advantage of desperate patients, Bartholet's criticisms are not true of the industry as a whole. Many clinics fully inform patients of all aspects of ART treatment—the potential problems, the chances for a successful pregnancy, and the costs they will have to incur in the process. In fact, we have found that most ART patients are well informed, not naive, uneducated couples pursuing an elusive dream, as Bartholet might have us believe.

The vast majority of infertile couples, however, are neither rigid Catholics (or fundamentalists) nor radical feminists. They do not have major ethical dilemmas with the technology of advanced reproductive medicine. Their desire is to have a family, and although they have traveled a great distance from where they began, they have not thrown good judgment to the wind in their desire to pursue their goal. We hope the discussion that follows will help couples considering ART treatment to feel even more informed, more prepared, and more able to ask the right questions. Knowing what to ask is the first step in getting the information needed to make the right decision. Information can also help couples determine when to stop treatment and move on to other alternatives.

Financial Issues

The average cost of an ART cycle in which egg retrieval is involved runs between $6,000 and $10,000, depending on the clinic, the geographical location, and the amount of medication used. Because ART is so expensive, cost is a major factor for many couples, particularly those whose insurance does not cover it, in deciding whether to pursue treatment. Frequently couples are forced to decide about whether to spend their money on an adoption, which may seem much more secure, or on one or more IVF cycles, a less certain outcome but a route that might lead to their long-awaited genetic child.

Unfortunately most companies that provide health insurance do not cover infertility, for it is not regarded as a 'legitimate' medical condition. Many insurers view treatment for infertility much as they view cosmetic surgery—unnecessary. Ten states, however, have mandates requiring health insurance providers to either offer or cover the costs of infertility treatment. These states are: Arkansas, California, Connecticut, Hawaii, Illinois, Maryland, Massachusetts, Rhode Island, New York, and Texas. Couples who live in the other states frequently find that their insurance does pick up a portion of their infertility bill, depending on their diagnosis and treatment. Some medical problems that cause infertility, such as endometriosis, are also legitimate medical conditions in themselves and are thus covered by insurance. As this book goes to print, the field of health care is being completely revamped, and it is not clear how the changes will affect infertile couples.

Couples finance their treatment in various ways: they take out loans, sacrifice expensive purchases, work longer hours, get second jobs, or stay in an unhappy work situation because their insurance is covering many of their infertility costs. Others who might choose to undergo high-tech treatment cannot because the price is too great. What is relevant here, however, is that for couples who are able to undertake one or more cycles, cost is generally an important consideration. Few couples without health insurance coverage can afford ART without financial sacrifice.

The ART Options

Many couples who decide to pursue an ART cycle find themselves bewildered by the various options. Although most laypeople are familiar with the term IVF, few would be able to explain the difference between IVF or GIFT or ZIFT or TET, or IUI, or any of the other variations of the new reproductive technologies. Some couples, depending on their medical diagnosis, are candidates for all of the procedures; others have only one or two options. Although much of an ART cycle is the same no matter what variation a couple is doing, there are some important differences. What they all share in common is the use of superovulatory medications (except in natural cycle IVF), and all (except IUI) involve an egg retrieval.

In vitro fertilization, the oldest of the new technologies, involves harvesting oocytes (eggs) from the ovaries and inseminating each one in a dish with up to 200,000 sperm (this mixing of eggs and sperm is what is meant by insemination). The sperm are carefully prepared by embryologists such that only the healthiest, most motile sperm are used. Two or three days later (depending on the clinic) the eggs that are fertilized (embryos) are transferred to the woman's uterus. Most clinics put back only between three and five embryos, depending on the woman's age and on the quality of the embryos. The more embryos that are transferred, the greater the likelihood of pregnancy. The trick is to avoid a multiple gestation, since multiples are considered to be high risk, while maximizing the probability of a singleton pregnancy. Among the advantages of IVF are that fertilization can be confirmed and the quality of the resulting embryos can be assessed.

Most clinics performing IVF have facilities that enable them to cryopreserve (freeze) extra embryos. Since many women, especially those who are younger, produce many eggs—often more than a dozen—extra eggs can also be inseminated, and those that fertilize can be cryopreserved and used in subsequent cycles. Cryopreservation was a pivotal development in the field of IVF. It is important to note, however, that not all embryos qualify to be frozen; many stop dividing before the point at which they can be cryopreserved, or they are too fragmented, or their quality is compromised.

Gamete intrafallopian transfer (GIFT) involves retrieving eggs and placing them directly into the fallopian tubes with large numbers of sperm. The eggs and the sperm are placed into the tubes almost immediately after they are retrieved. The unsolved part of the puzzle—unless pregnancy occurs—is whether the eggs fertilized but did not implant. The advantage of GIFT is that fertilization occurs in the tube, its natural site, which is assumed to be a better incubator than a petri dish.

Another advantage of GIFT is that, like IVF, extra eggs can be inseminated and cryopreserved for later use. When extra eggs from a GIFT cycle fertilize, it is presumed that fertilization occurred in the tube, but this presumption can never be truly determined. When extra eggs fail to fertilize, however, one never knows what actually happened in the fallopian tube. It is possible they did fertilize even though the inseminated eggs did not. There are two reasons for this possibility: the best-quality eggs are always selected for the GIFT procedure and are thus more likely to fertilize, and the tube is thought to be more efficient than the petri dish and a more likely site for fertilization to occur.

There are many variations on both IVF and GIFT. ZIFT—*zygote intrafallopian transfer*—is a combination of IVF and GIFT. Eggs are retrieved and inseminated as they are for IVF. Instead of being transferred to the uterus on the second or third day after insemination, however, the zygote (the fertilized egg that has not yet divided) is placed in the fallopian tube approximately one day after insemination. ZIFT has the advantages of both IVF and GIFT: fertilization can be determined and the fallopian tube is used as the incubator. But it also has the disadvantages of both: it is more costly, it involves two days of procedures including a laparoscopy, and although fertilization can be viewed, the embryo quality cannot be determined after only one day. Other variations involve putting eggs, zygotes, or embryos into the uterus or tubes at different points in their development, utilizing different methods of retrieval and transfer.

Intrauterine insemination (IUI) is the simplest of the new reproductive technologies and the least costly, since it involves neither egg retrieval nor zygote or embryo transfer. It is considered one of the ARTs because it usually involves superovulation and frequent monitoring in order to determine when ovulation occurs. When the timing is right, sperm that have been carefully prepared in the embryology laboratory are inserted directly into the uterus. Although fertility drugs are given, they are administered in smaller dosages, in hopes of producing no more than three or four eggs. Another advantage of IUI, besides its lower cost and absence of a surgical procedure, is that it may involve less monitoring. Its disadvantages are that fertilization cannot be determined, extra eggs cannot be harvested, inseminated, and the resulting embryos frozen, and, like the other ARTs, a multiple pregnancy may occur.

An IVF cycle in which superovulation is not induced is referred to as a *natural IVF cycle*. These cycles are offered by some programs and are appealing to many couples, particularly those for whom taking drugs is contraindicated by their medical history or who are worried about long-term side effects. A natural cycle means that a woman does not take fertility drugs to stimulate her ovaries. Her cycle is monitored carefully, so that just before she is about to ovulate on her own, the one egg she produced is retrieved and inseminated with her husband's sperm, in hopes that it will fertilize. Two days later, if fertilization occurs, the embryo is transferred into her uterus. Natural cycles are much easier for the woman, and they are much less expensive, but the odds that the one egg is of good quality, that it will fertilize, that the resulting embryo will be of good quality, that it will implant and result in a viable pregnancy, are not as high as in a stimulated cycle.

Women who have one or both fallopian tubes clearly open are theoretically candidates for any of the ARTs as long as adequate numbers of sperm can be obtained from their partner. Those whose tubes are blocked or absent have only IVF available to them. Couples with severe male infertility who want to determine whether fertilization can occur are probably best off doing IVF. If the woman is young, however, and particularly if she has not had a prior laparoscopy to view her pelvic area, GIFT may be the recommended treatment. She can undergo a diagnostic laparoscopy as part of the GIFT procedure and at the same time hope to obtain extra eggs in order to test fertilization. Different clinics, and different physicians, prefer different procedures, and each physician has a bias about which procedure is most effective for which condition. With the exception of blocked or absent tubes, in which the decision is clear-cut, research is equivocal about what works best for whom. Although physicians make recommendations based on their best judgments, the final decision rests with the couple, who must grapple with their choices. These final decisions may be based on medically minor but individually important issues. For example, a woman who does not tolerate anesthesia well may choose to avoid a GIFT procedure.

Short- and Long-Term Side Effects

The tragic effects of DES (diethylstilbesterol) have raised the consciousness of both medical personnel and infertile couples about the potential hazards of medications. The need to perform adequate controlled studies that speak to the efficacy and the safety of drugs, before they are made available to the public, is well recognized. Hence it is understandable that many patients are hesitant to take powerful agents that have a profound and potentially negative impact on their reproductive systems.

Pergonal, the mostly commonly used drug for ART cycles, has been on the market for approximately thirty years, and until 1993, no reports or published research indicated any possible harmful effects from using this medication. In January 1993, however, a publication by Whittemore and colleagues pooled data from three studies and reported that infertile women who used fertility drugs and did not become pregnant had a significantly increased chance of developing ovarian cancer. The results indicated between a three fold and twenty-seven-fold increase.[3] Whittemore's study appears to be flawed, in both its methodology and its findings, and it has been criticized extensively by researchers in the field of reproductive medicine. However, it cannot be easily dismissed, and despite its flaws, it must be taken seriously, as the basis from which to design better research leading to more valid conclusions.

Whittemore's study, which received wide publicity in the media, alarmed many infertile couples, as well as their families and friends. Some who were considering the new reproductive technologies may have even changed their minds. Others who attempted to understand how the study was performed, and how the conclusions were drawn, may have dismissed the findings as being unfounded or premature. One encouraging piece of information in the study is that women who had at least one pregnancy either prior to their infertility treatment or subsequent to it were exempt from the group who were more likely to develop ovarian cancer. Women who had used oral contraceptives prior to their infertility were also exempt from that group.

This study once again raised the question about whether fertility drugs may cause harmful (in this case life-threatening) side effects. This question is especially difficult for couples who are determined to do whatever is in their power to have a biological child. They wonder whether their perseverance is clouding their judgment. For them and others, the publicity surrounding Whittemore's study may have served an important function: it prompted them to pause in their treatment and question the wisdom of what they are doing.

There are documented side effects of the medications that are far less ominous than ovarian cancer but are unpleasant for many women taking them. Lupron, a commonly used drug in ART cycles, physiologically puts women into (temporary) menopause; the drug completely suppresses their estrogen levels by suppressing the pituitary hormones that stimulate the ovaries. These women frequently experience headaches and hot flashes. Side effects from Pergonal range from headaches to hyperstimulation syndrome in the physical realm, to mood swings, irritability, fatigue, and depression in the emotional realm. (It can be difficult to determine whether the depression felt during an ART cycle is due to the medications, the pain of childlessness, or the increased feelings of vulnerability that come with high-tech treatment.)

Hyperstimulation syndrome, when it occurs, is usually mild. However, it can become potentially serious, resulting from ovaries that are extremely responsive to the medications, thereby causing them to become quite large. Hyperstimulation can lead to severe weight gain (from fluid accumulation in the abdomen), low output of urine, and potentially serious changes in blood chemistry. Rarely, a woman experiences such severe hyperstimulation that she must be hospitalized and given intravenous fluids along with having her weight, urine output, and blood tests closely monitored.

The Physical Ordeal

Couples considering one or more of the ARTs must think about the physical aspects of the procedure. All of the new reproductive technologies use procedures that are physically invasive, time-consuming, and (to greater or lesser degrees) painful. Depending on the nature of the ART cycle and the protocols at the specific clinic, all cycles involve several days' worth of intramuscular injections, sometimes daily subcutaneous injections, as well, daily blood tests as ovulation approaches, and vaginal ultrasound monitoring to determine whether the ovaries are producing follicles. Since eggs grow inside the follicles, it is important that a sufficient number be growing so that several eggs can be retrieved.

Patients undergoing IVF procedures must have an egg retrieval, a minor but invasive, and generally uncomfortable, surgical procedure, performed vaginally via ultrasound guidance. Patients usually receive sedation or anesthesia to help with the discomfort. Patients who are undergoing a GIFT procedure also have a vaginal egg retrieval; in addition, they are required to have a laparoscopy in order for the procedure to be performed, because the eggs and sperm are placed directly into the fallopian tube via a catheter. A laparoscopy, which almost always requires general anesthesia, involves two incisions: one just outside the navel and the other lower in the abdomen where a probe is inserted. Although a laparoscopy does not require an overnight stay in the hospital or clinic, recuperation usually takes between two and four days.

The invasive nature of an ART cycle is not taken lightly by most couples. They have already been through several painful tests and treatments, and most women considering one of the ARTs know whether their pain tolerance is high or low. Some women, as part of their previous infertility workup, tolerated procedures such as an endometrial biopsy or a hysterosalpingogram with barely any discomfort; others found them unbearable, and when they learn what is involved in ART they become frightened. The amount of pain one is able or willing to undergo becomes an important aspect of the decision-making process.

Time Commitment

Another consideration for couples who are thinking about ART is the time commitment. There are three aspects of time that are important for couples to keep in mind: the distance to the clinic, the time they will need off from work, and the rigidity of the ART schedule. Depending on where the couple live, their work schedule, and their life-style, the time involvement can be easily manageable, nearly impossible, or somewhere in between.

Couples who live in or near large metropolitan areas have easier access to ART programs. Although frequent trips for blood draws and ultrasound monitoring can be inconvenient, most women, even those who have full-time demanding jobs, can manage to meet the requirements of both the program and their jobs, as long as the clinic is within reasonable driving distance of home (or of work).

Couples who do not live within driving distance of the clinic must put much of their lives aside in order to undergo an ART cycle. Not only do they incur added expenses (hotel rooms and restaurants), but they must also take time from other aspects of their lives. Some programs allow couples who live a great distance to have their blood drawn near home and couriered to the clinic; other programs have agreements with hospitals or clinics in different geographic areas to monitor a patient's cycle and fax results back to the home program. But even when much of the monitoring can be done close to home, living a long distance from the ART program complicates the process.

Certain jobs mix better with high-tech treatment than others. Women who work for themselves, work at home, or work part time have more flexibility than women who are teachers, for example. Women who work full time or whose part-time hours are rigid and conflict with the demands of the clinic feel more pressured by the time commitment.

An egg retrieval and embryo transfer involves two days. But exactly which two days it will be is not known until the couple is two days away from ovulation. For couples whose work involves frequent travel or other inflexible time demands, the unpredictability adds significant stress.

The requirements of an ART cycle are rigid. Clinics must carefully monitor each woman's cycle, adjusting her medications according to the results of daily blood tests and ultrasounds. Injections must be given at the same time each day so that the results accurately reflect how her body is responding to Pergonal. Thus, couples must sacrifice a great deal of spontaneity and adjust their lives according to the demands of the clinic, at least for the few weeks before egg retrieval or ovulation occurs. It is important for couples to know, however, that their social lives do not have to stop altogether. Many are remarkably resourceful during their ART cycles; some have been known to arrange to meet in a bathroom at a precise hour to do injections, even if it is in the middle of a dinner party. Others have given shots in the back seat of their car or in a restaurant parking lot. One couple reported doing their injection in a canoe.

ART Statistics

The Society for Advanced Reproductive Technology (SART) is a special interest group of the American Fertility Society. Its membership, though primarily physicians, includes those who have a professional interest in advanced reproductive technology. All ART clinics (in 1993 there were approximately 250) that are members of SART (most are) and perform at least forty ART cycles a year are required to report their data to SART. Any interested person can obtain copies of SART data by contacting the American Fertility Society in Birmingham, Alabama (see Resource List). (We urge all couples considering high-tech treatment to consider only clinics that are members of SART.)

In considering whether to do an ART cycle or where to do it, couples must understand the complicated nature of ART statistics. It is not enough to ask a particular clinic what its pregnancy rate is. The response is meaningless without all of the relevant information. Although it is not necessary to be a statistician or mathematician in order to understand what the figures mean, it is necessary to know what questions to ask and how to evaluate the answers. Couples should avoid clinics that do not willingly provide this information.

There are two pieces of information about a couple that are the most important in determining their prognosis: age of the woman and whether there is male factor infertility. Although the age at which women reach menopause is idiosyncratic (usually between forty and fifty-five), it is understood that fertility decreases as women get older, due to a decline in egg quality. Although some women may be quite fertile at age forty-five, most are not. Conversely, although most women are fertile at age thirty-five, some women are not. Statistics from all clinics indicate that women under age thirty-five have the best prognosis for ART; after thirty-five, pregnancy rates decline, and after forty they decline rapidly. Given this information, it is fair to assume that clinics that only accept couples if the woman is younger than forty should have higher pregnancy rates than those that accept older women. Couples must inquire as to what percentage, if any, of women being treated by ART are over age forty.

Some clinics use follicle-stimulating hormone (FSH) levels rather than age as a cutoff. FSH is the hormone released by the pituitary, along with luteinizing hormone (LH), that stimulates the ovum as well as the follicle (the sac of fluid that surrounds the ovum) to mature. The lower the FSH level, the more likely it is that the woman will respond well to the medication. Clinics that use FSH levels as a criterion for cycling rather than age have varying cutoff levels that they use to determine whether a woman can cycle. It is important to note, however, that an FSH level of, say, ten in a forty-year-old woman does not mean that she has the same prognosis as a thirty-five-year-old woman with the same FSH level. Thus, FSH levels are generally indicative of how well a woman will stimulate on the medication, but they are not in and of themselves a predictor of pregnancy rates.

IVF is frequently suggested as a treatment for male infertility. When sperm are placed in direct proximity with an egg (as in IVF), the numbers of normal-appearing motile sperm in a sample can be far fewer than they would need to be if the couple were attempting to conceive through coitus. However, even when the embryologist has carefully prepared the sperm for IVF, couples who have male factor infertility have lower fertilization rates than couples with no identified male problem. The greater the impairment is, the less likely it is that fertilization will occur. The point is that male infertility lowers success rates, and clinics offering IVF services to a large percentage of couples with male factor infertility (especially if they are willing to treat couples with severe male factor) should be expected to have lowered success rates.

Male infertility exists on a continuum. Some infertile men have semen parameters that are close to normal; others have numbers that indicate serious impairment. Couples entering IVF programs with a diagnosis of male infertility should ask questions about that program's success with problems like theirs. The couple needs to understand how the woman's age, in combination with the man's semen parameters, might affect their outcome.

The question about what percentage of women undergoing ART cycles get pregnant is not a simple one to answer. First, it is important to ask about the type of ART cycle one is considering. In general, IUI pregnancy rates, even with stimulated cycles, are not as good as GIFT or IVF, with some exceptions depending on age and diagnosis. Worldwide GIFT pregnancy rates tend to be higher than IVF, but that may be because women undergoing GIFT tend to have healthier reproductive systems or because not all clinics have the same level of embryology services. (Because the eggs and sperm are put back immediately in the fallopian tubes, GIFT procedures do not require the highly scrutinized manipulation and monitoring of eggs, sperm, and embryos as do IVF procedures.) Thus, some programs, in particular those that pride themselves on their embryology laboratory, may have better IVF success rates. When couples are comparing statistics from two or more programs, it is important that they compare apples with apples—IVF with IVF, GIFT with GIFT, and so forth.

Once a couple has isolated the statistics for the type of ART cycle they are considering, understanding the pregnancy rates can still be confusing. First, everyone who begins an ART cycle does not undergo an egg retrieval. Not all women stimulate sufficiently, and it is common in most programs for women to be cancelled prior to retrieval if there is reason to believe that only one or two eggs will be obtained. The older the woman is, the greater the likelihood that she will be cancelled. Programs that accept older women for ART cycles are likely to have higher cancellation rates, as well as lower pregnancy rates, than those that have more stringent age cutoffs.

Second, not all women doing IVF cycles who go through egg retrievals have embryo transfers. Usually only about 70 percent of eggs that are retrieved fertilize, even when the sperm is optimal. If a program accepts a large percentage of older women who produce only a few eggs and whose eggs are not as viable, fertilization may be very poor or not take place at all. Couples with male factor infertility also have lower fertilization rates and therefore more instances in which fertilization does not occur at all. Couples who do not achieve fertilization obviously do not have an embryo transfer, and those who do not have embryo transfer are not able to get pregnant (except in the rare instance in which the cycle was cancelled because of poor stimulation, but the woman ovulated and the couple conceived on their own or via an IUI.)

Understanding ART statistics is essential before choosing a program. To illustrate this point with actual numbers, we will use a hypothetical example of one hundred couples beginning IVF treatment at XYZ clinic. The clinic has a liberal age limit of forty-five, and it attracts more older women than other clinics. Let us say that fifteen of these women's cycles were cancelled, so that only eighty-five women actually went through an egg retrieval. Additionally, ten of the eighty-five couples did not have fertilization, and therefore only seventy-five of the original one hundred went through an embryo transfer. And fifteen of the seventy-five women who had embryo transfers had clinical pregnancies. If this clinic tabulates its pregnancy rate based on the original one hundred couples who began an IVF cycle, the rate is 15 percent (15/100). If it derives its rate from the number of couples who went through embryo transfer, the rate will be 20 percent (15/75). Both statistics are correct, but any comparison of programs must consider the actual numbers.

Two more explanations about statistics are important: the definition of pregnancy and the live birth rate. Pregnancy is measured by the amount of human chorionic gonadotropin (HCG) in the bloodstream, measured as the beta subunit of HCG (and therefore also referred to as the beta subunit). The first pregnancy test is given twelve to fourteen days after embryo transfer. In a viable pregnancy, the beta sublevels should double approximately every two days. Most programs require pregnant patients to come back for a second test a week after the first, in order to measure the HCG levels to see how the pregnancy is progressing. They will probably have the patient come back a week or so after the second test as well and will most likely schedule ultrasonography three weeks from the original pregnancy test in order to determine if the embryo is in the uterus (i.e., not ectopic) and has a heartbeat. The patient is considered to have a clinical pregnancy when she has rising beta HCG levels and the presence of an intrauterine gestational sac is confirmed by ultrasound. Although most clinical pregnancies end with healthy babies, some do not. Pregnancy loss occurs about 20 to 25 percent of the time, and its incidence increases with the age of the mother, reaching approximately 40 percent if the maternal age is greater than forty.

Although the majority of patients whose initial pregnancy tests are positive go on to have clinical pregnancies, many do not. Sometimes the hormones administered to induce ovulation (HCG) elevate blood levels such that the pregnancy test is unclear. In other cases, the embryo may have implanted for a short time, elevating blood levels slightly, but by the time the patient has a second blood level drawn, the numbers have tapered off. These situations are often referred to as biochemical pregnancies—a pregnancy that barely got off the ground. It is therefore important to learn how a particular clinic defines its pregnancy rates; biochemical pregnancies should not be included in statistics.

Live birth rates are also important—many feel they are the only important statistic—especially if there is reason to believe that a program is counting biochemical pregnancies in its success rates. If the difference between clinical pregnancy rates and live birth rates seems to be especially large in a program, it is wise to question these findings. It is important to learn once again, however, whether the live birth rate is calculated from all patients who began an ART cycle or from those who reached the embryo transfer stage.

The various ART clinics reporting to SART show consistent clinical pregnancy rates (as well as live birth rates) per cycle. In other words, the percentage of women who get pregnant on their fourth cycle is approximately the same as the percentage who get pregnant on their first cycle. Just as the chance of rolling doubles on one throw of the dice is not nearly as high as it is if one is allowed five throws, the cumulative chance of pregnancy increases if a couple (providing they have embryos to transfer) elects to do additional cycles. It is not clear, for how many cycles the cumulative data hold, but it appears to be true through at least five or six cycles. Some programs would argue more than that. This fact is most pertinent for couples who are assessing whether to do another ART cycle.

For couples deciding on ART, statistics provide cognitive information that is essential in decision making. In order for this information to be helpful, a couple must have a clear understanding about where they fall. Once they have all this information, they must make choices that are based also on subjective data, that is, on what feels right as well as on what is logical. For example, if a particular couple heard they had a 5 percent chance to become pregnant, it would be sufficient justification for them to say no to ART. For another couple, 5 percent might sound good, especially if their chances would otherwise be zero. The point is that couples differ in respect to what odds they feel make it worthwhile for them to proceed with ART treatment. What makes this issue even more confusing is that programs, as well as physicians, differ in the amount of encouragement they offer based on a couple's chance of pregnancy. Some physicians might encourage couples who have a 5 percent chance to keep trying; many others would strongly encourage them to move on. Each couple must search inside themselves to discover what they need to do—or not do—so they do not look back several years later regretting their choice.

Cryopreservation of Embryos

Once couples have decided to embark on high-tech treatment and have determined, in consultation with their physician, which form it will take, they confront a new set of decisions regarding the freezing and disposition of their embryos. Cryopreservation of embryos has been one of the most important developments of the new reproductive technologies, allowing many couples to get far greater mileage from an ART cycle and extending their reproductive possibilities.

Embryos are frozen one to three days after insemination in a cryoprotectant solution, stored in plastic straws or vials, and placed in liquid nitrogen. Depending on when they are frozen and whether they are viable, embryos contain between one and eight cells (occasionally more) when they are frozen. Programs that freeze embryos at an early stage most likely have a greater number of embryos to freeze from any one couple than do programs that freeze at a later stage. The reason is that many embryos stop dividing when allowed to continue past the first or second day. Embryos that are frozen earlier also have a lower survival rate when they are thawed than ones that are frozen later.

There are significant advantages to freezing embryos, for many women produce far more eggs than can be used in one cycle; eggs, unlike embryos, cannot be frozen. The extra eggs can be inseminated, and those that fertilize and are of sufficient quality to endure the freezing process can be stored (cryopreserved) for later use. If the woman does not conceive in that cycle, the couple can elect to go through a natural cycle in which she is monitored carefully via bloodwork, and when the timing is correct (her uterus is receptive), the embryos are thawed and transfered. Frozen embryo transfer cycles are much easier and less costly for couples than cycles in which fresh embryos are used, as the woman is not required to take fertility drugs (though some clinics do prescribe a hormonal regimen of estrogen and progesterone in order to achieve optimal uterine conditions). Additionally, if a couple does conceive during a fresh cycle and they would like more children in the future, they can return and go through a frozen cycle in hopes of achieving another pregnancy. One of the ironies of cryopreservation is that siblings can be conceived at the same time, but born years apart.

Many couples, even those who choose to freeze embryos, worry about the effects of the cryopreservation process on the resulting children. Although there is no evidence that children who are born from frozen embryos have any greater incidence of birth defects or physical or intellectual problems than do other children, the notion of being in suspended animation at the four-cell stage seems bizarre to many people. The oldest children resulting from cryopreserved embryos are just starting the primary grades. Although it looks highly unlikely that any long-term effects will appear, it is impossible to be certain of this for years to come.

The Catholic Church

The concepts of creating embryos outside the human body and cryopreserving them raise issues that reach deep into religion, philosophy, law, and science. Sometimes there is a meeting of the minds; at other times there are major debates. These issues center around the creation of embryos, the freezing of embryos, and the disposition of those that couples do not intend to use.

Although several religious groups have condemned the new reproductive technologies, the Catholic church has been the most vocal. Because Catholicism is one of the major religions and because the church has taken such strong stands on matters of reproduction, we will examine its position. In order to understand the church's position on the cryopreservation of embryos, it is neces-sary to understand its views on embryos in general, as well as its views about what may be done with embryos already created. In 1987 the Vatican published *Instruction on Respect for Human Life in Its Origin and on the Dignity of Procreation*, a document that has served as the basis for the beliefs of the Catholic church regarding IVF and the status of embryos. Because the process of IVF involves the joining of egg and sperm outside the conjugal union, the church does not sanction it. The *Instruction* states:

> The Church remains opposed from the moral point of view to homologous [both gametes come from husband and wife] in vitro fertilization. Such fertilization is in itself illicit and in opposition to the dignity of procreation and of the conjugal union, even when everything is done to avoid the death of the human embryo.[5]

Although the church is clearly opposed to IVF—and therefore op-posed to the creation of extracorporeal embryos—the *Instruction* goes on to elaborate in detail beliefs about both the freezing of em-bryos and the performance of research on embryos that have in fact been created. In this document, the church reiterates its belief that life exists on a continuum, beginning, according to the church, at fer-tilization and ending upon the death of that individual. The church believes that because an embryo has the potential to become a human being, it should be treated as such. The *Instruction* declares:

> Thus the fruit of human generation, from the first moment of its existence, that is to say from the moment the zygote has formed, de-mands the unconditional respect that is morally due to the human being in his bodily and spiritual totality. The human being is to be respected and treated as a person from the moment of conception; and therefore from that same moment his rights as a person must be recognized, among which in the first place is the inviolable right of every innocent human being to life.[6]

Regarding the issue of research on embryos, the *Instruction* states:

> Human embryos obtained *in vitro* are human beings and subjects with rights: their dignity and right to life must be respected from the first moment of their existence. *It is immoral to produce human em-bryos destined to be exploited as disposable biological material.* . . .

It is a duty to condemn the particular gravity of the voluntary destruction of human embryos obtained in vitro *for the sole purpose of research.*[7]

And regarding the cryopreservation of embryos, the *Instruction* states:

The freezing of embryos, even when carried out in order to preserve the life of an embryo—cryopreservation—*constitutes an offense against the respect due to human beings* by exposing them to grave risks of death or harm to their physical integrity, and depriving them, at least temporarily, of maternal shelter and gestation, thus placing them in a situation in which further offenses and manipulation are possible.[8]

The Warnock Committee Report

The position of the Catholic church thus bestows on the human embryo the status of a full human being. On the other side of the debate about what an embryo is are those who would treat it much as they would a piece of property—to be bought, sold, used, or disposed of as one sees fit. The vast majority of those who have any stake in this issue, however, take a point of view somewhere in the middle—that the status of the embryo is neither that of human being nor of property, but because it does have the potential to become a person if certain conditions prevail, it should be treated with respect and dignity, more so than if it were property.

In July 1984 in London, the Warnock committee, chaired by Dame Mary Warnock, published *Report of the Committee of Inquiry into Human Fertilization and Embryology.* The committee consisted of physicians, lawyers, scientists, social workers, and a theologian, and its report has been used by lawyers, ethicists, and physicians the world over in setting guidelines for particular programs regarding the new reproductive technologies. The Warnock report makes over sixty recommendations, including the use of embryos in research, the gathering of statistical information regarding infertility services, the use of donor gametes, and surrogate motherhood.

Regarding embryos, the Warnock report specifies that the use of human embryos in research must be regulated by law, and it recommends that fourteen days postfertilization be the outside limit to which embryos may be grown in vitro. The report also sets strict guidelines for what kinds of research on embryos may be permitted and to whom embryos may be transferred. Essentially, the Warnock report takes a middle-of-the-road position: that the use of embryos in research be restricted due to their special status as potential human beings. In recognizing the value of research, though, not only for infertile couples but for the purpose of curing genetic diseases, the committee allows for research on embryos if performed within well-established guidelines. Concerning embryo transfer, the committee declares that the transfer of an embryo from one species to another should never be permitted.[9]

The Disposition of Unwanted Embryos

Because the Catholic church does not approve of IVF, infertile couples who are practicing Catholics or have other strong religious beliefs, often struggle with whether they personally can participate in the new reproductive technologies, in particular IVF. Those who decide to do so then face another decision: whether to use cryopreservation.

Cryopreservation practice in ART clinics may reflect current legal statutes, which vary from state to state. Some states—Louisiana is one—have strict laws regarding the experimentation and disposition of embryos, implying that physicians who discard embryos can be prosecuted. These statutes may determine how many eggs a clinic is willing to fertilize, should the couple decide against cryopreservation. In other words, if a clinic will transfer only x number of embryos, they will inseminate only x number of eggs if the couple elects not to do cryopreservation.

Couples who cannot accept the idea of freezing extra embryos are at a statistical disadvantage if their clinic will not inseminate more eggs than they are willing to transfer. It is impossible to know ahead of time how many eggs will fertilize. Although approximately 70 percent of all eggs fertilize in a given cycle in which the sperm quality is normal, occasionally all or almost all will fertilize. Thus, if a clinic inseminated six eggs, in the hope that a couple would have four embryos to transfer, they could end up with five or six embryos, a number that is more than many clinics would transfer, because it puts the woman at too great a risk for multiple birth. Instead, the clinic would inseminate only four eggs, and most likely, even if there is no male factor present, they would end up with two or three good embryos, or possibly one or none. The fewer embryos transferred, the less likely it is that a pregnancy will occur.

Once couples have opted for cryopreservation—and the vast majority do—they are faced with a new set of decisions regarding future disposition of any remaining embryos. It may be that they end up with frozen embryos they do not want to use, as some fortunate couples eventually have the number of children they desire before they have used all their frozen embryos. Others discontinue medical treatment for various reasons, leaving frozen embryos in storage. There are three choices regarding these embryos: donation to another couple, donation to research, or discarding them.

Most clinics require couples to sign consent forms prior to beginning ART treatment that specify whether they will freeze extra embryos, how many they agree to transfer, and how they wish to dispose of any embryos they do not use. Some couples struggle at length with these decisions, attempting to anticipate all possible contingencies. These decisions are not irrevocable; couples are free to change their decision, should they have a future change of heart.

Embryo donation is a relatively new choice that allows a recipient couple to adopt embryos from a donating couple (see Chapter 9). The embryos are genetically unrelated to the recipient couple, though they will be gestated and birthed by the recipient/adopting mother. At IVF America Program–Boston the majority of couples initially choose to donate unwanted embryos to infertile couples. This clinic has found, however, that almost all couples who consent, prior to cycling, to donate embryos to infertile couples change their mind years later, when their families are complete, and decide to donate them to research instead.

The field of genetics is growing rapidly, as is the area of preimplantation genetics, and holds great promise for those couples—fertile and infertile alike—who may be carriers of genetic diseases that they do not wish to transmit to their offspring. Couples who donate for research purposes usually do so because they do not want to live with the knowledge that their genetic child was born to and raised by others. These couples are finding, in retrospect, that what they had previously thought would be a simple, easy, and altruistic gesture—donating their embryos to others suffering from infertility—is far more complicated emotionally than they imagined. Donating their embryos to re-search seems more palatable, as well as more beneficial to society, than merely discarding them.

Some couples do choose to discard their embryos, although state laws may or may not allow this option. Couples who opt to discard their embryos may do so themselves or, if the clinic is willing, designate someone to do it for them.

And sometimes even the best-laid plans can go awry. Couples who once agreed about what they wanted to do with their frozen embryos may disagree later, especially if their marriage is dissolving. The case of Mary Sue and Junior Lewis Davis of Tennessee illustrates the legal complications, as well as the emotional pain, that can ensue when divorcing couples disagree about what is to become of their once-joint embryos.[10]

The Davises had been through six unsuccessful IVF cycles and had seven cryopreserved embryos at the time they filed for divorce. Ms. Davis wanted to transfer the embryos into her uterus in order to have a child, insisting that they were living, and that she, as the mother, had a right to have them implanted. Mr. Davis no longer wished to become a father to these embryos/potential children and sought to prevent the clinic from implanting them in Ms. Davis or in any other woman. Although there were no precedents guiding the decision, the lower court judge ruled that the embryos were equal to human beings whose best interest was to be implanted and thus have the opportunity for life. Mr. Davis appealed this decision, and the Tennessee appellate court agreed with his argument that he should not be forced to father a child against his will. The court ruled that a man's right not to procreate outweighs a woman's right to procreate.

The Davis case points to the necessity of formulating prior agreements to which a couple must be held regarding the disposition of frozen embryos. John Robertson, a lawyer/ethicist and professor of law at the University of Texas, strongly recommends that couples declare in writing prior to cycling their instructions concerning disposition should they be unavailable or unable to agree when death, divorce, passage of time, or other contingencies occur. Regarding the Davis case and any other future cases in which couples have not signed prior agreements, Robertson, who agrees with the Tennessee court's decision, offers a formula in which to resolve such disputes:

> The party who wished to avoid offspring is irreversibly harmed if embryo transfer and birth occur, for the burdens of unwanted parenthood cannot then be avoided. On the other hand, frustrating the ability of the willing partner to reproduce with these embryos will—in most instances—not prevent that partner from reproducing at a later time with other embryos. As long as the party wishing to reproduce could without undue burden create other embryos, the desire to avoid biologic offspring should take priority over the desire to reproduce with the embryos in question.[11]

The appeal of the Davis case was important for two reasons. First, it dismissed the argument that embryos are human beings and therefore must be given the rights and privileges bestowed on humans. Second, it acknowledged the right of a person not to reproduce. In this instance, it was the man, who did not wish to become a father, but in future instances in which a couple divorces, it may be the man who wishes to have the embryos implanted in another woman and his ex-wife who wishes to dispose of them.

The ART Process

Couples who decide to undergo IVF treatment find themselves in a place that they never expected to be. Few, if any, could have imagined when they set out to have a child together that they would take this intimate process out of their bedroom and into a doctor's office, let alone into an operating room and adjacent IVF laboratory. Even when they accepted their infertility, most hoped that their problem would be resolved long before they faced decisions regarding the new reproductive technologies. Now they find themselves at a crossroads, about to embark upon the complex journey that is IVF.

Before describing the medical and emotional journey of IVF, it bears reminding that for many infertile couples—perhaps most—it is a strange, science-fiction-like process. When they are in the midst of ART, couples can easily lose sight of how far they have come, and they can minimize the complexities and demands of their experience. Margarete Sandelowski, a nurse and researcher who has worked extensively in the field of infertility, describes the experience of ART couples as "forcing conception." She captures their experience well and contrasts it with the experience of fertile couples who conceive effortlessly:

> Pain, not pleasure; struggle, not ease; separation, not unity; public exposure, not intimacy; and artifice, not naturalness, comprised the phenomenology of getting pregnant in infertile couples. In contrast to their fertile counterparts, these couples felt compelled to fight body, nature and convention to achieve conception.[12]

Becoming an IVF Patient

Every IVF cycle begins with emotional and financial decisions. There are important ethical questions to consider, as well as medical decisions to make about what treatment to try, when to try it, and which program to use—if there is a choice. Many of these decisions take time and careful planning, and the wait required along the way can be frustrating for couples who have already been waiting far too long to have a family.

Once a couple has decided to try ART treatment and has entered or chosen a program, there are still many tasks and preparations they face prior to beginning a cycle. First, they may have to wait several months—perhaps longer—before they can begin cycling. The application process may take time to complete; most clinics require that all prior medical records be sent. Some programs have waiting lists that can be up to a year long, before a couple is even able to have a consultation, while other programs accept couples almost immediately. Most programs also require additional testing as a prerequisite to cycling, which can include various hormonal screens as well as hepatitis and rubella screening and a semen analysis for the man. Most ART clinics require a test for the presence of human immunodeficiency virus (HIV) antibodies, which increases anxiety for most couples.

Once couples have had a medical consultation (many programs also require a consultation with a mental health provider and/or a nurse), the woman will probably undergo a complete physical examination, including measurement of uterus size (for IVF patients), so the physician will know how far to insert the embryos during the transfer. Once all the testing is completed, the woman can begin ART on the appropriate day of the cycle, which is determined by the protocol she is following.

For couples moving on from their gynecologist or infertility specialist or transferring from another ART program, there are new people to meet and a new system to learn. In addition to getting to know the staff and learning the ropes, couples must adjust to the waiting room and its special culture. Some clinics proudly display pictures of babies born from the program; others avoid anything that would remind patients of what they do not have. Some programs provide RESOLVE literature, post flyers from adoption agencies, or offer reading material about infertility; other programs are striking in their absence of all reference to the topics of pregnancy or parenthood.

No matter what a particular program's philosophy about waiting room environment, there are certain to be patients who are uncomfortable there, as well as those who are appreciative of the environment. One of the inevitable occurrences, however, is that whether or not clinics encourage or discourage communication among patients, it happens anyway. It is common for patients to overhear that someone is receiving less medication (or more) than they are, had far more (or less) follicles on their ultrasound, better- (or worse-) quality embryos, and so forth. Some patients appreciate being able to talk to others about their cycle, comparing and contrasting results. Other patients find that it increases their anxiety, especially if they perceive that others may have a better chance of success.

Couples also need to make arrangements to fit ART into their schedules, although more often than not it feels as if their lives are being fit into the cycle. Many women and men need to rearrange their work schedule, especially if traveling is a job requirement. Hence, couples are also faced with difficult decisions about whom to tell and what to tell them; if they do not tell their employer about their treatment, they may be accused of being lazy or irresponsible if their work attendance falls. However, telling colleagues and/or employers about ART treatment opens them up to questions that can feel intrusive, especially around the time of a pregnancy test.

Couples need to decide whether they will tell family members or friends, or both, that they are attempting IVF. Some couples are private; others tell almost everyone that they are involved in high-tech treatment. Having other people to talk to, complain to, and cry with can help make the ART experience less lonely for both husband and wife. The drawback to being open is that everyone who knows wants to know the outcome, and when couples receive bad news, they do not necessarily want to discuss it with others. It can help to make an arrangement such as, "Don't call us, we'll call you if it's good news," with those who know about their ART cycle.

As couples prepare themselves emotionally for ART treatment, it is important that they balance feelings of hope with feelings of caution. Many try IVF in order to feel they have done everything possible to have a biological child, so they will not have to look back with regrets. They do not want to be overly optimistic about their chances for pregnancy, but at the same time they wonder whether there is something to the "mind over matter" theory, and if so, whether it applies to ART treatment. Hearing tales of couples who claim that "IVF worked because I knew it would" can be upsetting to those who are trying to remain only cautiously optimistic.

Most couples do seem to cope with the high emotional stakes inherent in IVF by finding an adequate balance of optimism and caution. After all, they would not be going through the emotionally exhausting, time-consuming, physically invasive, and financially draining ordeal of ART if they believed there was no hope that treatment would work. At the same time, however, couples know—or should know—that the odds, even in the most optimal situations, are against them. Most conclude that to have no hope is senseless, but to have too much is also a mistake—one that potentially sets them up for even greater disappointment. It can help—providing a couple is able to make embryos and has the financial and emotional resources to undertake at least a few cycles—to temper long-term optimism with short-term pessimism.

The Role of Stress. Just as some ART couples wonder whether thinking positively will "make it happen," others wonder whether too much stress will negatively affect their outcome. They wonder if they should take a leave of absence from their job while undergoing a cycle or plan a vacation. Others avoid certain foods, change their diets, or learn yoga or meditation.

Stress, once thought to cause infertility, is now understood to be a serious and unfortunate by-product of it. (If stress did indeed cause infertility, then almost no one who ever experienced long-term infertility would be able to conceive.) Practically all physicians acknowledge, however, that there is a connection between the mind and the body, although the strength of the connection in regard to infertility is unclear.

We feel that it is extremely important that couples not add a mandate to relax or to reduce stress to their list of ART requirements. Stress is part of life and cannot be willed away. We have each known several highly stressed women who had successful ART pregnancies. In fact one psychiatrist/patient said, upon hearing that his wife was pregnant, "This proves it. Stress causes *fertility*. This was one of the most stressful months my wife has experienced." Another patient coincidently also a psychiatrist, said, upon giving birth to IVF twins, "Please tell couples not to worry about stress. I was a total wreck during my IVF cycle and my pregnancy, and I had two healthy babies." Finally, we are reminded of the woman who was so terrified during the blood drawings that she had to have three nurses hold her arm down each day. She too, went on to have a healthy and uneventful (but extremely anxious) pregnancy and delivered a healthy baby.

Loss of Control. Prior to encountering infertility, many people believe they have some measure of control over their lives—that if they identify realistic goals and work hard to achieve them, they can accomplish almost anything they set out to do. This belief gives them a sense that they are in charge of their lives. The loss of control over life is one of the major losses of infertility. Couples soon learn that hard work does not necessarily ensure success.

By the time couples get to ART treatment, they feel that they have lost a large measure of control. In many ways, ART reinforces this notion. Undertaking an ART cycle means that a couple must be able to allow others to be in charge; they must be prepared to tolerate uncertainly on a daily basis; and they must be able to endure the agony of waiting, knowing that their best efforts probably will have nothing to do with the outcome. Couples must wait for test results, ultrasounds, and blood levels. They must wait to see if fertilization occurs and, if so, once embryos have been transferred, they must endure the wait to see if the pregnancy test is positive.

In vitro fertilization, the most commonly performed ART procedure, paradoxically makes couples feel both more and less in control of conception. On the one hand, a cycle provides important information. A couple learns whether fertilization has taken place. They learn whether the woman's ovaries produced follicles, how many eggs they produced, and how many cells the embryos divided into before they were transferred to her uterus. In addition, they can get a rough estimate of the quality of the embryos transferred, at least from the eye of an embryologist. This is far more information than they have ever before had. On the other hand, the fact that others are involved in such an intensive effort to help them get pregnant—something most couples can easily do on their own— promotes a sense of feeling out of control.

In the course of a typical IVF cycle, there are predictable times in which couples feel more or less in or out of control of their bodies. During the first part of the cycle, patients tend to feel very much in control; although the daily requirements can be grueling and couples must be rigid about following the protocols, there are specific tasks that rest in the couple's hands: injections must be administered at roughly the same time each day; blood must be drawn and ultrasounds performed on schedule; the patient (or partner) must call in daily to get instructions about medications; the egg retrieval must be performed at exactly the right time (when the eggs are fully ripe but before the woman ovulates on her own). Most patients make sacrifices (eliminating alcohol, caffeine, and other medications, eating well; resting; exercising mildly) in order to feel that they have given the cycle their best shot.

But once the eggs are out of the woman's body and in the embryologist's hands, IVF couples feel out of control. Many wonder whether the "right" sperm and the "right" egg were put in the same dish, or whether the "right" embryos were transferred. It is a time when couples may be especially fearful, remembering the case of Julia Skolnick who in 1986 gave birth to a child of a mixed race, presumably because of a mixup in the laboratory. If fertilization is poor—or, worse, does not occur—they may think that the embryologist was incompetent or that a toxin accidentally destroyed their embryos.

The fact of the matter is that most clinics have extremely high standards. Eggs, sperm, and embryos are labeled and relabeled, checked and double-checked. It is understandable that couples might worry about mistakes in the laboratory, but of everything that could go wrong in a cycle, using the "wrong" gametes or transferring the "wrong" embryo is probably the last thing about which couples should have concerns.

Following embryo transfer, women typically struggle with attempting to regain control. Perhaps because they feel so out of control, some go to extraordinary efforts to take charge of their bodies: they meditate, take naps, or refrain from rigorous exercise to decrease stress or tension. If nothing else, they know these actions will prevent, or at least reduce, self-blame, making it harder to look back and be critical about what they did not do to nurture the embryos. Yet despite their best efforts, most do not get pregnant, at least in a given cycle. Commonly those whose cycles have failed feel helpless, hopeless, and depressed.

Waiting is a fact of life throughout the entire ART experience, and it enforces the sense of not being in control. Much of the waiting involves minimal time—for example, waiting to get the results of daily blood drawings or ultrasounds to see if the medications are working. Other waiting periods are longer—waiting to see if there are enough eggs to retrieve or awaiting the results of fertilization. The wait that seems endless to most couples, though, is the wait to find out about pregnancy. Most women report that despite the daily demands of ART, the first half of the cycle proved easier than they expected. Most are able to continue with their jobs, their social life, and their hobbies. The time tends to go by quickly, as they are keeping busy doing injections, going for blood draw and ultrasounds, and telephoning for results. On the other hand, the last two weeks of the cycle—post transfer—can seem endless.

Stimulation and Monitoring: The Daily Ordeal

Although the specifics of a medication protocol vary by program and by patient, all ART cycles (with the exception of natural cycle IVF or GIFT) involve several days of medications that are given by injection. The injections must be timed precisely (generally in the evening) and are administered daily (in some cases twice a day). Husbands typically are taught to give the shots. If he does not feel able to do so or travels a great deal, a close friend or neighbor can learn. Some women give themselves the shots, but most—including physicians and nurses who are patients—find the idea too difficult.

For many couples, the daily injections are a central stress of IVF treatment. Sometimes the stress is focused on the needles themselves. Men are troubled that instead of conceiving a baby in pleasure, they are forced to inflict pain on the woman they love. Although they initially worry that they will cause real physical harm—hitting a vein or a vital organ—most realize soon enough that it is not a complicated task, and they develop confidence in their ability to do the job. Men with male factor infertility, whose partners are undergoing IVF solely because of the male factor, have a particularly difficult time "hurting" their mates and watching them suffer as a result of "their" problem.

Women dislike the injections for different reasons. Their buttocks become black and blue and very sore, so that they are constantly reminded of IVF every time they sit down. Some women say they begin to feel like drug abusers. A small but significant percentage of women have a longstanding fear of needles, which makes the injection process even more difficult. Frequently hypnosis or relaxation techniques can be helpful when a woman has severe anxiety about injections.

Although most women say they get used to the shots, the process remains upsetting. Prior to ART, their bodies had been poked and prodded extensively. The pain from the needles, though it may be minimal, reminds them of the pain they have already endured and the reality that their ordeal is far from over.

The two main medications that are used in the stimulation phase of an IVF cycle are Lupron and Pergonal. Lupron is given by injection and administered subcutaneously (just under the surface of the skin), which makes the shot less painful than the Pergonal injection, which is administered intramuscularly, usually in the buttocks. Lupron, also referred to as a GNRH (gonadotropin-releasing hormone) agonist, suppresses the ovaries by shutting down the body's normal production of LH and FSH, both essential in triggering ovulation. Pergonal, which consists of a combination of LH and

FSH, or Metrodin (pure FSH) is given in order to stimulate the ovaries to produce eggs in a controlled but hyperstimulated manner. Physicians strive for the dosage that will produce the most number of good-quality eggs without unduly increasing the risk of hyperstimulation syndrome. Lupron is given to shut down the ovaries completely, so that when Pergonal is introduced, the follicles will mature evenly. In the early days of IVF, before Lupron was used, cycles were frequently cancelled when one follicle became dominant. Since follicles grow at a constant rate, if one becomes dominant the others cannot catch up to give the desired cohort of multiple follicles maturing together. Another frequent cause of cancellation, before Lupron suppression was commonly used, was a premature surge of the woman's LH, which can trigger premature ovulation.

Some medication protocols (those referred to as *down regulation*) require that Lupron begin in the luteal phase of the previous menstrual cycle. Although downregulation prolongs the number of days in which medication is given, thereby increasing the number of days of injections, some programs feel that it yields the best results in the majority of women. In other protocols (referred to as *flare-up*), Lupron is begun almost simultaneously with Pergonal, on the first day of the cycle.

The injections of Lupron and Pergonal are not the only instances in which a woman must be stuck with a needle during her ART cycle. In order to have her blood levels checked (which will determine whether she is being properly stimulated and whether her medication dosage needs to be changed), she must make several trips to the clinic to have blood drawn. Programs differ in the number and frequency of blood drawings required, but most programs insist on daily monitoring of the cycle in the week prior to egg retrieval.

For some women, especially those with small veins or veins that are difficult to find, the blood drawing is one of the most upsetting aspects of treatment. Relaxation or hypnosis can be helpful tools for coping with blood draws in such instances. Other women have found that asking for a particular nurse whom they trust, lying down, looking away, or applying hot compresses to their arm are simple requests that help ease their anxiety.

In the first part of an ART cycle, couples are involved in an ongoing drama that centers around the question of how they are responding to the medications. Patients must have frequent ultrasound monitoring in order to determine whether the medications are doing their part and causing a good number of follicles to grow. Eggs ripen inside the follicles, and although not all follicles produce an egg, most do.

No matter which ART protocol a woman is involved in, the same questions are crucial: how big the follicles are, how many follicles there are, and when the retrieval is likely to be. Each day the tension builds as the couple nervously awaits the report, hoping the news will be good yet fearing that something might go wrong. Commonly couples find they have irrational thoughts, such as "maybe all the follicles disappeared" or "perhaps they shrunk." It is also tempting (though not necessarily helpful) to compare one's progress with the progress of other women who are cycling at the same time.

The number of follicles is tracked via ultrasound, and they are carefully measured by the ultrasonographer because size is one of the gauges, along with blood levels, used in determining when the eggs will be retrieved. The follicles, which produce eggs, are the first visible sign that a couple is on their way to producing a child. And because couples are able to view their follicles on the ultrasound screen and to monitor their progress over time, they are likely to become attached to them, viewing them as the beginning of their child.

Although women undergo frequent blood tests and ultrasounds, with most medication protocols couples must wait several days before they know how well the medications are working. Not all cycles go smoothly, and many need to be cancelled because a problem occurred with stimulation. Although couples are generally warned that this event can happen, many are still stunned when it actually does.

There are two situations that might cause physicians to cancel a woman's cycle. One situation occurs when the woman overresponds to the medications, putting her at high risk for hyperstimulation syndrome. This type of problem can almost always be corrected in a subsequent cycle, and although it is upsetting when it happens, it does not signal future doom.

Another cause for cancellation is that a woman's ovaries did not stimulate adequately, most often due to aging. Although couples are generally warned that age is a major factor in pregnancy rates, some couples do not attach much importance to this information, especially if the woman is having regular menses and knows she is ovulating monthly. If the woman perceives herself to be in good physical shape and feels that her body is younger than her years, she may not attend to these warnings. News of poor stimulation, and hence cancellation, can be shattering, especially to the woman because it brings up fears that she may be facing the end of her reproductive life.

Couples in this situation feel defeated. So much effort went into their decision making, and yet the cycle barely got off the ground. Most clinics do not give up at that point, however, because other protocols can be tried, some of which may work better on older women. Some couples do decide to stop treatment, though, regarding the cancelled cycle as a sign that it was not meant to be. Once a woman has experienced two or three cancelled cycles, it is generally recommended the couple discontinue ART because the chances of yet another protocol's yielding different results are very slim.

Egg Retrieval, Insemination, and Embryo Transfer

The egg retrieval and subsequent embryo transfer are the focal points of an IVF cycle. Couples, especially those undergoing their first cycle, approach those events with anticipation and anxiety. Even women whose cycles have gone smoothly, wonder if they will ever get to the retrieval. They also wonder when it will be, which physician (in the case of larger programs) will do the procedure, and how many eggs will be obtained. In some instances, particularly if there has been a problem in the past, women worry that their husbands may not be able to produce sperm on demand.

Many couples, especially those who have had feelings all along about the "unnaturalness" of ART and regard it as "forcing nature," experience anxiety and fear about the egg retrieval, although the procedure is usually easier than they anticipated. The retrieval, which is performed vaginally via ultrasound guidance and is physically invasive, is considered to be a minor surgical procedure. For many women it is uncomfortable; in most clinics the pain is mitigated by sedation, administered intravenously, and generally performed in an operating room if the program is affiliated with a hospital. In some programs, a spinal or epidural anesthesia is used; others administer minimal sedation to women just prior to the procedure.

Most programs do not allow partners to be in the room when the retrieval is performed; they are concerned that should he become faint or require attention in some way, there will be no one available to attend to him, and his presence would be disruptive to the process. Some clinics do let partners be present, however, and wives whose husbands are allowed into the retrieval room tend to feel comforted. Husbands are usually happy to be able to offer support to their wives and to feel more involved in the process. One man commented that being there allowed him "to pretend they were not having sex in separate rooms."

During the retrieval, an ultrasound probe is inserted into the vagina. The probe guides a needle, which pierces the back of the woman's vagina, and is then inserted into the follicles one by one. Follicular fluid is aspirated from each of the follicles and brought to an embryologist, who puts the fluid into a dish and looks for an egg under the microscope. The retrieval usually takes between a half-hour and an hour, depending on several factors, including the number of follicles, the experience and dexterity of the physician, and whether the ovaries are easily accessible.

When a woman undertakes a GIFT procedure, she must undergo a laparoscopy so that the eggs and sperm can be placed directly into her fallopian tubes. A laparoscopy is done under general anesthesia and requires two small incisions, one just outside the navel and the other deep in her abdomen, where a probe is inserted. An overnight stay in the hospital is not required, but recuperation usually takes two to three days.

Although most men have had numerous experiences producing a semen sample prior to the ART procedure, many claim they never truly get used to it. The drama of IVF and the emotional buildup leading to the retrieval can cause even the most nonchalant of men to feel anxious about producing on demand. In addition, the IVF process, with its emphasis on precision and timing, tends to make husbands fearful that after all their wives have been through, they could ruin everything if their physiology fails to cooperate. In reality, eggs can live several hours before they must be inseminated, so there is more time available than most men realize. Occasionally men do have difficulty producing sperm on the day of retrieval, but if problems are anticipated, it is usually possible to come up with a contingency plan—perhaps freezing samples beforehand or asking his mate to be present in the collection room. Occasionally couples have arranged to stay in a nearby hotel, collecting the sample there and rushing it to the clinic.

Once eggs are removed from the woman's body they are inseminated with her partner's sperm. The couple must then wait another day (or two depending on whether the clinic transfers embryos two or three days after egg retrieval) to find out if fertilization occurred. This is another period when the time can pass painfully slowly, especially for couples with male factor infertility or for couples who have never had a pregnancy together and therefore do not know if fertilization is possible. If only a small percentage of eggs fertilize or the embryo quality is poor, couples are understandably upset because their odds of getting pregnant are greatly reduced.

If fertilization does not occur at all, it is devastating, even for couples with male factor infertility who may have been prepared, at least intellectually, for this outcome. After all their hard work and effort, there is no possibility for pregnancy to occur. Worse, since fertilization results tend to be relatively consistent from one cycle to the next, assuming a sufficient number of mature eggs to begin with, it is possible, even likely, that another cycle may not fare any better. Couples with failed fertilization must decide, with their physicians, whether it makes sense to try again, perhaps altering the procedure in some way, in the hope of obtaining a different result the next time.

The embryo transfer is truly the high point of the IVF drama for couples who have achieved fertilization, especially if they have many embryos to transfer and/or freeze. Embryologists rate the embryos according to the number of cells into which they have divided, their uniformity, and the degree of fragmentation. Although some clinics may not routinely convey much information to couples for fear of getting their hopes up (or, conversely, shooting them down), that information is probably available should couples ask for it. However, each laboratory has different standards, and to a great extent, the ratings are subjective; two embryologists may disagree about the quality of a particular embryo.

Furthermore, having excellent-looking embryos does not mean a pregnancy will occur, nor does poor embryo quality mean that it will not. An embryo may appear perfect forty-eight hours after fertilization, but there is no way of knowing whether it will ultimately survive. Conversely, an embryo may get off to a slow start but transform into a viable fetus. The embryo quality is only one measure of a couple's chances. (It may be obvious yet is important to mention that embryo quality has nothing to do with "baby quality.")

Prior to cycling, couples are told that ART treatment results in a multiple gestation approximately 25 to 30 percent of the time. Because multiples are considered to be a high-risk pregnancy, IVF practitioners try to avoid it. Many couples, however, are confused by their physician's caution regarding multiples and feel thrilled about the prospect of having more than one baby. Although most multiples are twins, about 5 percent of ART pregnancies result in triplets or greater—and the more babies, the riskier the pregnancy, and the greater the likelihood of premature birth and its attendant risks, including the death of all the babies.

Programs differ about the maximum number of embryos they will transfer. The more that are transferred, the more likely it is that a pregnancy will occur but also the greater is the chance of a multiple pregnancy. The goal is to maximize the possibility of pregnancy while minimizing the possibility of a multiple birth. Since multiple births are more likely to occur in younger women (they tend to have better-quality eggs and higher pregnancy rates per embryo transfer), some clinics have a cutoff age below which they put back fewer embryos. The IVFAmerica Program, for example, recommends transferring three embryos in women under age thirty-five and four for women over age thirty-five but will put back fewer embryos if their quality is good and more if the quality is fair or poor.

The question of how many embryos to transfer is perplexing to many couples. After years of feeling barren, they can hardly believe that any babies will grow inside them, let alone two or three. Yet we have witnessed the shock and disbelief on many faces when the ultrasound shows more than one strong heartbeat.

If a couple has gone through a few cycles without a pregnancy, their physician may suggest transferring more embryos in the next cycle. It is important to remember, however, that the odds of getting pregnant are approximately the same per cycle, so a couple who has gone through a number of failed cycles may still become pregnant with multiples in the following cycle. We are reminded of a couple who completed five IVF cycles without getting pregnant, each time having three good-quality embryos transferred. On the sixth cycle (which they had predetermined would be their last), after also having three embryos transferred, the woman became pregnant with triplets, delivering three healthy babies eight months later.

The embryo transfer itself is a relatively painless procedure, feeling similar to an IUI, a treatment many women experienced prior to undergoing IVF. In an embryo transfer, a thin catheter containing the embryos is inserted through the woman's cervix, and the embryos are placed into her uterus. She is required to lie still for a short period of time (two to four hours in most programs).

Although there is no evidence showing it makes a difference, some physicians believe that because it may take an IVF embryo up to three days to implant, patients should be on bed rest for several days following transfer. This recommendation, which is not the norm, is usually met with resistance. After already having to adjust their daily schedule to the demands of an IVF cycle, most women have no desire to stay in bed for long and are eager to get back to their normal routine. However, the occasional woman who is exhausted by the emotional and physical rigors of the first half of the cycle is pleased to have a mandated rest period.

The Endless Wait

The twelve- to fourteen-day wait before getting pregnancy results is a test of emotional endurance. With little to do but wait and with hopes, dreams, and sometimes even life savings at stake, couples look toward the pregnancy test with tremendous anticipation. The days crawl by as it approaches, and two weeks can feel like two months. Many report feeling helpless. In the days before embryo transfer, there was daily involvement, now they are on their own, having minimal, if any, contact with program staff.

Because there is nothing specific to be done unless progesterone support is prescribed, women find themselves at a loss, focusing on their emotional, spiritual, and physical state. Many hope that a positive attitude will help; some even talk to their embryos, play quiet music, avoid conflict—in short, do everything possible to provide a soft, nurturing habitat in which their embryos can settle. Others try to maintain life as usual, perhaps modifying any strenuous activities or experiences that might cause them to blame themselves should they not become pregnant.

Women typically check their body each day for symptoms— some sign that will reveal whether the embryos "took" to their uterus. Unfortunately, the medications or hormones administered to help stimulate egg production and those given after embryo transfer to help maintain a potential pregnancy can produce symptoms that simulate early pregnancy. Women who have not been told about these side effects begin to think they are pregnant and allow their fantasies to take over. If they have a negative pregnancy test—and most do—the disappointment is jolting.

Approximately twelve to fourteen days after the embryo transfer, patients return to the clinic for a blood test to determine whether they are pregnant. It is not uncommon for women who are not pregnant to have begun their menses before having the blood test. They come to the clinic reluctantly, because they were instructed to do so, but they feel they are wasting their time. Although most women who have begun to bleed are not pregnant, some actually are pregnant: what they assumed was their period was implantation bleeding, or a small portion of their endometrial lining that got sloughed off. For this reason, all patients are required to come in for a blood test, regardless of whether they have begun to bleed. Patients who have started to bleed know it would be rare for the test to be positive, and many say they prefer getting the bad news ahead of time in the form of their menses.

As difficult as it is to wait the requisite number of hours, it is even more difficult to make the call (or to answer the telephone if a particular clinic prefers to telephone patients, rather than vice versa). Many women describe walking around all day with a pit in their stomach. The hours crawl by, the tension builds, and couples muster their courage to deal with the news, whatever it is.

The Results

When the Pregnancy Test Is Negative. There is no good way to give bad news. It is the one aspect of their job that nurses dread; some say they never get used to it. Nurses, who have the most day-to-day contact with patients, get attached to the couples they treat and often feel like their cheerleader. When the test is negative, it is hard to know what to say to a woman or man who has invested so much effort to become pregnant. Some patients prefer a straightforward, matter-of-fact response when they call for the results; others appreciate consolation. Knowing the patient helps to determine how to best deliver the bad news.

All ART couples, even those who are "ideal candidates," and who participate in the most successful programs, have the odds stacked against them in any given cycle. Most are probably aware of their chances of success before beginning an ART cycle and are also aware that another cycle can yield very different results. Yet despite this awareness, if they are not pregnant, the news is still devastating.

When infertile couples attempt any new treatment, they usually have a great deal of hope that it will be the 'magic formula' that will produce their longed-for child. Failure to conceive with any treatment results in enormous disappointment and disillusionment. When couples embark on high-tech treatment, however, they are even more likely to view it as the magic answer to their problem. Frequent accounts in the media about "miracle babies" help perpetuate the idea that if nothing else works, high tech will.

The fact is that couples have been invested in a pregnancy long before they physically began their ART cycle. Once they began, they followed the progress of their cycle from the early follicular stage through transfer, when they learned the characteristics of their embryos. For many, experiencing an embryo transfer is as close as they have ever come to being pregnant. Some women talked to their embryo during the two weeks subsequent to transfer; others prayed that the embryo would remain viable and healthy.

It is almost impossible for couples not to feel attached to their embryos and not to feel devastated if the pregnancy test is negative.

Thus, the news that ART did not work is unfathomable to many couples. To some—especially those who viewed their embryos as potential children—it can feel as if they had a miscarriage. For this reason, it is important that ART couples who feel this way take time to grieve the child they did not have but in whom they invested so much of themselves.

When the Pregnancy Test Is Positive. For most couples who carefully plan their families—at least for the fertile majority—the reality of pregnancy begins when the chemical solution in the home pregnancy test changes color. These couples may celebrate their pregnancy with a glass of wine, a candlelight dinner, or perhaps in a more casual way, as if saying to themselves, "What's the big deal? We wanted a baby. We knew what to do. And it worked." For ART couples, it is never quite clear exactly when a pregnancy becomes reality or when they can allow themselves to celebrate—and surely not with a glass of wine! A minority, however, do allow themselves to rejoice, and although they may experience moments of disbelief, they have faith that their prayers have been answered.

For ART couples, pregnancy is seen as a process, and when it actually begins is rarely clear. Some believe that pregnancy began when their embryos were transferred into the mother's womb. Others feel it began when they received the news that the test was positive. Still other couples declare that it was not until they saw the embryo on ultrasound and witnessed its heart beating that the pregnancy began.

Although there is no good way to give bad news, there are many ways to give good news. No matter how it comes, ART couples frequently experience a range of reactions that they did not expect. Some find that in addition to joy, they also feel fear. Others feel shocked or are in disbelief. It is common, after so much disappointment and heartache, to think that an error was made—perhaps a mix-up of the blood samples. One woman commented, a week after learning her test was positive, that she now knew what it must be like to have manic-depressive illness. At moments she felt so excited she could burst, and at other moments she experienced waves of terror that she would wake up and it would all be a dream. The terror would send her into depression, and it was only her husband who could calm her down.

Questions and fears are part of the early pregnancy experience for couples who are expecting after assisted reproductive technology. They wonder, whom should they tell—if anyone? Can they make travel plans or are they better off staying close to home where they feel safer, should something go wrong. Did more than one embryo implant, and, if so, how will they feel if they are having multiples? Did the embryos implant in the uterus or must they confront the threat of ectopic pregnancy?

Although they knew prior to trying ART that miscarriage is always a possibility, many women pregnant after ART are surprised at how terrifying this prospect is. Just as there are several hurdles over which couples must leap prior to getting pregnant, they now realize they have several more hurdles to face before they can bring home a baby. Yet the majority of women—approximately two-thirds—whose first test is positive will bring babies home eight and a half months later.

Pregnancy is monitored by the levels of beta subunit in a blood test. In early gestation the numbers are low, though in a healthy pregnancy they should double approximately every two days. Estradiol levels as well as progesterone levels can also indicate whether a particular pregnancy appears to be getting off to a good start or whether there is reason to be concerned.

Couples are often confused by the pregnancy tests. A first pregnancy test, though positive, may produce low numbers because it is so early on and because implantation may have occurred late. If the numbers are very low, clinics caution couples immediately that the pregnancy is precarious. These cautions, while necessary, are often difficult for couples because there is nothing they can do except wait the prescribed number of days before having another test. A second test may reveal whether the pregnancy is progressing normally—or the results may be equivocal again, and the couple is sentenced to another week of endurance testing.

Even when everything looks good the first time, couples suffer through an excruciatingly long wait—usually a week—before returning for a second test, which will reveal more information. If the second test again yields good results, it is a great relief, yet the couple is still a long way from their goal. A third pregnancy test, again about a week later, is another marker that can help couples relax if the news is good—or feel devastated if it is bad.

While the focal point of the IVF cycle is the embryo transfer, the high point of pregnancy after ART for most couples is the ultrasound, done approximately three weeks after the original pregnancy test—five weeks from conception. They hope the ultrasound will reveal the presence of a normal-size gestational sac that has an embryo with a heartbeat and is located in the uterus. When the unmistakable flicker appears on the screen, it is truly a time of celebration. Although couples are still eight months away from their dream and pregnancy loss can occur at any stage, they are much closer than they were just a few weeks earlier.

Pregnancy after infertility—even after a positive ultrasound—is a time of mixed emotions, and high-tech treatment adds even more intensity to the experience. No matter how good the odds are that a pregnancy will result in a baby and no matter how smoothly the pregnancy is going, women feel very anxious that something will go wrong. They are constantly tuned in to their body, looking for any clue that might tell them whether they should relax or remain vigilant.

Like other pregnant women, those pregnant after ART treatment usually have some symptoms: morning sickness, frequent urination, fatigue, or sore breasts. Most are grateful to have these symptoms and consider them reassurance that all is going well. However, because of all the medication taken, a woman pregnant as a result of ART may be confused, wondering whether what she is feeling is actually a side effect of the medications rather than a sign of a healthy pregnancy. Furthermore, any lessening of these symptoms, however slight, can frighten her. In fact, when symptoms do disappear suddenly in the first trimester, it may be a sign that the pregnancy is in jeopardy.

As unpleasant or as inconvenient as the symptoms of pregnancy are, women who do not experience them, even if their pregnancy is perfectly healthy, worry that it is not viable. They may require extra monitoring via blood tests or ultrasounds, depending on how far along the pregnancy is. The monitoring can be reassuring to them, in the way that side effects are to those who have them, that all is well within their womb.

As thrilled as they are to be pregnant, women who are pregnant after high-tech treatment also feel cheated. They cannot be normal, pregnant women. Their feelings of disbelief, confusion, anxiety, and even isolation are unique to their experience. And although many are able to relax to some degree after their first trimester, most remain vigilant throughout their pregnancy.

Most clinics follow ART patients through their ultrasound—four to five weeks after embryo transfer. If the pregnancy is normal, the couple then transfers to the care of an obstetrician. This can be a momentous time for couples—mostly exciting but difficult in some ways. They are leaving a situation where they never wanted to be in the first place but that has become familiar and usually a source of support. They are leaving staff who served as their cheerleaders and understand how special this pregnancy is. Most patients are extremely grateful to all who assisted in bringing them what they have wanted and worked for, for a very long time. It is with somewhat mixed emotions (but mostly with sheer joy) that they say good-bye.

Evaluating the Cycle

Why a Cycle Fails

When normal, healthy-appearing embryos are transferred and pregnancy does not occur, couples and physicians wonder what went wrong. In many instances everything seems to have gone right: the stimulation went well, the sperm quality was good, and the embryos looked excellent—but the pregnancy test was negative. And although ART staff know very well that the odds in any cycle are always against a pregnancy occurring, they find themselves perplexed at how often the test results are negative.

Although the reasons why a particular cycle failed will never be known for sure, there are two possible and probably obvious explanations: the embryos stopped dividing or there was a problem with implantation. In these situations, there is every reason to hope that another cycle will yield a pregnancy. Although this information can be consoling to some couples, it is frustrating to others who cannot afford more ART treatment or found the protocols too rigorous.

Physicians review ART cycles that fail. In some instances, there are obvious reasons why pregnancy did not occur, such as poor stimulation or poor embryo quality. Women who are older tend to stimulate more slowly and require larger dosages of Pergonal than do younger women. It is more likely that their cycle will be cancelled prior to egg retrieval or that the quality of the eggs will be compromised, sometimes resulting in lower fertilization rates or poor-quality embryos. These are explanations that physicians offer, and although they can advise couples as to whether they believe a change in the medication protocol will yield different results, patients remain baffled.

There are some couples who consider the first cycle a trial run, not expecting it to work though secretly hoping they will be successful on the initial attempt. These couples are aware that it may take a cycle or two to adjust the medications correctly. They know that to some extent guesswork is involved in finding the best medication protocol, and they are prepared for a longer haul. These couples usually experience their greatest disappointment and grief following a second or third unsuccessful cycle.

What Next?

When an ART cycle fails, couples consider what to do next. This decision is based on a series of questions that they ask themselves and their physician:

• Was their treatment a good one that simply did not work the first time?
• Would another treatment be better—or at least as good—and perhaps less expensive?
• Can they afford (financially and emotionally) to try again?

Assuming that finances are not a deterrent, some may decide to try the same treatment, coming to the conclusion that one failed cycle is by no means an indication of future failures. Other couples will try something different because of financial considerations, stress, the desire to try something new, or their physician's recommendation.

If the woman has one or more fallopian tubes open, her physician may recommend switching to another type of ART cycle. Some couples who did an IVF cycle in part to learn whether fertilization could occur (and it did) might decide to attempt GIFT next, believing it might work because the fallopian tube is a better incubator. Or they may opt to do IUI, avoiding an egg retrieval, as well as reducing their expenses. On the other hand, couples who began high tech with GIFT and did not become pregnant may be advised to attempt an IVF cycle next, in order to be certain that fertilization is possible. Still other couples may elect to try ZIFT, which involves more physical effort and more expense than the others but offers the benefits of both GIFT and IVF. The high-tech possibilities are numerous, and couples frequently feel overwhelmed by their choices. Some physicians are more vocal about what they feel a couple should do; others prefer the couple themselves make the final determination if more than one option appears to be a good choice.

Different programs specialize in different treatments. One clinic may believe GIFT is the treatment of choice as long as at least one tube is open. Other clinics, priding themselves on their embryology laboratories, may believe strongly in IVF as the treatment that yields the most information and the best results. Researchers and clinicians are constantly debating the question of what is the most effective treatment, comparing and contrasting all the possibilities. The point is that each couple's medical situation is different, and in the absence of definitive data, couples, in consultation with their physician, must choose the treatment that seems right for them.

When fertilization does not occur, especially if the egg quality was poor or there were few eggs to inseminate, another try may be recommended. However, if there were several eggs to inseminate and none fertilized, programs might not encourage couples to recycle, unless they believed that a change in the way the eggs or sperm were prepared might lead to conception in another cycle.

In situations where fertilization does not occur due to male factors, the decision about where to go is more complicated. Some ART programs are better equipped than others to deal with male infertility and are able to alter the way they prepare sperm for insemination, in hopes of obtaining fertilization on another try. A few (and the numbers will increase as the technology becomes more available), move on to micromanipulation.

Micromanipulation

As we have attempted to note throughout this book, infertility in the nineties is a time of new opportunities—and new dilemmas. Couples frequently comment that there is always a new 'carrot' dangling in front of their eyes. Each new treatment option brings new hope, but at the same time it contributes to the fear couples have, that since there is always something new to try, they will never know when to stop.

The newest treatment option for couples suffering from male infertility is micromanipulation, sometimes referred to as microinsemination. This new technology is a treatment for couples who have not been able to achieve fertilization through standard IVF or who are ineligible for IVF because the sperm quality does not meet the clinic's requirements. Micromanipulation is an astounding treatment—when it works—offering the hope of fertilization for certain couples who previously had no hope of achieving it.

Microinsemination of human eggs was first performed in 1985; by January 1993, approximately 250 babies had been born as a result of this procedure. Micromanipulation uses sophisticated tools and equipment for the purpose of facilitating fertilization. It is very costly, extremely painstaking, and offered only in a few clinics. The largest, and best known, is Cornell Medical Center in New York City. Because of the cost and limited availability, this technology is open only to a small percentage of couples with male infertility.

There are many couples who welcome the possibility that something might help the husband's sperm. Reluctant to adopt or to try donor insemination, they want to exhaust every other possibility before seriously considering those two options, or before moving on to child-free living. Unless the cost precludes the treatment, they are enthusiastic about pursuing this very latest advanced reproductive technology.

Other couples, especially those who had come to some degree of comfort with a second choice, are troubled to learn about micromanipulation. They feel the pull, once again, for a biogenetic child and want to feel that they did their best to make that happen. Nevertheless, having moved 'forward' in the direction of alternatives, the idea of 'moving backwards' into more high tech treatment, is unappealing.

If IVF and GIFT etc. are considered to be high tech treatment, then micromanipulation techniques can be considered to be super, high tech treatment. In micromanipulation the embryologist attempts to induce fertilization by various methods: injecting the sperm directly into the egg or making a slit or hole in the shell of the egg (zona). In the first process, referred to as subzonal injection (SZI), several sperm (usually four or five but sometimes more or less depending on the quality) are injected just underneath the shell into what is called the perivitelline space. In a more recently developed process—intracytoplasmic sperm injection—(ICSI) a single sperm is injected directly into the center of the egg—its cytoplasm. The second method, known as partial zona dissection (PZD), involves making a slit in the zona through the use of a microneedle, thereby allowing the sperm easier access into the ovum.

Research published in 1993 indicated that of all the micromanipulation techniques, ICSI appears to be the most promising. Researchers in Belgium were able to successfully fertilize 54% of the eggs they injected, which resulted in a 31% pregnancy rate per treatment cycle. (More recent research presented at the 1993 annual meeting of the American Fertility Society, unpublished to date, indicated even higher fertilization rates).[13] Thus, if a woman is able to produce a large quantity of eggs, it is likely that she will have embryos to transfer, an obvious precondition for pregnancy. Once the embryos are transferred, pregnancy rates in most programs tend to be about the same as they are for IVF patients in that particular clinic who have the same number of embryos transferred.

Some couples who consider microinsemination are worried about potential medical problems in the offspring. They fear that a defective sperm may have been used unknowingly, causing a problem in the child that may or may not be evident at birth. Geneticists, however, claim that sperm that are unable to fertilize on their own do not carry defective genetic material; rather a biochemical problem impedes them. To date, the children born from microinsemination procedures appear to be normal. However, it is too early to draw definitive conclusions.

We began the second half of this chapter by discussing the issue of what it means to force conception. There are probably few couples who struggle with the issue of "forced conception" more than those who turn to micromanipulation. Many—even those who feel comfortable with the process of IVF—wonder whether the literal injection of sperm into egg is going a step too far. The idea of forcing nature feels morally wrong to many couples. They ponder such questions as, What has happened to medical science? Are people trying to play God? Are we tampering with the natural order? Other couples, by contrast, do not draw such strong distinctions between micromanipulation and the other ARTs. They regard it as one more astonishing advancement of reproductive medicine. They may have concerns about the long-term effects of the technology, because it is so new, but they do not have ethical problems with it.

Couples who have been unable to achieve fertilization in vitro and who move on to microassisted fertilization techniques feel they have done everything humanly possible to try to conceive a child together. Those who do not get pregnant, although extremely disappointed, are generally able to move on to family-building alternatives with no regrets about stones they have left unturned. Those who do become pregnant and later give birth to a child believe that they are the recipients of a miracle—a child who never would have existed if it were not for modern reproductive technology.

When is Enough, Enough?

It would be much easier emotionally for couples if ART either worked or did not work on the first cycle. As upsetting as it would be to get the bad news, couples would be able to grieve their disappointment and loss and move on, without wasting more time, money, and energy chasing a dream that can never be. But because a couple's chances of pregnancy, assuming they reach the embryo transfer stage, are consistent through several cycles, it is impossible to know whether the next cycle will be the one to work.

Since ART treatment is covered by medical insurance in only a few states, many couples know before setting out to do ART that they can afford only one cycle. Others know that they can afford two or perhaps three cycles. Still other couples, regardless of their economic situation, decide at the outset that they wish to try only one time. Because ART is available, they feel they must try it, but they have no desire to immerse themselves for a lengthy period.

Most couples who have health insurance or can afford treatment and whose first cycle went well but did not result in pregnancy, do decide to continue ART treatment. In Massachusetts, where infertility treatment (including ART) is a mandated insurance benefit, couples who undergo ART do an average of about two and a half cycles. That statistic takes into account all couples who begin an ART cycle regardless of whether they get as far as embryo transfer and those couples who get pregnant on a first or second cycle but would have continued had they not been pregnant.

Most ART couples set a reasonable number—commonly between three and six cycles—at which point they will stop if they have not become pregnant. Unless given definitive reasons why additional cycles would not be fruitful, most feel inclined to continue, hoping to avoid regrets later. It is important, however, for all couples to remember that continuing or ending treatment is an individual decision and that they must decide for themselves when they can stop without feeling regretful.

Most women have an easier time managing ART than they anticipated. There are, however, a small number of women who have extreme reactions to the medications or some of the procedures and decide to end treatment after a single cycle rather than put themselves through another endurance test.

Although most couples can find a reasonable end point to treatment, some cannot. They continue to undertake ART cycles long after it seems unlikely that treatment will work. They include women who adjust to the protocols and regimes quite easily, who claim that the injections do not hurt, the blood draws are no problem, and they have become used to the daily drives to the clinic. Also included in this group are those who appear unable to grieve, those who cannot—or will not—pursue a second choice, and those who disagree with their spouses about what to do next. For these continuous cyclers, ART has become a way of life. Although physicians may have advised them after eight, ten, or a dozen or more cycles that their chances of getting pregnant are probably miniscule, they refuse to give up. One patient made the following declaration to the social worker at her clinic: "I've decided to stop counting and just do cycles. I'll keep cycling and cycling as long as I can until it either works or I'm in menopause."

Sometimes a pregnancy that ends in miscarriage makes a couple rethink their plan to discontinue treatment. For instance, if they were planning to do four cycles but a pregnancy loss occurred after one of them, they may be understandably tempted to try additional times. After all, since ART worked once, there is reason to believe it might work again, this time with a better outcome. A pregnancy that ends in miscarriage is like a carrot that is held out, signaling their goal is in sight but not unless they are willing to venture forward.

Couples are not only confused by how many cycles to do but also how frequently to do them. There are couples who want to put high-tech treatment behind them. Their aim is to do back-to-back cycles for an identified period of time and then move on. Consecutive cycles means six a year at the most, since clinics require a month of rest between ART treatments. Some programs may require an even longer rest period, either because they believe the woman's body will function better after at least two normal cycles or because they have too many patients to accommodate.

Couples who prefer to cycle consecutively usually live within a reasonable distance from the clinic and adjust to the rigorous protocols fairly easily. They incorporate ART into their schedules with as little disruption as possible. Most of them have a plan that sets a certain number of cycles, and when they have reached that point, they end treatment and consider alternatives to biological parenting.

Many other couples who are prepared to cycle several times know that they need a reasonable rest period in between. ART is enough of a disruption, and they need to renew their strength and their relationship and return to a normal life for a period of time. Although the prospect of dragging out high-tech treatment interminably is not appealing, the alternative—back-to-back cycles—is even less appealing. These couples may do anywhere from two to four cycles in a year, depending on their pacing.

Older women may not have the luxury of being able to take much time off in between cycles. Every month that passes may reduce their chances of getting pregnant, especially if their FSH levels appear to be rising. Older couples who would ordinarily choose to rest between cycles must weigh the potentially negative effects of waiting with the extent to which frequent or back-to-back cycles impinge heavily on the quality of their life.

Still other couples, especially younger ones, are choosing to discontinue treatment temporarily and pursue an alternative path to parenthood, knowing they have the option to return to ART later and knowing that the technology will be even better. These couples have figured out that their primary goal is to become parents and that being biological parents is a secondary goal, one they are prepared to forgo. Others take a lengthy break from high-tech treatment, not to pursue an alternative family-building method but to reassess their goals and to take an extended vacation from the grueling demands of ART.

The field of high-technological reproduction has grown enormously since the birth of Louise Brown. In vitro fertilization, which forms the basis for all the ARTs, has become a widespread and multipurpose tool, having redefined reproduction. ART enables couples to procreate without having sex, and bypasses previously insurmountable reproductive problems. Cryopreservation has revolutionized the process of conception by allowing embryos to be frozen, a phenomenon that greatly expands reproductive possibilities. Even physicians specializing in the ARTs cannot keep up with the developments and the vast amount of research that has proliferated as a result. What is clear, however, is that once the ball began rolling it could not be stopped, and although IVF and all its variations have supporters and detractors, the new reproductive technologies are here to stay.

The new reproductive technologies do have critics, among them Elizabeth Bartholet, who after years of IVF attempts eventually ended treatment and adopted two sons. Bartholet is critical not only of the ART industry but also of those who pursue biological parenthood relentlessly. Although we strongly agree with her that adoption should be far easier and much more affordable and we understand well that family bonds are formed by love and nurturing and not by genes, we also realize that Bartholet came to these conclusions only after she went through the emotionally arduous process we describe in this chapter. Many of the happiest and most enthusiastic adoptive parents we have known were, like Bartholet, among the most persistent ART patients. Experience tells us, however, that they too needed to go through the exhausting process of infertility and come out the other side in order to reach these conclusions.

For every couple who faces infertility, there is a difficult and painful journey, often through the rocky terrain of the ARTs. For some couples, that journey leads to the birth of a child or children; for others it leads to a different resolution. As clinicians working in the field, as authors, as parents, and as women who have experienced infertility, we firmly respect every couple's right to say no to ART—whether for personal, financial, religious, ethical, or emotional reasons. Our experience has taught us, however, that couples who try the ARTs have few regrets. Those for whom ART does not result in a successful pregnancy feel the satisfaction of knowing that they have done their best. And for others—those who are fortunate to have successful pregnancies—they have a living, growing reminder of the miracle of modern science and the mystery of creation.

Pregnancy Loss

We have no voices to remember. We have no occasions or activities to remember. We have no recollections of smiles or kisses to comfort us. We have only pictures of our two dead babies. We have birth and death certificates of our daughters who were born only to die. Why did this happen to us? We laid down our lives for this pregnancy. We did everything that was humanly possible to be parents. Now we are parents but we have no children.

—*A couple whose stillborn twin daughters (at twenty-two week's gestation) were conceived with GIFT after five years of trying.*

If life were fair, all infertile couples who achieved pregnancy would go on to have healthy babies. Far too often, however, long-sought, hard-earned pregnancies end in loss. In this chapter we look at the experiences of couples who endure pregnancy loss—miscarriage, ectopic pregnancy, stillbirth, and loss in multiple gestation—all after turning to the new reproductive technologies. We will also discuss multi-fetal reduction, an extraordinarily difficult form of pregnancy loss that is primarily an outgrowth of the new reproductive technologies.

Early Pregnancy Loss

For several weeks I replayed the scene of the ultrasonographer telling me the bad news. I can picture the screen and the room and the sounds, and most of all, her words. I know that just before she told me, after performing both a vaginal and an abdominal ultrasound, she turned for a moment and faced the sink, while carefully rinsing off the probe—turning her back to me. I remember how her back stiffened, and she raised her shoulders and sighed. I knew, at that instant, that it was over—that she was building the resolve to tell me. She was trying to find a way to say that all that we had sought for so long and attained—was lost.

Miscarriage is almost always a painful and difficult experience, even for those who conceive easily. Women, in particular, feel grief, fear, guilt, and confusion. When loss occurs following treatment with the assisted reproductive technologies, these feelings may be greatly intensified. ART couples experience a special kind of anguish as they ask: Why did this happen? Did we do the wrong thing by forcing nature? Did I somehow cause this loss? Could something have been done to prevent it? Is pregnancy really a matter of what is meant to be?

Medical Facts

In order to understand the anguish that couples feel as they ask and attempt to answer these questions, it is important to begin with some medical facts, for although there is no single and definitive explanation for early pregnancy loss, miscarriage is no longer the mystery that it once was. Physicians have identified a number of factors that can cause or contribute to miscarriage. We begin with a brief discussion of these factors because we have found that medical information helps couples to grapple with what is often the most puzzling and troubling question: Why did this happen?

Miscarriage, also known as spontaneous abortion, is usually defined as the loss of a pregnancy in its first twenty weeks. The vast majority of these losses occur within the first twelve weeks, making miscarriage after the first trimester less common. In fact, most miscarriages actually occur within the first six to eight weeks of pregnancy. However, since some women miscarry before they even know that they are pregnant and others experience the physical signs of miscarriage several weeks after the fetus actually dies, the prevalence of very early miscarriage is underreported. Although technically an embryo does not become a fetus until its eyelids fuse (usually about sixty days past conception), the word *fetus* is commonly used when a pregnancy has been confirmed. Thus, we will use the term *fetus* to avoid confusion.

Miscarriage can be caused by problems in the fetus or by problems in the maternal environment. The current understanding is that most early pregnancy losses are caused by problems inherent in the fetus; estimates are that 60 percent of miscarriages in the first half of the first trimester and 15 to 20 percent of miscarriages in the second half of the first trimester are caused by chromosomal abnormalities.[1] These defects in the fetus prevent it from growing beyond a certain point.

Problems in the maternal environment, although more varied, are a less common cause of early pregnancy loss. For example, there can be uterine factors. Some women suffer from Asherman's syndrome, a scarring of the uterus that can occur after a dilatation and curettage (D & C) or abortion or following an infection. Asherman's syndrome can cause miscarriage by preventing an embryo from implanting properly.

Another maternal cause of early pregnancy loss is a progesterone deficiency. However, since most women who become pregnant through the ARTs have their progesterone levels monitored regularly, it is unlikely that a woman will lose an ART pregnancy due to progesterone deficiency. Women whose progesterone levels are low, are given supplemental progesterone preventatively, and many programs prescribe it for all their ART patients.

Placental problems are occasional causes of early pregnancy loss, but more often they cause later losses. Placenta previa is a condition in which the placenta attaches to part or all of the cervix. Abruptio placentae is a condition in which the placenta separates from the uterine wall. Pregnancy losses also occur when the placenta does not function properly and denies the fetus essential nutrients.

Early losses can be caused by infections or by systemic disease in the mother such as diabetes, thyroid disease and autoimmune conditions. However, these are thought to be infrequent causes of miscarriage.

Another potential cause of miscarriage is embryo toxic factor. Dr. Joseph Hill at Brigham and Women's Hospital in Boston has investigated the possibility that some women have a toxin that destroys their embryos. (Some promising results have been reported when these women are treated, in subsequent pregnancies, with very high dosages of progesterone. The theory is that the high dosages will overcome the potency of the embryo toxin and permit the fetus to survive.)[2]

Finally, there is a new form of early pregnancy loss that is a direct outgrowth of the ARTs: biochemical pregnancy. In a biochemical pregnancy, the first pregnancy test (two weeks after ovulation) indicates a low but positive beta subunit number, but subsequent tests reveal that the pregnancy never got off the ground. Some physicians feel that a biochemical pregnancy does not constitute a pregnancy at all. They say that a woman is pregnant (sometimes referred to as clinically pregnant) only after her pregnancy hormone levels have risen twice and a gestational sac has been confirmed. Hence, from a medical standpoint, a biochemical pregnancy is not always considered a pregnancy loss. We feel, however, that it is important to include this experience in our section on pregnancy loss since, from an emotional standpoint, a very real loss has occurred.

Feelings

Couples are frequently plagued by questions following the loss of an ART pregnancy. As they confront the questions and struggle to find answers, they face an array of emotions.

Grief. When infertile couples learn that their hard earned pregnancy has ended in loss, most feel profound grief. Even those who tried to shield themselves from disappointment by postponing any sense of celebration feel shattered. They realize that once they learned that the pregnancy test was positive, they began to feel attached to the growing life inside them. Now, the fetus, on whom they had begun to focus their hopes and dreams, is gone.

The grief that couples experience is often intensified by the fact that others rarely acknowledge the significance of their loss, especially when it occurs very early in the pregnancy. Instead, friends and family tend to focus on the "good news" aspect: now the couple knows they can achieve pregnancy. Physicians also try to comfort them by telling them that they are excellent high-tech candidates because they have now achieved pregnancy.

Although there is usually some truth to the "good news" aspect of a pregnancy loss, couples who miscarry hardly feel like celebrating. Rather, they need to grieve and to know that their grief is acknowledged and respected. When others focus on their potential for success in future attempts, they feel that their sorrow has been "disenfranchised." Worse are those instances in which couples who cannot afford the costs of another ART cycle are told, "At least you can get pregnant." Such predictions heighten their sense of loss.

By making a pregnancy visible early on, ultrasound monitoring can foster early attachment. Hence, this technology may contribute to the sorrow couples feel when the pregnancy is lost. They focus on the photographs that they receive from the ultrasound technician and experience them as concrete proof that a baby is beginning to grow. When a pregnancy is lost, the photos that were treasures at six, seven, or eight week's gestation become unexpected signs and symbols of their grief.

Fear. Many people react to the miscarriage of an ART pregnancy with fear. Even those who can afford, both financially and emotionally, to try again will do so with keen awareness that treatment may not work. They may fear that this was their only chance at pregnancy and dread returning to a treatment process that they fear will only result in failure.

A fear that arises with a vengeance is that of another pregnancy loss. Even when there is no medical reason to see this loss as anything other than a random event, some couples worry that it is likely to happen again. Infertile couples know of repeated pregnancy loss and fear that this problem will turn out to be their next hurdle in their difficult path to parenthood.

Isolation. Because many couples do not plan to tell friends and family about their pregnancy until it is well established, those who miscarry often feel alone. When they tell people after the fact that they were pregnant, others seldom grasp the full impact of the loss.

Friends and family tend to react with confusion. Since little is written in the popular press about pregnancy loss with the ARTs, there are many people who assume that women who conceive with IVF or GIFT have a successful pregnancy. Assuming that the loss was a highly unusual event, they expect that the couple can try again and count on a successful pregnancy. Women's magazines and other popular journals contribute to this perception by featuring articles about "miracle babies." Hence, families and friends are often unprepared to offer support and compassion to the couple experiencing pregnancy loss.

Grieving couples also feel isolated from their caregivers. Some say that they sense the nurses and physicians are disappointed in them—that they have suddenly gone from being a success story to a symbol of failure. They experience their caregivers' withdrawing from them and conclude that this withdrawal is a sign of disappointment. In fact, caregivers do feel disappointment, but this disappointment is not in the patients but rather in the outcome. They are attached to their patients, they have served as their cheerleaders, and they experience a sense of defeat when everyone's enormous efforts end in loss.

We have found that caregivers are often better prepared to handle the disappointment that follows a failed cycle than that which occurs with a pregnancy loss. This is not surprising since failed cycles are an integral part of ART clinical work. By contrast, pregnancy loss is a less common and more dramatic event. Caregivers, finding themselves at a loss for comforting words, may appear to be withdrawing.

Guilt and Self-Blame. Among the questions that plague couples who miscarry an ART pregnancy are the following: Did I do something to cause this loss? and Was there something that could have been done to prevent it? The struggle to answer these questions often prompts intense feelings of guilt and self-blame, especially in women.

It is hard to convince a woman that miscarrying was not her fault. Although infertility is a shared problem, pregnancy can feel like a solo experience. Women focus on the fact that the fetus was in their body when it died and conclude that there must have been something they did to make this happen. Some are merciless in their self-scrutiny.

Men as well may struggle with feelings of doubt and regret. They look at the outcome of their experience—and especially at their wife's suffering—and wonder if they made a mistake by "forcing nature." Is this loss a punishment, they wonder, for their decision to try the ARTs? Some are haunted by past words of well-wishers who said, "If you're meant to become pregnant, you will." Memories of such pronouncements are especially painful for observant Catholics and others whose religious teachings oppose IVF: they worry that God is now punishing them for going against their faith.

Some of the guilt that people feel following a miscarriage seems to be their attempt to gain control over a situation that is beyond their control. Many scrutinize their past behavior, trying to find explanations. Women who went through IVF are especially vigilant in this process, focusing on everything that they did—or did not do—during the cycle. They revisit their activities—what they ate and drank, how far they walked, how often they showered, the number of times they carried groceries—in search of the cause of their pregnancy loss. Since the medical process is managed precisely and carefully, it is easy for women to assume that whatever went wrong was their fault.

Women scrutinize their thoughts as well as their deeds. They may torment themselves with thoughts such as, "If I was really a good person, this would not have happened." Some worry that they were not appreciative enough of their pregnancy, that they may have jinxed themselves by feeling ambivalent or by worrying that they were carrying multiple fetuses. Some condemn themselves for the envy and jealousy that they felt of pregnant friends and relatives in the past. Still others reexamine the degree of optimism or pessimism that they brought to the process: "I didn't think positively enough," or "If we hadn't gotten our hopes up ... ," or "Maybe the stress I felt and the constant worrying I did made me lose the baby."

Women who lose an ART pregnancy may examine their past for clues about why this has happened. Those who chose to terminate an unwanted pregnancy years earlier are prone to look back on this event and feel that they are now receiving their just punishment. Those who delayed parenting in order to pursue other life goals may feel that had they tried earlier, they would have been spared the trials of infertility and pregnancy loss.

Some women feel that they have a fundamental character defect. They may have no idea what it is but simply believe that if they were a "better person," the miscarriage would not have happened. Women whose low self-esteem predated their infertility are especially vulnerable to believing they have a character defect. It is as if their pregnancy loss is proof of what they knew all along: that they are not "good enough" to be mothers.

Some IVF programs inadvertently promote guilt in their patients. Those that recommend a lengthy bed rest following embryo transfer, may prompt women to feel that any movement, however slight, could harm their fetus. Moreover, the bed-rest prescription implies that the well-being of the pregnancy is within the patient's control and that she has an obligation to curtail her activities if she wants the embryos to implant and to stay implanted.

Anger. Infertile couples who miscarry ask another question: Why us? Having endured the unfairness of infertility and the physical, emotional, and financial trials of the ARTs, they feel unjustly teased as well as cheated when the pregnancy ends in miscarriage. Some feel that they were never properly warned about the percentage of ART pregnancies that end in miscarriage.

Some of the anger that couples feel is directed inward, in the form of guilt and self-blame. Other angry feelings are directed outward—at physicians and nurses. Couples sometimes wonder if there was something that their physicians could have done to prevent miscarriage. For example, should they have been given more progesterone to support the pregnancy? Others are less specific in their questions but have a sense that if the physician had paid closer attention to their pregnancy, the outcome might have been different.

Couples with strong religious beliefs may express anger toward God and their religion. Some conclude that their faith has betrayed them. Once again, they raise the questions that reverberated throughout their infertility treatment: Why is this happening to us? What did we ever do to deserve this? Why are our best efforts to "be fruitful and multiply" being stymied?

God, religion, and spirituality are forces that help many people get through their infertility, but some reach a point when they feel they have been tested unfairly. Pregnancy loss after ART often represents that point at which the "test has gone too far." Angry and confused, people sometimes turn away from their religion, feeling that their faith—once a source of great comfort—has abandoned them.

The Burden of Technological Monitoring

Many couples who experience a pregnancy loss following ART describe their experience as technologically confusing. Not only was their conception the result of advanced technological interventions but the course of their pregnancy was immediately monitored and predicted by laboratory tests and by ultrasound. Having mastered the language of high-tech treatment, from Lupron to

Pergonal to estradiol levels, newly pregnant patients now face new terminology that they feel obliged to learn and understand: HCG levels, progesterone levels, and ultrasound measurements. Although many couples find this monitoring helpful, appreciative of the up-to-date information that it provides, occasionally there are those who find the technology confusing and intrusive.

ART couples are often troubled to discover that early pregnancy testing can raise more questions than it answers. Unlike their fertile friends, who do a home pregnancy test and learn that they are pregnant or not pregnant, infertile couples undergo an early blood test that frequently renders confusing information. Dramatic examples of this are biochemical pregnancies; couples may be told that the pregnancy test is positive but low. When this happens, even the most knowledgeable and sophisticated patients are unsure how to react.

Since most clinics measure more than one hormone level, couples may be confused to learn that one or more assays may be high (signaling a probable "good" pregnancy), yet others may be low (signaling caution). Another possibility is that the hormone levels will be "somewhat" low and rise "somewhat" slowly. When this occurs, weeks may pass before it is clear whether the pregnancy will be ongoing or is doomed to end in loss.

When the numbers are equivocal, infertile couples may begin to feel that there are degrees of pregnancy. This is inconsistent with what they have always been told—that they can't be a little bit pregnant—and leaves many with a sense of confusion. For some, this confusion subsides over the weeks that follow, as blood tests first confirm the pregnancy is probably viable and ultrasounds identifies the number of gestational sacs (there may be more than one) and their location (uterine pregnancy needs to be ruled in and ectopic ruled out). Further confirmation can come at approximately seven weeks (five weeks after retrieval) when ultrasound can identify whether there is a fetal heartbeat.

Miscarriage can still occur after a fetal heartbeat has been confirmed on ultrasound. Although some couples have a warning—they are told that the heartbeat is weak—most do not. In fact, they are usually told that it is extremely rare; only about 5 to 10 percent of women with confirmed fetal heartbeats go on to miscarry. Nonetheless, we have each known several couples who have lost a pregnancy after a confirmed fetal heartbeat. The experience is a devastating one in which couples feel cheated by technology: the monitoring that they counted on for accurate information has instead promoted false hope.

Miscarriage after finding a fetal heartbeat is puzzling to physicians, as well as to their patients. Some point to advanced maternal age and the greater likelihood of chromosomal abnormalities in older women. Others suspect that the fertility medications can cause changes in the uterine lining that make it difficult for the embryo to implant properly and may contribute to miscarriages throughout the first trimester.

Whatever the cause, miscarriage after several weeks of close monitoring is a devastating experience. Although most couples feel that the monitoring is still more of a help than a hindrance, we have also known couples who feel that the high-tech monitoring made their experience more difficult. They say that they would have preferred to go through the physical and emotional pain of a miscarriage at ten or eleven weeks (physicians remind them, however, that the pregnancy could have been ectopic and this needs to be identified early) rather than to suffer the agony of "roller coaster monitoring." Some feel that the frequent tests robbed them of any opportunity to enjoy being pregnant and contributed to their sense that they had forced nature. One woman described her experience as like the "Chinese water torture—a cruel, slow process."

Late Pregnancy Loss

During my eighteenth week, I went in for a routine exam. Everyone told me how well I was doing and they signed me up for childbirth class. The doctor told me that I could expect to feel life in another two or three weeks. Then she said, "And now for the fun part—let's hear the heart beat.

Silence. There was only silence. They tried several times, several ways. Finally, they did an ultrasound. I didn't want to look. I knew. Then the doctor said she was sorry—that it looked like the baby had died three or four weeks earlier.

I can't believe that all the while that I was busy rejoicing—busy buying maternity clothes and signing up for childbirth class—my baby was dead.

Unlike their fertile friends, who typically breathe a sigh of relief when they complete their first trimester, infertile couples, being so accustomed to loss, never feel entirely out of the danger zone. Nonetheless, the likelihood of pregnancy loss greatly diminishes in the second trimester, and many infertile couples feel somewhat more relaxed as they enter it. This increased comfort, together with the increased attachment that they feel toward their unborn child (despite the fact that many try hard to avoid it), makes later miscarriage all the more startling and difficult when it occurs.

Second trimester losses are accompanied by an intensification of the questions and feelings we have already discussed. In addition, most couples experience an overwhelming sense of shock; even those who had remained cautious and anxious are stunned when a pregnancy is lost in the second trimester. As with early miscarriage, we have found that some understanding of the medical causes helps couples to cope with their loss.

Medical Facts

Late miscarriages, like early ones, can be caused by either maternal or fetal factors. The most common cause of late miscarriages is a maternal factor, unpleasantly termed an incompetent cervix, referring to a premature dilation of the cervix, sometimes as early as eighteen or nineteen weeks. If the problem is detected early enough a cerclage (suture) can be placed around the cervix to keep it closed. However, if significant cervical dilation is present, little can be done to prevent pregnancy loss. For those women with an incompetent cervix, in future pregnancies a cerclage can be put in place at 12–14 weeks of pregnancy. When done prophylactically, the success rate is 80–90%. Sadly, many women must suffer a late pregnancy loss before the need for this prophylactic treatment is identified.

Fibroid tumors and uterine abnormalities are other maternal causes of late miscarriage. A small percentage of women with fibroids will have a tumor that grows so large and so rapidly that it causes the uterus to contract prematurely. A small fibroid located near the uterine cavity can also be detrimental. However, since many infertile women who have fibroids undergo myomecto-my—the surgical removal of a fibroid tumor—prior to ART treat-ment, it is unlikely that a rapidly growing fibroid will compro-mise an ART pregnancy. Similarly, since most infertile women undergo hysteroscopy—an internal viewing of the uterus—it is unlikely that uterine abnormalities will be undetected prior to ART treatment.

Immunological problems, related to the father or to the mother, are another possible parental factor in late miscarriage. These caus-es are currently being investigated, and we will review them later in this chapter when we discuss repeated miscarriage.

Chromosomal abnormalities are the most common fetal cause of late miscarriage and are thought to account for 10 percent of these losses, for although most chromosomally abnormal fetuses do not survive beyond twelve weeks, some do. The fetus can appear to be developing normally but, as with many early miscarriages, there is something inherently wrong with it that causes it to abort. When this happens several weeks into the pregnancy, after a heartbeat has been detected and after fetal growth has been followed on the ul-trasound screen, it is a bewildering experience.

Finally, many second trimester losses are of unknown etiology. In this situation, when no explanation can be found for the loss, women are plagued with doubt and self-blame. Since many women assume that if the pregnancy is ongoing, the fetus is normal, those who suffer late miscarriages are frequently convinced that they "did something to the baby." Some are tormented by this belief; they look back to identify the thought, action, or behavior that "caused" the loss.

Feelings

In addition to self-blame, late miscarriage prompts feelings of anger and a sense of injustice. Infertile couples know that life is not fair, but losing a pregnancy after they had finally begun to believe it was real feels immeasurably cruel. Couples wonder why so much em-phasis is placed on getting through the first trimester if a pregnancy remains vulnerable in the weeks that follow.

Couples who go through infertility frequently feel defective;

their bodies do not work right. A pregnancy after long-term infertility, even if it ends in early miscarriage, may help repair some of these feelings. Couples are comforted to know that conception can occur. However, when a long-sought pregnancy is established, progresses, and then ends in loss, the experience may accentuate a woman's sense of defectiveness.

One woman who experienced two second trimester miscarriages following GIFT cycles, said:

> I found that my relationship with other women changed when I found that I was infertile, and then it changed again when I miscarried. I feel like an infertile woman with a very dark rain cloud over my head. It is as though my burden of infertility was lifted and then returned, with even more weight and force. I feel that I am now a walking symbol of the precariousness of good luck.

Some women who have late miscarriages after ART despair that even the most sophisticated technological assistance cannot repair something fundamentally wrong with their bodies. As we noted earlier, the close monitoring that most receive can contribute to the anguish; they saw an actual fetus on the ultrasound screen and now wonder what they "did to it."

The "character defects" that we decribed in relation to early miscarriage also plague women who suffer late miscarriages, especially after the ARTs. When others pronounce, "Maybe it wasn't meant to be," they think, "Maybe God knew that I would be an unfit mother [or father] and this was God's way of telling me." Some extend their self-blame to their decision to use IVF or GIFT, feeling that if they were of stronger moral fiber they would have known enough not to try to "force nature."

Repeated Miscarriage

Although many infertile couples fear that a single miscarriage following the ARTs means that there will be others, most are spared this devastating experience. But some couples become pregnant after long-term infertility, only to face the frustration and devastation of repeated pregnancy loss. For some, the losses are interspersed with long periods of infertility.

Medical Facts

Women who have repeated miscarriages were once called "habitual aborters," an unfortunate term that implied (unintentionally) that the women were responsible for their miscarriages. Psychologists practicing a generation ago frequently offered psychodynamic explanations for the losses. For example, Helene Deutsch, a well-known and well-respected psychoanalyst, offered two interpretations of multiple miscarriage in her 1945 work, *The Psychology of Women II*. She stated that some women miscarry because they fear motherhood. Other women became habitual aborters because they are so traumatized by their first pregnancy loss that they develop an unconscious compulsion to repeat the trauma.[3] Thus, in the absence of medical knowledge, elaborate psychological theory was created that served to exacerbate guilt rather than shed light on the phenonmena.

Now we have several medical explanations for repeated miscarriage. Although they should relieve women of some of the burden of self-blame, some women, especially those who are still labeled habitual aborters, may wonder if this new problem is definitive proof that they were not meant to be mothers after all.

The possible causes of repeated miscarriage are varied, and as time has gone on, more explanations are being found. Current investigation of multiple miscarriage is focusing on embryo toxic factor and potential immunological factors, both alloimmune and autoimmune.

Some physicians feel that alloimmune problems are responsible for multiple miscarriage in some couples. They theorize that in normal pregnancy, a woman develops a blocking factor that prevents her from making antibodies to her fetus, which would cause rejection of the fetus because it would be experienced as a foreign body. Some women who suffer multiple miscarriages, it is thought, fail to develop this blocking factor, thereby allowing their immune system to kill the fetus. Experimental treatments in which the woman is injected with her husband's white blood cells are being used in a few treatment centers. The theory behind this treatment is that the presence of the husband's white blood cells will help a woman to develop the absent blocking factor.

Another possible immunological cause of repeated miscarriage, and one that is more widely accepted, is an autoimmune problem known as the antiphospholipid antibody (or anticardiolipin antibody) syndrome. The presence of these antibodies increases the likelihood that blood will clot. If these clots occur in placental vessels, blood flow to the fetus will be altered.

Physicians are experimenting with treatment that involves taking one baby aspirin daily. An alternative protocol is to use a baby aspirin in combination with a steroid, usually prednisone, and heparin, a blood thinner. These treatments aid circulation, thereby enabling the fetus to receive its needed nutrition from the placenta.

Feelings

It is unusual for a couple to move from long-term infertility to repeated pregnancy loss. Nevertheless, there are couples who manage to cross one new frontier—conception—only to find themselves on another—repeated pregnancy loss. The treatment for this second new frontier is even newer and more experimental than the ARTs. It takes remarkable perseverance, stamina, and hope for a couple to enter into the experimental treatment of multiple miscarriage when they must endure so much to first achieve pregnancy.

Ectopic Pregnancy

Ectopic pregnancy, one that occurs somewhere other than the uterus, is almost always a confusing and traumatic experience. We have found that couples can get a better handle on the experience when they have some understanding of the medical facts.

Medical Facts

Ectopic pregnancy is rare in the general population; only an estimated 1 percent of pregnancies are ectopic. Of these, the vast majority (probably 90 to 95 percent) occur in the fallopian tubes. The remaining 10 percent can occur in the cervix or the abdominal cavity, or an embryo can attach to an ovary.

An ectopic pregnancy constitutes a medical emergency. If it is caught early, before rupturing, it may be treated by medical or surgical intervention. Once it ruptures, emergency surgery is required to remove the fallopian tube.

Ectopic pregnancy is more common in the ART population, accounting for 5 to 8 percent of IVF pregnancies. This comes as a surprise to many people, who assume that because in vitro fertilization bypasses the fallopian tubes, it cannot possibly result in an ectopic pregnancy. However, if an embryo is placed in a portion of the uterus near where it meets the fallopian tube, it can migrate up into it and become trapped inside the tube, especially if the tube is damaged or malformed.

Although women who experience ectopic pregnancies following ART treatment usually have preexisting tubal disease, this is not always the case. Some women turn to the ARTs because of unexplained infertility or because of a male factor and still end up with an ectopic pregnancy. When this happens, they are understandably confused. Most are quite startled to learn that ART treatment, in and of itself, put them at slightly increased risk for an ectopic pregnancy.

Reproductive endocrinologists have several explanations for why ectopic pregnancy is more common in infertile women, especially those using the ARTs. In addition to the fact that many turn to ART treatment because of tubal disease, there are other explanations for why the embryo may migrate to the tube. One is that fertility medications alter the hormonal environment of the fallopian tubes, making it more likely that an embryo will implant there following a GIFT procedure. Also, since there is often more than one embryo transferred in IVF, or several eggs in GIFT, there is increased potential for something to lodge in the fallopian tubes.

Because ectopic pregnancy is rare, fertile women who conceive without difficulty are seldom alerted to the possibility. Some suddenly find themselves in excruciating pain before they even know they are pregnant. Others may suspect pregnancy but have no idea that an embryo can implant outside the uterus. Both groups, as well as those who may be somewhat more prepared for the possibility of an ectopic pregnancy, are often startled to find themselves en route to or coming out of emergency surgery. Pregnancy has suddenly turned into a life-threatening condition.

The Difficulty of Diagnosis

Because IVF and other high-tech patients are carefully monitored via ultrasonography, ectopic pregnancies that are the result of the ARTS are generally diagnosed early. This is almost always an advantage, since early diagnosis can save the tube as well as spare the patient some of the physical and emotional trauma. However, there are some instances in which it is difficult to diagnose an ectopic pregnancy, even with close monitoring:

- Blood HCG levels that remain low or rise irregularly can indicate an ectopic pregnancy, as well as an impending miscarriage. However, blood levels may be ambiguous. When this happens, the patient is usually monitored more closely, but even then, several days may elapse before it is clear whether the pregnancy is ectopic.
- Pregnancies in the proximal portion of the tube (the part closest to the uterus) cause early tubal rupture. This area, the isthmus, is more muscular and does not distend as well as the midportion of the tube, thus making it more vulnerable to rupture. Even close monitoring may not identify the pregnancy as ectopic in time to avoid rupture.
- There may be more than one implantation site in the tube or a simultaneous intrauterine and ectopic pregnancy in which the ectopic pregnancy was not found because the uterine pregnancy was obvious. In this, case hormone levels would probably be rising appropriately, obscuring the problem.
- Physicians and patients usually base their calculations about what the hormone levels should be on the timing of the GIFT or IVF procedure. However, physicians know that sometimes delayed implantation occurs, and they may assume the laboratory numbers are slightly off but that the pregnancy is probably fine.
- Since gastrointestinal and ovarian symptoms are common after ovulation induction and can mimic ectopic pregnancy, it is difficult for physicians to make a differential diagnosis based on a woman's physical discomfort alone.
- Although bleeding may occur with an ectopic pregnancy, it is not uncommon for women to bleed early in normal pregnancy. Some mistake this bleeding for either their menses or, if they know

they are pregnant, for breakthrough bleeding, perhaps indicating an impending miscarriage. This may delay the diagnosis of an ectopic pregnancy.

- Some patients who develop acute pain are rushed to an emergency room and seen by a physician (probably not an obstetrician) who completely misses the diagnosis. Although ectopic pregnancy is a common cause of acute abdominal pain in women of childbearing years and should be suspected in infertility patients (whether or not they are known to be pregnant), some physicians do miss the diagnosis.

The intense pain of a ruptured ectopic pregnancy and its rapid onset are some other reasons why it is such an upsetting experience. Women report finding themselves in sudden and debilitating pain. The degree of this pain, together with the fact that its origins may be misdiagnosed or dismissed, intensifies the crisis.

Women who have had ectopic pregnancies and later return to treatment have remarked that they will never forget the pain. Some say that it makes them feel ambivalent about becoming pregnant again; they long for a baby but are terrified that the pregnancy will be another ectopic one. They may postpone treatment until they feel more equipped to deal with this possibility.

Treatment. Ectopic pregnancy can be treated surgically or medically or by both methods. No matter which method is used, however, the treatment can add to the trauma of the experience. Women and their husbands are often startled by the urgency with which surgery is presented to them, especially when it may follow hours, or even days in which the seriousness of their condition was not recognized. Many are confused and angry when they feel that doctors suddenly turn from minimizing their problem to indicating that they are in a life-threatening condition.

An ectopic pregnancy is treated medically with chemotherapy. This news can be shocking to a couple who associate chemotherapy solely with cancer. However, chemotherapy is an effective non-surgical, and hence less invasive, treatment for ectopic pregnancy. Unfortunately, recovery can be especially protracted, and patients sometimes require several weeks of monitoring. It is also not uncommon for pregnancy hormone levels to decline slowly or incompletely and for patients to require a redosing of medications. This prolonged treatment and surveillance can be very stressful for a woman who wants to end a traumatic ordeal.

Surgical treatment of ectopic pregnancy is also traumatic, especially for those who have only recently gone through oocyte retrieval in an IVF procedure or a laparoscopy for a GIFT procedure. Even women whose ectopic pregnancies were diagnosed early, making their surgery less emergent, are distressed to find themselves back in the operating room.

Prognosis. Women who experience an ectopic pregnancy may be frightened of what may lie ahead. A history of one ectopic does not necessarily mean that another will follow, but these women are at greatly increased risk. The prospect of a second ectopic pregnancy is frightening to many patients, especially those whose pregnancies have ruptured and have experienced emergency surgery.

The degree of risk of a subsequent ectopic pregnancy depends on the original diagnosis and on how the first ectopic was treated. Physicians estimate that 10 percent of women who have had one ectopic pregnancy will have another. However, women who lost a tube when the ectopic pregnancy ruptured and have a healthy remaining tube may be at less risk for a second ectopic than someone who has two partially damaged tubes remaining. Some women in this latter group may wonder why their doctors bothered to save either tube, since the surgery may have left them at increased risk for another ectopic pregnancy.

Feelings

Women undergoing the ARTS are usually aware of the possibility of an ectopic pregnancy. Those who spend any time around an infertility clinic may hear from other patients about their experiences with ectopic pregnancies, especially when those pregnancies caused or contributed to tubal disease. However, those who do not have tubal disease may not realize that the treatments they are undergoing put them at an increased risk. When these women are confronted with an ectopic pregnancy, they may be confused, especially after undergoing IVF. It is difficult to understand how embryos that were placed carefully in the uterus could end up in the tubes. They may also feel doubly punished, having entered treatment with one problem, only to acquire another, limiting their future treatment options. In other words, intrauterine inseminations and other less costly and invasive treatments may no longer be viable options for them. They wonder whether they would have been better off, both physically and emotionally, had they not become involved in the ARTs. This dilemma must be especially painful for those who turned to the ARTs because they wanted to avoid looking back with regret.

Whatever the cause of an ectopic pregnancy, we have found that infertile women are devastated by the experience, especially after treatment with the ARTs. They cannot believe that they have gone from one medical ordeal to another, usually in the space of a few weeks. Nor can some believe that they went through so much to create embryos, only to have them implant in the wrong place.

The Role of Caregivers

Caregivers play an important role during and after pregnancy loss. When an ART pregnancy appears to be in trouble, caregivers frequently find themselves walking a fine line: they may need to warn the couple that the pregnancy is at risk but must avoid predicting loss. Not only have caregivers been known to be wrong—even high-tech monitoring can be misleading—but couples are often upset even when the prediction is correct. Some say they felt intruded upon, that everything about their pregnancy, including its loss, involved technological intervention. Most couples, however, appreciate the warning because it diminishes the shock.

Because caregivers are so intimately involved in miscarriage after ART, an involvement that often spans several weeks, it is crucial that they remain involved after the loss. Couples may feel abandoned, fearing that the program now regards them as failures. Caregivers can convey to a couple that they share in the loss and that they are not disappointed in or angry at the couple. They can let the couple know that they will welcome them back for another treatment cycle and help them to sort out decisions about when to return to treatment. Should the couple decide not to recycle, for emotional or financial reasons, caregivers can support their decision to move on.

We have found that nurses and physicians who genuinely feel optimistic about a patient's chance to have a successful pregnancy often have difficulty accepting a decision to end treatment. Caregivers become attached to patients and may have difficulty separating what they personally would do from what might be in the best interest of the couple—a couple who has just gone through a major loss. It is important to let patients know that they are welcome back, as patients or visitors. Those who decide to adopt should be encouraged to send pictures and announcements to the clinic. This overture will assure them that the staff does not view pregnancy as the only successful resolution to infertility or regard their decision to move on as settling for second best.

Caregivers play an important role in helping couples determine when to resume treatment and in determining the appropriate treatment. They should assure patients that there is no rush (unless the woman is older, in which case time is an important factor) and that they will be welcome back whenever they feel ready. Healing is often a lengthy process after pregnancy loss and couples may need to hear this from their caregivers.

Loss in Multiple Pregnancy

Couples undergoing ovulation induction are at increased risk for a multiple pregnancy. In fact, multiple gestation occurs in about 30 percent of IVF or GIFT cycles. Although couples are told of the possibility of twins or triplets—or possibly more—many are unprepared for the realities of a multiple pregnancy. Having come to regard themselves as barren, women cannot imagine even one fetus growing inside them, let alone two or three.

Childless couples often react to the news that they may be having more than one by saying, "Terrific—we'd love an instant family" or, "That's fine with us—the more the merrier." Those who are paying out of pocket feel especially blessed that they are getting "two for the price of one" when they learn they are expecting twins. Such enthusiastic reactions lead physicians—and the couples themselves—to minimize or forget about the risks and difficulties of multiple gestation and birth.

Many couples are not prepared for the challenges of a multiple pregnancy. Although some are thrilled, others become upset and confused when they learn they are carrying multiples, especially when there are three or more fetuses. These couples are confronted with a troubling paradox: their infertility treatment has resulted in a risky form of superfertility. They face the threat of severe prematurity and its associated problems or the disturbing option of multifetal reduction—the process of aborting one or more fetuses in order to decrease the risk to the remaining one(s). Those who thought they wanted instant family may look back with guilt and regret, angry at themselves—and possibly at their physician—for forcing nature.

Couples who learn that they are carrying twins tend to feel a mixture of delight and caution. Most are pleased with the prospect of two babies but are also concerned about prematurity and other complications of a multiple gestation. Some realize that they were naive when they hoped for a twin pregnancy, since a singleton pregnancy usually poses fewer risks.

Physicians do not consider a multiple pregnancy a blessing. Rather, it is a high-risk pregnancy, carrying with it an increased risk of miscarriage. Loss in multiple gestation can happen early in the pregnancy or later.

Early Loss in Multiple Pregnancy

Since any woman who has more than one embryo or more than one egg transferred is at risk for multiple gestation, she is usually followed closely by blood tests and ultrasounds to determine how the pregnancy is progressing and the number of embryos that have implanted. The purpose of the ultrasounds is not only to determine how many sacs are in her uterus but also to rule out that any embryos have implanted outside her uterus.

When a heteroectopic pregnancy (embryos in the tube and in the uterus) is found early, it is often possible to save the uterine pregnancy since the ectopic pregnancy can be surgically removed without disturbing the intrauterine pregnancy. If the ectopic pregnancy ruptures (usually not the case in ART pregnancies due to the close monitoring), the tube is removed and the patient is followed.

Another kind of early pregnancy loss occurs when early ultrasounds reveal two or more gestational sacs but later ultrasounds fail to detect heartbeats in all of them. Frequently the sac (or sacs) that does not have a developing fetus in it vanishes on its own. Little is usually made of these experiences, and couples sometimes express relief when they occur, especially if the "lost" embryo was a third (or fourth) one. But it is common for couples also to feel a great deal of sadness. Viewing on ultrasound an embryo (or two) without a heartbeat and at the same time seeing at least one embryo that does have a heartbeat can be both an upsetting and a joyous experience. Couples may be confused by their conflicting emotions, frequently feeling they do not have a right to feel sad when they have one healthy pregnancy.

Some parents comment that it is not until much later, perhaps after the birth of the surviving fetus(s), that they experience a sense of loss. Some say that years later they will occasionally look at their twins and wonder what the third would have been like had the embryo survived. If they have a single child, they may be even more likely to wonder about the twin.

In other instances, two or more sacs are identified, all with heartbeats, but on a subsequent ultrasound, one or more heartbeats are undetectable. This loss, frequently described as the vanishing twin, is very upsetting, especially if the doctor has not prepared the couple for this possibility. However, even those who know that losing a twin is always a possibility still experience varying degrees of sadness and loss, coupled with a fear that they will also lose the healthy fetus.

Although the loss of a multiple gestation is frequently discovered by ultrasound, there are times when an actual miscarriage occurs without warning, accompanied by bleeding and cramping. When this happens, couples become terrified, assuming they are losing the entire pregnancy. This is sometimes the case; however, many women do go on to successfully carry and give birth to the one or more remaining fetusses.

Late Loss in Multiple Pregnancy

Many losses in multiple pregnancies come in the second and even third trimesters, when the parents are attached to each of the fetuses and to the idea of parenting twins or triplets. Prenatal testing and monitoring frequently reveal that a fetus has died in utero or that he or she will not survive long past birth because of congenital problems. In these instances, a couple is told that the pregnancy must be carried as long as possible for the sake of the other(s). Women then find that their joy has turned to anguish as they must carry a dead or dying fetus for several weeks.

When a couple experiences a later loss in a multiple pregnancy, family, friends, and even physicians frequently fail to understand the significance of it. Instead of acknowledging how painful it is to lose a child who is so wanted, they focus on the well-being of the surviving twin(s). The expectation is that the couple will feel so grateful to have an ongoing pregnancy that they will be able to dismiss the death of their other baby.

The Center for Loss in Multiple Birth (CLIMB) is a support network for parents throughout the United States and Canada who have experienced the loss of one or more fetuses in a pregnancy. In its newsletter, CLIMB members chronicle the pain they have experienced on losing one or more multiples. Their writings emphasize that the survival of one or more babies does not erase their pain. Rather, their enduring feelings of loss make the survival of another child bittersweet. One CLIMB member stated, "Two out of three or one out of two is NOT good when it's your baby who has died." Following is a brief excerpt from an essay by Sandy Lee, a CLIMB member, that appeared in the newsletter:

> We had visions of watching Erin smile while riding her tricycle down the street. We had visions of her going to the prom (after carefully checking out her date!). We had visions of watching Erin and Kristen growing up together. So it's with unfulfilled hopes and dreams for this little girl and "our twins" that we grieve. . . .
> Taking Kristen out in her stroller, we think about the twin stroller we almost bought. When the three of us drive off for a ride in the car, we often feel as though we're leaving someone behind.[4]

Jean Kollantai, president and founder of CLIMB, notes that CLIMB members often go through a great deal medically and emotionally with their surviving child(ren), who frequently require lengthy stays in the neonatal intensive care unit for prematurity or other problems that affect multiples. She adds that this experience, difficult for all parents, is made much more painful by the previous infertility and by the death of one or more of the babies. Kollantai notes that many of the babies who survive are medically fragile or handicapped, adding to the tremendous parenting challenge and providing another ongoing reminder of their loss. She observes that these parents face a complex grieving process that includes mourning the loss of their special status as parents of twins or multiples.[5]

Loss of An Entire Multiple Pregnancy

Couples are not always prepared for the difficulties that women can encounter carrying a multiple pregnancy. Even some mothers who are in the care of highly skilled obstetricians are shattered to find that they cannot carry their babies long enough. All too often, multiples are born so early that none survives. When this happens, the loss is shattering. Often it follows a long, difficult period of bed rest, as well as the use of medication to postpone labor.

The CLIMB newsletter is filled with testimonies to the attachment that parents feel for their lost babies. The essays that describe the collision of joy and sorrow experienced by those who lost one or more babies and have given birth to a twin are deeply moving. The accounts that tell of the death of both twins or of all three triplets speak to the overwhelming grief of couples whose children are with them for too brief a time. Most of these couples lose their babies in the late second or early third trimester of pregnancy. One woman found these words to describe her loss:

> When we found out that I was carrying twins, it felt like our wish for "instant family" had come true. I had had a very hard time with the fertility drugs, even to the point of being hospitalized for hyperstimulation, and so we felt especially grateful to be able to put the "getting pregnant" part behind us. Little did we know the difficulties and the pain that would follow.
>
> Our daughters were born at 24 weeks and each lived for just over an hour. During that small window of time, we tried to give them the love of a lifetime. When they died, it felt like our whole family had died. All our dreams. All our hopes. All our expectations. All our children gone before their time.

Kollantai has observed that parents who lose both or all of their babies often feel angry at the technology that was successful in helping them conceive their babies but was unsuccessful in saving them. Parents also feel guilty for having wanted children so much that they resorted to using the ARTs, and they may even blame themselves for conceiving children who were put at such risk. Although the trauma of this experience makes it easy for them to conclude that they were "not meant to have children," most go on to try again. Kollantai offers the following explanation for this phenomenon: "Seeing their own offspring for the first time, even though tiny and dying, is the experience of a lifetime and propels many into further efforts to conceive."[6]

Multifetal Reduction

Infertile couples who turn to the ARTs and other new paths to parenthood find themselves in places that they never expected to be. Perhaps no subset of infertile couples experiences this more poignantly and more powerfully than those who undergo multifetal reduction. Few, if any, could have imagined that they would find themselves faced with the unimaginably cruel dilemma: the elective abortion of one (or more) fetuses for the good of the others.

Multifetal reduction was originally developed to reduce risks to mothers and babies in some instances of multiple gestation. Although it was highly unusual before the use of Pergonal, women did occasionally become pregnant with four or more fetuses. When this occurred, physicians sometimes recommended reduction of one or more of the fetuses, so that the remaining ones would have a better chance for survival. Multifetal reduction was also used sometimes when prenatal testing revealed that one fetus in a multiple pregnancy had congenital defects.

The ARTS, in which three, four, or even more embryos/oocytes are commonly transferred, have led to increased use of multifetal reduction. Because it is often difficult for a woman to carry three or more fetuses safely to term (and because the ARTS result in triplet or larger gestations in about 5 percent of ART pregnancies), multifetal reduction is now used to reduce a pregnancy to one or two babies. This procedure, performed primarily to obviate health risks to either the mother or the babies, carries with it a high emotional price. Couples who consider multifetal reduction find themselves confronted with a profoundly troubling dilemma: aborting one of the fetuses they endured so much to conceive or putting all of the fetuses at risk if they reject the procedure.

The decision to undergo multifetal reduction is always agonizing, fraught with questions, doubts, and fears of regret. Regardless of how many fetuses a woman is carrying, couples wonder if they are making or have made a mistake. Even when it seems clear that multifetal reduction offers the only hope, for a "good outcome", the decision to undergo the procedure is painful. The fetus being reduced is neither unloved nor unwanted. Rather, it is the beginning of a long-sought and greatly cherished child.

A risk of multifetal reduction (although it happens infrequently) is that the remaining fetuses will accidentally be terminated. Aware of this enormous risk, couples feel unclear about what is the right decision. Most are terrified that they will decide on multifetal reduction, lose the entire pregnancy, and then be tormented with regret.

The decision to undergo this procedure is especially difficult for those who are carrying triplets. Triplet pregnancies represent that gray area in which it is neither clear that a reduction is necessary nor that it will improve the outcome of the pregnancy. Many women do carry triplets successfully, and reductions do not always ensure the health and survival of the remaining babies. Yet women who carry triplet pregnancies are in a much higher risk category than those who carry twins, for premature birth, which can result in neonatal death or in potentially serious physical, psychological, or neurological problems for the offspring. Consequently, couples expecting triplets find themselves in even more of a dilemma than those carrying larger multiple pregnancies: will multifetal reduction help or hurt their efforts to build a family? (It appears to us that most couples expecting triplets do not elect to reduce the pregnancy. Rather, they live for many months with both fear and excitement about the outcome.)

Couples who decide to undergo multifetal reduction—and this is often the case with those who are carrying more than three fetuses—do have a tremendous sense of loss following the procedure, undoubtedly intensified by their feelings of guilt. Many couples blame themselves for pushing nature beyond its limits, feeling that they are now getting the punishment they deserve. They may feel guilty also in the company of other infertile couples who long for a pregnancy and are astonished that anyone could electively abort a fetus that was so hard to come by.

Couples who endure a multifetal reduction may feel angry toward their physician, whom they perceive as having inadequately prepared them for the possibility of conceiving triplets or quadruplets. Those whose physicians encouraged them to transfer four or more embryos sometimes feel betrayed, fearing that their doctors cared more about their success rates than they did about the couple and their offspring. Sometimes couples may even suspect that they were not told the truth about the number of embryos/oocytes that were transferred. They may imagine that the clinic, in an effort to have a high pregnancy rate, transferred "extra" embryos (or eggs). (This fantasy may be an irrational displacement for their anger and fear about having the procedure performed.)

The experience of infertility profoundly changes people's attitudes and beliefs about life and death, including their feelings regarding elective abortion. Thus, couples confronted with multifetal reduction face a moral dilemma: If it is not medically necessary, then is selective reduction an elective abortion? Since many infertile couples, regardless of their religious beliefs or support of a woman's right to choose, feel that they could not personally undergo an abortion, the decision to reduce electively is extremely disturbing. One woman writes this about her experience:

> If I had been pregnant with four or more, there would have been no questions about reducing the pregnancy. But triplets was such a gray area. In my three IVF cycles, I had never taken a casual view of embryonic life. I had always frozen the extra fertilized eggs for potential (and once, actual) use later, because I could not bear simply to throw them out. And now I was dealing not with a two day old, microscopic embryo in a petri dish, but an eight-week old fetus already implanted and growing in my womb.[7]

The period following a reduction procedure is an anxious time. Its outcome, the well-being of the remaining fetuses, may be unclear for several weeks or months; unplanned fetal loss can occur a long time after the actual procedure.

Couples who lose their remaining fetuses following a reduction procedure, whether or not the procedure actually caused the loss, suffer intense self-blame and recriminations. Although this suffering will probably be strongest for those whose religious backgrounds oppose abortion, others, including those who are pro-choice, find themselves agonizing not only over the multifetal reduction decision but also over prior decisions that they made. One woman expressed it the following way:

> I look back and wonder if I should have taken fertility drugs in the first place. After all, no one forced them into me. I took them voluntarily and knew all along that they brought with them the possibility of multiples. Later, when we moved on to IVF and I agreed to have four embryos transferred, I was, in a sense, agreeing to carry a multiple pregnancy. Having made this series of decisions, I can only hold myself accountable for the death of my babies.[8]

Finally, there are those couples who have a successful multifetal reduction, ending up with a healthy twin or singleton pregnancy, and then find themselves experiencing a collision of emotions: delighted to be expecting a healthy baby but guilty about what they did. Many did not anticipate that it would affect them so much.

Sometimes the reduction procedure is successful, but one or both of the remaining babies dies later in pregnancy, at birth, or after birth. It may seem logical that some of the events of these pregnancies would prove that the multifetal reduction was indeed a necessity (given the problems that still developed with fewer babies), but the death of a baby (or babies) is inherently filled with grief, pain, and guilt for the parents. The couple may fantasize that some aspect of the selective reduction procedure caused problems in the remaining fetus (es) or that God is punishing them for going through with it. Although that explanation is medically (and spiritually) improbable, the guilt that couples feel allows them to conjure up all sorts of unrealistic possibilities. Parents who are left with no surviving babies feel extreme pain and guilt over the decisions that they have made.

The Grieving Process in Multiple Gestation after ART

Partial Loss

Couples who suffer the death of one or more of their babies in a multiple pregnancy usually find that others do not understand or appreciate their loss. Instead, people tend to say, "You're lucky to have ended up with a healthy baby" or, worse, "Imagine how difficult it would have been if there had been two [or three]'!" Couples need to remind themselves that these comments, although intensely painful, are usually not ill intended; others want to help them to feel better and believe that these remarks are supportive. Moreover, some family members and friends may be unaware of what it means to lose a fetus in multiple pregnancy.

To the extent that they feel able, parents can serve as educators. As long as they are grieving the loss of the baby who dies, they may need to explain to others that the survival of one fetus does not erase the loss of another. They may wish to explain that if a triplet dies in utero and two survive, the two are surviving triplets, not twins. Similarly, the single baby that survives when a twin dies in utero may actually remain a twin in his or her parents' eyes.

Parents need to seek support from others who do understand and to take all the time and the opportunities they need to grieve for their baby—for "our twins" or "our triplets." This is seldom easy, both because parents are busy caring for their surviving baby and because their family and friends are likely to take a "let's move on" approach. However, we have found that parents who are able to grieve enjoy their newborn and find meaningful ways to remember those children who did not survive. Sometimes what helps is to set aside some time or times during the day to grieve. It can be planned, for example, when the baby sleeps or when someone else is caring for him or her.

Since most of the people in the couple's lives will want to celebrate the arrival of the child who survived, rather than grieve the child who did not, caregivers can play an especially important role in helping couples. Those who participated in their medical care knew, first hand, that other babies were expected and they should acknowledge this. Rather than avoiding the subject for fear of opening a wound, caregivers should be open and direct, aware that the parents will appreciate someone's thoughtful acknowledgment of their lost child.

Loss of an Entire Pregnancy

Couples who lose an entire multiple pregnancy, especially when the loss occurs late in the pregnancy, often feel as though they have lost their family. They realize that the instant family they may have joked about was a reality to them. They had come to expect and anticipate the juggling that comes with twins or triplets and instead feel a huge void in their lives.

When the couple feels ready to attempt another pregnancy, it is important that their goal not be instant family. Although the arrival of two or three healthy babies would have been a joyous event, they have learned the difficulty of carrying a multiple pregnancy. More important, they need to be prepared for a singleton pregnancy (or no pregnancy, since the odds per cycle are always against success, even when the couple has been pregnant previously). Although a singleton pregnancy is more likely to have a successful outcome, it would not offer them "instant family."

Parents who attempt another pregnancy should give careful consideration to whom their caregivers will be. Some remain confident in the physician who cared for them the last time; others will feel a need to change doctors. Those who do will want to know how their new physician treats multiples. Although their next pregnancy may not be another multiple gestation, they will want to be prepared for this possibility and to know how the new physician manages a multiple gestation. Some physicians are more active in their treatment, watching patients very closely, and others are less so, taking the approach that they will wait to see whether signs of a problem arise before intervening. The latter approach is, understandably, difficult for someone who has lost one or more multiples. It is also important to know how the physician feels about multifetal reduction: is he or she likely to pressure them to reduce the pregnancy or does he or she feel confident managing multiple gestation.

It is not uncommon for couples who have lost all their babies in a multiple gestation to consider themselves parents and to refer to themselves in this way. Since much of the world will not know or understand this, caregivers can be especially helpful to the couple. They must communicate their clear awareness that nothing can take away the fact that the couple conceived, carried, and gave birth to children, whether or not those children were born alive or dead.

Caregivers can help couples to sort out their complex feelings regarding another multiple pregnancy. It will be important to help them with their feelings regarding selective reduction, especially if it was an issue in their last pregnancy loss (either because they lost the pregnancy following a multifetal reduction or decided against it and subsequently lost the pregnancy). It is also important that caregivers acknowledge that the couple may have fears about a singleton pregnancy as well. Just as they had no way to know what was normal or not in their multiple pregnancy, they do not have a way to know whether their problems were due to the fact that it was a multiple gestation or whether it was a matter of bad luck (and they know, all too well, that even bad luck can occur more than once).

Some couples experience multiple pregnancy loss again, but many go on to have a successful pregnancy—with a single or multiple babies. Some couples face more years of infertility. They know what it is like to experience pregnancy, labor, and delivery, as well as what it means to expect biological offspring. These couples, who have come so near and yet so far, may have a more difficult time moving on to alternatives to biological parenthood.

Stillbirth

Stillbirth after infertility is the unthinkable. How can a pregnancy, hard earned and now well established, end in fetal death? Sometimes there are medical explanations; rarely are there ways of understanding this trauma emotionally. Stillbirth is testimony to the fact that life is often unfair. Couples who would make wonderful parents, and who arrive at the threshold of the finish line, are occasionally struck down in their tracks. Stillbirth is always a devastating loss, but after long term infertility that includes high technological treatment, it is unfathomable.

Stillbirth or intrauterine fetal demise is a relatively rare occurrence in a singleton pregnancy. Nonetheless, there are infertile women who have healthy pregnancies following IVF or GIFT, only to have them end tragically in severe prematurity, a cord death, from unexpected obstetrical complications, or from unknown causes. Our experience has taught us that even in the face of these heartbreaking losses, couples find the strength and resilience to move on.

When a pregnancy goes to completion and then is lost, there are many *what ifs*. Grieving parents look back and wonder what they could have done differently. Could another obstetrician have provided better care? Should they have called the doctor or gone to the hospital earlier? Was there anything damaging about either their attitude toward the pregnancy or their activities? These unanswerable questions and self-blame are very painful, especially in the months following the loss.

The Feelings

Anger. As much as people will look back and scrutinize their own actions and judgment, they will also feel anger toward their physician, nurses, and other caregivers. It is also common to feel angry at God. In this age of scientific advances and medical miracles, it is difficult to comprehend how this tragic event could have happened at all, especially to them, when they had already been through so much.

When family and friends' lack recognition of the enormity of the loss that these couples feel, it adds to their pain. By contrast, couples who perceive that others understand and acknowledge their loss seem to have an easier time healing than those who feel that others minimize what happened. A woman whose son was born at twenty-nine weeks and lived only a short time spoke to us about how much it meant to her when others came to his funeral. She saw their attendance as acknowledgment that her son was a person, whose life, though very brief, had meaning. There was nothing that others could do to erase her pain, but their presence at the funeral certainly served to ease the sorrow.

Isolation. Couples undergoing infertility treatment inevitably meet others who are also struggling to have a baby. Similarly, those experiencing a miscarriage tend to find others in the same boat. By contrast, a couple who loses a baby late in the pregnancy or at birth is likely to feel alone in their experience. This isolation is heightened for those who experience fetal demise following ART treatment.

Couples feel isolated not only as a result of the relative uniqueness of their experience but also because others tend to withdraw from them. Finding words to comfort a couple who has struggled to have a baby and then loses it at birth or just prior to birth is indeed difficult. Yet any expression of concern is better than withdrawal. Many people, however, feel awkward and inadequate to provide comfort. When this occurs, couples feel hurt and abandoned, and the abandonment exacerbates the pain of their loss.

The Role of Caregivers

Caregivers, especially the nursing staff in labor and delivery, are essential in helping a couple endure the trauma of stillbirth after the ARTS. These nurses are instrumental in helping a couple make the decision to hold their dead baby, a decision that most couples find difficult at the time but look back upon with appreciation. Nurses who take photos of the couple holding their baby provide a great service to grieving parents. These photos, together with a lock of hair and a birth and death certificate, offer many couples important evidence of the significance of their child's short life.

Nurses and other caregivers can also help grieving couples plan a memorial service. This is especially important when there was no warning of trouble; some couples who enter a hospital filled with anticipation leave in grief. Couples experiencing shock, as well as those who had some advance preparation, usually need and welcome assistance with funeral arrangements and with decisions about when and where to bury their child.

Although labor and delivery nurses play the most critical roles at the time of the actual loss, other caregivers are instrumental in a couple's grieving process in the weeks and months following a stillbirth after ARTS. These caregivers, including the couple's infertility physician and office staff, can help the couple take the time to grieve their loss, as well as begin to make decisions about if and when they will return to treatment. Some couples will need to go through an extended period of mourning; others will be comforted by active plans to renew medical treatment.

Finally, physicians play an essential role in stillbirth after ARTS by helping couples to understand the experience from a medical standpoint. There will be many questions to be asked, not all of which have answers, yet patients who feel that their physician takes time with them will be prepared to move on, from both a cognitive and emotional standpoint.

The pregnancy losses we have described testify to the depth and breadth of life's apparent random unfairness. It is difficult to comprehend how a couple can go through so much to establish a pregnancy and then endure the excruciating pain of losing it. Yet we have witnessed—over and over again—the resilience of such couples, as well as their strong determination to move forward.

4

Moving Forward
Deciding to End Treatment

When is enough, enough? This is the question that tortures and confounds infertile couples in the 1990s. Many wonder how they will ever know when it is time to stop treatment when there are always new and ever expanding reproductive options. For unlike those who struggled with infertility in earlier times, when there were fewer treatments available, couples today are hardpressed to say, "We've tried everything. Now we know that we've done our best."

As we have seen throughout the first half of this book, couples who become involved in the ARTs find themselves in a place that they never expected to be. Having first approached parenthood with the assumption—in most instances—that children would come easily, many were surprised and confused when 'doing what comes naturally' did not work. With fear, caution and sadness, they eventually made their way out of the bedroom and into a doctor's office. Later, many moved on to more high tech, "state of the art", treatments—treatments which were impersonal, intrusive, costly, time consuming and sometimes, physically painful. With courage and fortitude ART couples committed themselves to doing "whatever it takes" to have a child.

For many couples, the journey through ART treatment, though difficult and unexpected, proves rewarding. Some try one IVF or GIFT cycle and go home with a baby (or babies) nine months later.

Others travel a bumpier road—through failed cycles and pregnancy losses—but eventually accomplish their goal. For each of these couples, the ARTs are miraculous.

But what of the other couples? What happens to those who also travel through the treacherous terrain of high tech treatment, but who do not end up with a successful pregnancy? How and when do they say, "We have come to the end of this road and we are ready now to travel down a different pathway."? Living in a time of rapid and promising medical advances, how do these couples arrive at a point that they can move on without regret?

Guidance From the Heart

Most couples say that deciding to end treatment would be easier if a physician were to tell them that pregnancy was a hopeless goal. Such news, though devastating, would be clear and would offer them the opportunity for closure. But few couples are given such a definitive prognosis; most are forced to make a decision for themselves. They do so each in their own style and at their own pace. What is enough for one couple is too much for another and not enough for yet a third. The following considerations are subjective ones that are important for couples to think about in making their decision.

Feelings About Genetic Continuity

For some couples the decision about when to end treatment revolves around the feelings that one or both of them have about genetic continuity. As we have seen—and will continue to see throughout this book—people have different feelings about genetic continuity and about the significance of parenting a child with whom they have a genetic connection. For some, genetic continuity forms the cornerstone of the parenting experience: without it, there is no compelling reason to raise children. Such couples (or individuals) often come from families that emphasize lineage; they have grown up with a sense of pride and connection to an ancestry celebrated in family trees, family stories, and, possibly, written family histories.

Individuals also have feelings about their genetic makeup. Some believe that their genes are unique. Because no one else in the world is exactly like them, they consider their genes to be priceless. Others see nothing unique about the genes they possess; after all, there are many people who have blue eyes, or red hair, or a talent for music or mathematics. Those in the first group want to pass on and preserve their genes; the latter group tends to view their quest for parenthood in broader terms.

There is no right point of view about genes. Rather, each person must examine his or her own feelings about this complex subject. Those with a powerful longing to pass on their genes will probably have difficulty leaving treatment. It may feel easier for them to remain in treatment—even with only bleak hope for success—than it is to try to let go of their longing. Those who feel that a genetic connection is neither necessary for nor central to a satisfying parenting experience move more easily to alternative paths to parenthood. Couples in the former group come to a point when they realize that remaining in treatment is only serving to postpone (or prevent) them from achieving their real goal, which is parenthood.

Couples may not be in agreement about the significance of genetic ties. Sometimes they resolve their differences by pursuing a parenting alternative that offers them half a genetic connection (donor insemination, ovum donation, or surrogacy). This solution works best when the person for whom genetics is more important is presumably fertile. However, because none of these second choices comes with a guarantee of success, some of these couples encounter further difficulties ending treatment.

The Nature of the Gamble

ART treatments demand enormous commitments of time, energy, and money. For some couples, the decision about when to end treatment revolves around their feelings about what it means to have committed such substantial resources to this effort. Some feel that having done so much, they cannot quit. Attempting pregnancy can begin to feel more like gambling than like medicine. One woman who was struggling with whether to try IVF for the fourth time stated, "'Having a chance' sounded good at first, but now it is beginning to feel like winning the lottery. It's beginning to sound like 'stuck.'"

Couples who find they cannot quit may be stuck for two reasons. Some feel that quitting would mean that all their efforts had been in vain. Only by remaining in treatment—and achieving success—will they feel their efforts were worthwhile. Others who feel that ending treatment is quitting prematurely view ART as much more of a gamble and feel that their odds of success increase the longer they remain in treatment. (In fact, IVF pregnancy rates support this perspective as long as couples produce embryos). Such couples wonder how they can end treatment now when the next cycle might be the one that works.

There are also couples who, despite the disappointments they have endured, persist in believing that good people are eventually rewarded. They view their bad luck as time limited; if they continue a little while longer things will work out. These couples manage to keep a positive outlook throughout treatment, refusing to believe that life—or their faith—will let them down.

By contrast, still other couples look back on the time, effort, and money that they have committed to treatment and see it as evidence that enough is enough. These couples feel that they do have a great deal to show for their efforts; the thickness of their medical file is enough proof that they have done all that they can. They perceive continued treatment efforts as a waste of valuable resources best spent on adoption or on an alternative path. Such couples know that one more cycle—or two or three—holds no guarantee that they will "hit the jackpot". In addition, their infertility experience has taught them that life is not always fair and that often those who have suffered the most are called upon to suffer again.

Avoidance of Grief. There are some couples who appear to be cycling indefinitely. Consciously they believe that persistence will eventually equal success. Unconsciously, however, they are avoiding grief. Couples who stay in treatment because they are reluctant or afraid to face the grief they will feel if they end treatment recognize that they will have to experience a long mourning process before they are able to move on. Exhausted and depleted by infertility, some feel too vulnerable to face their grief. Paradoxically, they remain stuck in the very treatments that perpetuate their sorrow and self-blame. They do so because each new cycle offers them some small kernal of renewed hope, and as long as they possess that kernal, they are able to avoid their loss.

Difficulty Saying Good-bye

Closely related to the difficulty that some couples have in facing the loss of their dream is the sadness and fear that they often surprisingly feel about saying good-bye to treatment efforts. We refer to the separations that occur when couples leave a treatment facility. They must say good-bye to the physicians and nurses to whom they feel attached and to their role as ART patients.

Although couples (and in particular the women) know they will not miss unpleasant procedures and treatments, most realize they will miss their physicians and nurses. Having at times felt angry and disappointed with their caregivers, these couples may be puzzled to realize they also feel attachment to them. Many are further perplexed when they recognize that they will miss being ART patients; it was not an identity that they sought for themselves, but they have mastered it.

Many couples never say good-bye formally. Instead, they never make another appointment and try to walk away without looking back. They may be afraid their caregivers will be disappointed with them or that the caregivers themselves will feel like failures. Sometimes they are correct.

Physicians and nurses are not always able to help patients with the grief that accompanies saying good-bye. Perhaps they feel a sense of failure and disappointment as well as guilt; these are the patients for whom the miracle treatments have not worked. Understandably, caregivers find it easier to celebrate with their successes than to share the pain of those who recognize a need to move on.

Physicians and nurses who understand the sense of failure and disappointment that many couples feel upon ending treatment can help reduce such feelings by expressing positive sentiments about adoption or other alternatives, including the decision to remain child free. They convey to their patients a clear sense that their decision marks a successful resolution to infertility.

Feelings About Second Choices

In the course of infertility treatment, many people identify a "light at the end of the tunnel". Recognizing that they may not succeed in having their first choice—a genetic child—they look to alternatives. Most find that although they may not like the idea, they can imagine another pathway to parenthood—or a satisfying child-free life.

Individuals and couples have different feelings about the light at the end of the tunnel. These feelings are determined by their experience with a given option (i.e. a man whose best friend was adopted may have very positive associations to this option), as well as by their feelings about the significance of genetic continuity. What is most important in deciding to move on is that a couple be able to reach agreement about this second choice. For some couples, this is relatively easy; for others, it seems nearly impossible.

Some couples are unable to identify a second choice, but most can engage in this emotionally charged and complex decision-making process and eventually arrive at a decision. Many are relieved to discover that they were never as far apart as they had initially feared: each needed to be able to make the decision in his or her own style and individual pace. Additionally, couples tend to balance each other: one member may be able to move forward with more determination because the other is cautiously holding back. Similarly, the partner who expresses reluctance may be doing so because he or she has confidence that they will still continue to move forward as a couple. Sometimes they switch positions at a later date. It is common for couples considering adoption, for example, to take turns advocating for this parenting option. When one feels enthusiastic about it, the other may think of several reasons that it is a bad idea. Later, each may change his or her viewpoint. In short, delicate balancing often occurs as couples prepare to end treatment, and this balancing can be a necessary part of deciding that enough is enough.

In examining their second choices, some couples focus their attention on their feelings about the pregnancy experience, while others look more carefully at genetics or at the social aspects of parenting. Couples who feel strongly about experiencing a pregnancy together, even if it will not result in their full genetic child, will look more carefully at options that offer a shared pregnancy: donor insemination or ovum donation. Those who focus more on a genetic connection may consider gestational care. However, the majority of couples, even among ART veterans, tend to look to adoption, finding it the most familiar, successful, and predictable second-choice path to parenthood.

Couples who, after considering parenting alternatives, conclude that genetics and gestation are too important to give up often decide not to pursue alternatives, determining that being child free will be more satisfying for them. Many begin by identifying other ways that they can have children in their lives. Some have nieces or nephews they hope to spend time with; others think about becoming a big brother or big sister to a child in need. Although most could not have imagined that they could go from being childless to embracing being child free, they emerge from a period of exploration and mourning with a renewed sense of optimism and energy.

Sadly, there are some couples who are unable to reach a decision about a second choice. They find themselves at an impasse, with a strong desire to move on but without a place to go. These couples are in crisis. Counseling can be useful in helping them sort through their feelings, attitudes, beliefs, and prejudices about the alternatives that are available to them, and one spouse may eventually come to feel more comfortable with his or her partner's preference.

Couples who cannot come to any agreement have a bleak future. Their inability to identify an alternative increases their sense of isolation from each other, as well as from both the fertile and infertile world. Sometimes these couples fear for their marriage, and some infertile couples' marriages do end in divorce (as do the marriages of many fertile couples). Nevertheless, many clinicians agree that couples who struggle through the pain of infertility often find that the struggle has brought them closer to each other. Many feel comforted by this evidence of that resiliency as individuals and as a couple.

Couples select their second choices based not only on feelings about genetics and gestation but also on the availability and accessibility of other options and on the degree to which their outcome is predictable. Some couples might find the idea of a particular alternative appealing but will not pursue it because geography, cost, or some other factor makes it virtually inaccessible. Conversely, they may decide against an option, even if it is readily available to them, because it is unlikely to result in a successful outcome. Having been on the roller coaster ride of infertility for too long, they are reluctant to enter into another process that may result in disappointment.

Adoption. When they are in the midst of infertility treatment, many couples receive unsolicited, and often unwelcome, advice about considering adoption. In addition to ignoring what the decision to adopt means for couples from an emotional standpoint, these well-meaning but unknowledgeable individuals may believe that it is always easy to adopt. In fact, the adoption of a healthy infant, is an expensive process if done through a private agency (often between twenty and thirty thousand dollars). Independent adoptions (in which couples attempt to locate birthparents themselves), though less costly, may involve a long wait as well as a series of disappointments, before couples achieve their goal of parenthood.

Finances aside, adoption can still be a difficult process. International adoption often means traveling to another country and may also require staying there for a prolonged period of time. Moreover, adoption too is a process filled with uncertainty; birthmothers sometimes change their minds, leaving adopting couples with yet another loss.

Another reason why adoption can be difficult is that couples are not always eligible for the adoption program of their choice. Some agencies, as well as some foreign countries, have age restrictions (which may be considered discriminatory) or requirements for length of marriage. Others take extensive medical and psychiatric histories and may exclude certain couples because of past problems. However, there are no universal requirements for adoption and most couples can identify a viable route to adoption.

Donor Insemination. Donor insemination (DI) is available and accessible to virtually all couples with male factor infertility. The process is neither costly nor especially time-consuming to pursue. In fact, some couples with male factor infertility who might otherwise lean toward adoption decide on donor insemination, at least in part because of financial factors. Another important consideration for these couples is that donor insemination is an alternative that offers a high probability of success, especially for couples with no identified female problem. Although it can take several months to achieve a pregnancy, most fertile women conceive in less than a year. Despite its convenience, however, there are many reasons why couples who are eligible for DI elect not to pursue it. (Donor insemination is the subject of chapter 5.)

Ovum Donation. Ovum donation is available and accessible to some couples in whom the woman has ovarian failure or the inability to conceive is thought to be a function of aging eggs. Those who have a known donor, as well as those who have access to an anonymous donor program and live near a medical center that offers this treatment, may decide to try this option. Others will be deterred from pursuing it for financial, geographical, or emotional reasons. (Ovum donation is explored in detail in chapter 6.)

Surrogacy. Surrogacy is available to couples with documented female infertility but whose partner is fertile. It generally has a predictable outcome: the vast majority of surrogates become pregnant in a reasonable period of time (under six months) and go on to have successful pregnancies. And only in the rarest of circumstances do surrogates have problems relinquishing the child they bore. However, surrogacy is not accessible to many couples because it tends to be a very expensive option, with fees often ranging above $30,000. In addition, most couples do not live near a professional surrogacy program, and many are reluctant to travel or to become involved in a long-distance arrangement. Furthermore, historically surrogacy has been surrounded by controversy; of all the parenting options, it is the most objectionable to the greatest number of people. Couples pursuing surrogacy must be prepared to face criticism for their decision. (Surrogacy is covered in chapter 7.)

Gestational Care. Gestational care is available to couples who can produce healthy embryos (through IVF) but cannot carry a pregnancy. This too is costly option and one that does not come with a high probability of success (although the younger the biological mother, the more likely the carrier is to become pregnant). In addition, gestational care is not easily accessible to many couples since it relies on highly specialized legal and psychological services, as well as on a skilled medical team. (Gestational care is the subject of chapter 8.)

Child-free Living. Child-free living is available to all couples. Like adoption, it is not discussed in this book because it does not involve medical intervention. However, from an emotional perspective, it can be a satisfying resolution to infertility and thus deserves mention. We encourage readers who are interested in considering this resolution to read *Sweet Grapes*, (by Jean & Michael Carter, (1989)), a well-written and uplifting book about one couple's process of resolving their infertility through child free living.

In examining second-choice options, infertile couples are often influenced by other infertile couples whom they come to know in the course of their treatment. Relationships that begin spontaneously in a physician's waiting room or are outgrowths of RESOLVE and other support group experiences are often instrumental in helping couples begin to take steps to end treatment. Many couples gain the confidence to pursue a particular option when they hear about the experiences of their friends. There is no better "advertisement" for adoption, for example, than a couple who is bubbling over with enthusiasm over their newly adopted infant.

For many couples, one of the hardest parts of moving on is facing the fact that their second choice, with the exception of those who decide to be child free, poses some uncertainty and that sometime they may have to identify and pursue yet a third choice.

Couples moving on must think about how they will—or will not—tell others about their decisions. Those who are adopting will face a variety of reactions from others, and those who feel tentative about the decision are likely to be especially sensitive to others' questions or criticisms. Positive reactions from family and friends will help reinforce the rightness of their choice, but the inevitable insensitive comments are likely to bring renewed questions and doubts.

Those who are moving on to donor gametes tend to be more private about their plans and may have difficulty telling others that they have decided to end treatment leading to a biogenetic child. Those who prefer to maintain privacy about their use of donor gametes may decide to camouflage the fact that they have ended one form of medical treatment and entered another.

All couples who are embarking upon a new option should take some time to renew their relationship and to look back with some perspective on where they have been and where they are going. Although there may be pressures to move on without delay, those who are able to take even a short treatment-free time may benefit from the break.

Guidance From the Mind

Another set of factors helps determine how and when couples decide to end treatment. These are factors based more on rational facts than on feelings or emotions. They are objective rather than subjective considerations. Thus in deciding whether to end treatment, it is important that couples pay careful attention to the wisdom of the mind as well as the heart. Each offers a different perspective, yet both are important in guiding couples about when to move on.

Among the key determinants in any couple's decision to remain in treatment or to leave it are the treatment opportunities. Depending on their geographical location, financial or insurance situation, diagnosis, prognosis, treatment history, and age, they will have more or fewer treatment options available to them.

Availability and Accessibility of Treatment

There are over 250—and perhaps as many as 300—clinics in the United States offering ART, most located in major metropolitan areas. Couples who live near these clinics can seek or continue treatment without having to travel long distances or relocate temporarily. By contrast, couples who live far from treatment centers face significant decisions about travel each time they try another cycle or a new treatment.

Living far from a treatment center means taking time off from work—often for several days or even weeks at a time. Usually this time constitutes leave without pay or hard-earned vacation time. Neither option is appealing and can contribute to a couple's decision to end treatment.

Cost is another major factor—often the most significant one—in determining whether a couple has access to treatment. Infertility treatment is very expensive and is not covered by medical insurance in most states. (It is common, however, for insurance companies to cover certain aspects of treatment, particularly if the diagnosis relates to a medical problem such as endometriosis). Consequently, many couples need substantial financial resources in order to pursue high-tech treatments. Some arrive at the decision that enough is enough when they find that they are unable to afford additional treatment. For some couples this forced decision brings relief; to others it adds to the injustice of their experience.

Considerations regarding the costs of adoption also influence couple's decisions about remaining in treatment. Some couples decided, in the midst of treatment, to put aside money for adoption, and they may end treatment when they realize that additional medical expenditures will dip into or more seriously deplete their adoption resources. Other couples who have insurance coverage for medical treatment may prefer to stop treatment and embrace adoption but cannot afford its high costs. Although eager to adopt, they remain in treatment for financial reasons.

Access to treatment may also be restricted by the policies of a particular program. Some IVF programs limit treatment to women under a certain age or to couples with certain types of infertility problems. Some programs refuse treatment to unmarried couples, lesbian couples, or single women, although such policies can probably be challenged as discriminatory.

Diagnosis and Prognosis

Couples focus on their diagnosis, and even more so, on their prognosis, when they face the question of whether enough is enough. Although there are occasionally couples who have a conclusive diagnosis—documented ovarian failure or azoospermia—most do not have a clear marker that indicates they are at the end of the line. Instead, most have been given diagnoses that carry with them some hope.

Physicians can be helpful to couples attempting to assess their chances for future success. Reviewing their diagnosis, the results of previous treatment (a couple who has achieved an ART pregnancy but suffered a miscarriage will often have more hope for future success than one whose treatment efforts have never resulted in pregnancy), the treatment approaches that have already been tried, and their age can offer a couple a clearer sense of whether additional treatment is likely to prove worthwhile.

The physician's task involves challenges far greater than trying to make a rational assessment of a couple's prognosis. Experience has taught every physician that infertility brings surprises and that sometimes the most hopeless situations bring unexpected success, while the ones that appear most promising can end in disappointment. Experience has also taught physicians that some couples are looking for guidance and permission to leave treatment, while others want their doctor to offer them yet another treatment opportunity. These factors and others cause many physicians to avoid the difficult topic of discontinuing treatment.

Physicians who are able to discuss ending treatment often find that their patients appreciate the guidance. Some cautiously introduce the topic by asking a couple whether they have considered adoption and sensing, from their response, whether they welcome the opportunity to discuss alternatives to treatment. Couples may feel relieved by their physician's cautious approach and view his or her questions as evidence of caring about them. Moreover, these couples may long for some confirmation of their own growing sense that it is time to move on.

Sometimes couples feel that their physician is giving up on them when he or she mentions adoption. Initially, this discussion can be upsetting, especially for those who feel a strong connection to their physician and sense they are being abandoned. Nevertheless, many couples come to appreciate their doctor's willingness to talk about adoption and realize, in retrospect, that broaching the subject, although jolting, introduced them to the possibility of ending treatment. Moreover, their physician's mention of alternatives serves as endorsement of other options.

Treatment History

The length of time that a couple has been infertile and the success or failure of past treatment efforts influence their feelings about when to end treatment, regardless of their diagnosis. Most couples can put their lives on hold only for so long and subject their relationship to the stress of infertility. Most women are willing to undergo physically invasive and painful procedures only for a limited time. This length of time varies considerably among couples but eventually most find that they are running out of energy. Their exhaustion is the result of their experiences and is not necessarily reflective of prognosis or duration of infertility. Some couples stay in treatment upwards of ten years; others stop after two or three.

Sometimes couples may want to stop treatment but are reluctant to do so because their physician assures them they still have a good chance of conceiving. This reassurance is confusing. On the one hand it is wonderful news, after all their physician is the "expert". On the other hand, they feel exhausted and depleted by their past treatments. Although their physician's optimism is encouraging, they wonder how they can reconcile two conflicting perspectives: pregnancy is possible, but the energy necessary to pursue it is vanishing.

Couples who have had a pregnancy as a result of ART treatment and have subsequently suffered one or more miscarriages are especially uncertain about whether to stop treatment. They often feel saddened and defeated by their experiences and long to avoid further suffering, but at the same time, their pregnancy offered hope. They may have been told that the pregnancy loss was a random event and should feel encouraged by the knowledge that they can become pregnant. Those who have suffered two or more pregnancy losses are in a more difficult situation; they do not know if they can become pregnant or, if they do, whether they can carry a baby.

Couples coming to the end of treatment may attempt to set a deadline on their efforts to have a baby: if they are not pregnant by the new year, by next Mother's day, or some other defined date they will move on to an alternative. Others set a limit on the number of IVF attempts they are willing to do, or on how many more months (or years) they will continue treatment promising themselves that they will move on once they reach that designated point. A deadline can help couples regain a sense of control, especially if they recognize that they can always alter it if their medical situation or their feelings change.

Age

Because the woman's age plays a significant role in fertility, many couples focus on age when they try to determine whether enough is enough.

Women in their twenties or very early thirties and their husbands sometimes fear that their treatment could go on forever. With all the dramatic advances in reproductive medicine and years of potential fertility ahead of them, there may always be something new to try. Some feel torn between their desire to stop treatment and move on and their awareness that they have not tried everything and that for medical reasons they do not feel pressured by time.

One way couples solve this dilemma is to decide to abandon efforts temporarily, taking an alternative path to parenthood but with the assumption that they will return to treatment in the future. Others abandon the effort totally, never intending to turn back.

Women in their late thirties or early forties and their husbands usually have a different outlook. They may be exhausted by their treatment efforts but know that this is their last opportunity to bear a child together. Faced with declining fertility, they feel that they had better push themselves now.

Often women identify a maximum age for having children, although they may revise that number from time to time. For example, a woman may have assumed that she would have had her first child by age thirty. When she married at twenty-nine, she moved her anticipated childbearing age upward, perhaps to thirty-three or thirty-four. Upon encountering infertility, it may have moved still upward. But not all women who specify a maximum age are comfortable revising it, believing that it is unwise for them to have a child past a certain age. When they reach their targeted age, they conclude that it is time to move on.

The situation for older women is confounded by the fact that their chance for a successful outcome, whatever their diagnosis, is limited. They wonder if it makes sense to take powerful medications or to undergo invasive, uncomfortable procedures when their odds are so poor. They are also aware that age brings with it an increased chance of miscarriage—sometimes estimated to be as high as 40 to 50 percent in women over forty.

When a women is in her mid-thirties and has been attempting pregnancy for an extended time, the decision to end treatment can be even more perplexing. Unlike younger women, who can pursue other options and return to treatment a few years hence, women in their mid-thirties know that stopping treatment now probably means ending it forever. If they decide at some point in the future to try again, it will be with diminished chance of success.

Although most couples focus on the age of the woman in deciding how long to pursue treatment (and her age is reproductively much more significant than her partner's) some couples pay attention to the age of the man, but for social rather than medical reasons. For example, if the husband is significantly older than his wife, they may decide that in fairness to the child—and to each other—he should not be past a certain age when his wife conceives a child.

More so than in the past, there are couples in which the woman is older than her partner, and her husband's relative youth can influence treatment efforts. Some couples try longer for a pregnancy than they might if he were the same age as or older than his wife, feeling secure that the child will have the benefits of a young father. One forty-one-year-old woman whose husband was thirty-one commented that she had never felt odd about being an older wife until she began dealing with infertility. Although her husband reassured her many times that he did not marry her in order to have children, nevertheless, she felt she was letting him down and feared he might leave her for a younger woman.

Grief, Resolution, and Celebration

Couples sometimes extend their treatment experience in an effort to avoid grief about their inability to have a bio-genetic child. Although this effort may temporarily spare them some pain, the truth is that most couples feel worse about themselves if they prolong treatment in order to avoid their grief.

The grief that comes at the end of infertility treatment takes different forms for different couples, depending on their past history and current life circumstances and their feelings about genetic continuity. Individuals who have had earlier losses in their families often find that leaving treatment prompts them to revisit those losses. For example, a man who had looked forward to naming a son after his deceased father may feel that the loss of his expected son adds to the depth of his earlier loss.

Couples whose lives are otherwise rich and full may find that their grief paves the way for relief; it frees them up to enjoy and celebrate other aspects of their lives. By contrast, couples who are experiencing frustrations and disappointments at work or with family and friends may find their grief more burdensome.

Personality styles also influence the ways in which couples grieve at the close of treatment. Some couples tend to be passive, accepting their sorrow as something that will end when it will end. Others take a more active approach, trying to create rituals and cere-monies for moving on. They may plant trees in memory of their unborn children, write poems, create a religious ceremony, or hold a private memorial service.

When couples decide that they have truly had enough of treat-ment and that they have successfully identified a second choice, they commonly combine grief with celebration. Although this sounds contradictory, joy and sorrow can be two sides of the same coin. As sad as couples feel upon ending treatment, because it sig-nals the end of shared genetic parenthood, they also feel a sense of relief that the medical ordeal is over. One woman describes this merging of grief with relief.

> Our grieving took the form of celebration. Alex and I went out to dinner, had a bottle of wine, went home and threw out the remaining vial of Pergonal and all the ovulation predictor kits. Then we made love. For the first time in nearly four years, our love-making felt like a sign of our success as a couple, rather than our failure. We still felt profoundly sad that we would not "make a baby" together, but there, in bed together, that sorrow was not with us. We were too busy en-joying the love and tenderness that remained strong between us.

PART II

Third Party Parenting

5

Donor Insemination

Donor insemination—the process in which a woman is artificially inseminated with the sperm of a man other than a husband/partner—is not a new reproductive technology. Dating back approximately one hundred years, donor insemination can more aptly be considered an 'old' reproductive technology for couples with male factor infertility. Over the years, however, donor insemination has been mistakenly identified as a treatment for male factor infertility, yet it has never been a treatment in the way that surgical procedures or pharmacological regimens are. The latter are designed to improve the quality and quantity of sperm so that conception can occur; the former is an alternative path to parenthood.

One of the problems with presenting donor insemination (DI) as a *treatment* for male infertility, is that the word 'treatment' implies 'cure,' and donor insemination, though a cure for childlessness, is not a cure for infertility. The question—one which is not often acknowledged—is why donor insemination is presented to infertile couples as a treatment, rather than an alternative childbearing method. In order to answer this question it helps to reflect back on the history of DI and on the history of male infertility. By looking at these separate, but intertwined histories, we can better understand why this case of "mistaken identity," occurred, and how, along with many other factors, it has shaped the history and the practice of donor insemination.

Setting the Stage: A Climate of Shame and Secrecy

The history of male infertility begins with the Bible. The Old Testament commands men to produce heirs to inherit their property and carry on their name. Barren women were pitied and held responsible for their condition, but men who did not have offspring were seen as tragic figures and were shamed. They were out of compliance with God's law.

The importance (and necessity) of paternity in biblical times is illustrated by the fact that a man whose marriage was childless after ten years was instructed to find a concubine to bear children for him. Even more extreme measures were mandated posthumously for a man who died without children: his brother was obligated to marry the dead man's wife and have children with her. The resulting offspring were considered the dead man's children, bearers of his name and evidence that he did not die without heirs.

The process in which a man impregnates his dead brother's wife is referred to as a Levirate marriage. Although some biblical scholars have pointed to such arrangements as the earliest form of donor insemination, there are obvious differences between the two. Nevertheless, the concept of creating a child from another man's sperm and raising the child as the legal offspring of the husband is similar to the concept of donor insemination.

Although our biblical ancestors realized that semen is necessary to achieve pregnancy, they did not understand why. Not until thousands of years later, in 1677, did Anton van Leeuwenhoek, inventor of the microscope, discover the presence of sperm. Even after his discovery, however, it took two more centuries before the mechanics of reproduction were known.

Van Leeuwenhoek subscribed to the preformationist school, believing that a single spermatozoan contains all the elements essential to create an adult human being and that during the embryonic period that individual would emerge. The woman was necessary, he thought, because she provided the gestational environment, but she did not have a role in the conception of the child. Van Leeuwenhoek therefore believed that the man plants the seed of his future child in much the same way that a farmer plants seeds in the ground. If the soil is not fertile, the land will be barren. Thus, it is easy to understand why our ancestors believed that women alone are responsible for infertility. Since sperm could not be seen in an ejaculate—let alone be counted, as they can today—our ancestors must have assumed that if a man ejaculated his seed, he was fertile.

Over the past hundred years and especially in the last few decades, much has been learned about infertility, including that both men and women have an equal stake in the creation of their children and that infertility can occur in either partner. Knowledge about the causes of male infertility and the ways to diagnose it has increased severalfold, especially in the last decade. Understanding a problem, however, does not necessarily mean it can be cured. Although physicians are often able to identify why a man is infertile—low sperm count, poor motility, too many abnormal forms, the presence of antibodies—treatment for male factor infertility is limited.

Efforts to treat male infertility have focused on ways to improve the numbers of normal, motile sperm thought to be necessary for conception. Although some couples with male infertility are helped by medicine or surgery, treatment has lagged far behind treatment for female problems and has been largely unsuccessful. When surgery or pharmacology fails to improve sperm count, efforts to expedite the process of fertilization—bringing the sperm closer to the egg—have been attempted. These treatments, known as artificial insemination (AI), refer to the process whereby sperm is introduced into the female reproductive tract through the use of instruments or other artificial devices.

Historically, artificial insemination was used with animals long before it was used for human beings. The practice dates to the fourteenth century when Arabs used AI to breed horses. Yet it was not until 1799 that the birth of a human, conceived via artificial insemination (with the husband's sperm), was recorded in London. The first such birth in the United States was recorded in 1866, and since then the technique has become increasingly popular among physicians.

Artificial insemination is performed by placing the sperm in the woman's vagina, cervix, or uterus. Placing it in the vagina is effective only when a mechanical problem precludes semen from being deposited there. Placing sperm in the cervix (intracervical insemination) brings it closer to its ultimate destination, the fallopian tube, where it is hoped that an egg awaits. Whether conception rates actually improve as a result of intracervical insemination was a topic frequently debated among reproductive endocrinologists. This technique has been largely replaced by intrauterine insemination (IUI).

Placing sperm—rather than semen (which may cause severe cramping)—directly in the uterus, thereby bringing it even closer to the egg, is a treatment that has been widely available since the early 1980s. This treatment, known as intrauterine insemination (IUI) has not been especially successful; many couples with male factor infertility undergo years of IUI treatment without having a pregnancy. Some of these couples turn to IVF.

As we noted in the first half of this book, the development of in vitro fertilization revolutionized the field of reproductive medicine. This development was of special significance to the treatment of male infertility since it presented an opportunity to truly bring sperm and egg together. IVF was also a revolutionary diagnostic tool, providing clear evidence of whether fertilization could occur. When eggs do not fertilize via in vitro fertilization, some couples then turn to donor insemination.

Although artificial insemination was performed for several decades using the husband's sperm, it was not until the late 1800s that the first case of AI using a donor was documented—by William Pancoast, who claimed to have performed the procedure in secret. Thus began a trend that continued for one hundred years and still continues today for most couples choosing DI: that of secrecy. The theme of secrecy, as we will see throughout this chapter, has governed the theory and practice of DI, from the way donors are selected, to the way in which physicians speak to couples about this option, to the way in which DI parents conduct their relationships with their children. Unfortunately, as we will also see, shame is a byproduct of secrecy, yet shame only serves to increase men's feelings of being defective—not real men.

Over the years donor insemination has been used with increasing frequency by couples with male infertility. When placing the sperm alot closer to the egg—even on top of it—does not result in conception, a 'logical' next step might be to substitute another man's sperm. Thus DI could be considered the "ultimate bypass." As we noted earlier, this concept is not new; it dates back to Biblical times and reinforces the importance of paternity. And because sperm is easily obtainable and easily storable (see "The Selection and Practice of Anonymous Sperm Donation" on page 178 of this chapter) this process of 'substitution' is easily performed.

Current donor insemination (DI) statistics are difficult to gather; physicians' records are confidential, and many couples are beginning to perform their own inseminations without using a physician as an intermediary. An estimate of the number of births per year resulting from donor insemination is approximately 30,000. Thus DI plays a prominent role among family-building options for couples with male factor infertility.

Because male infertility is considered shameful, and because donor insemination is usually presented as a treatment, physicians do not often speak to couples about the emotional aspects of this problem. Accordingly, most do not address the overwhelming sadness that infertile men and their partners feel upon learning their diagnosis. Thus many couples find themselves DI parents without having grieved their loss—and without having explored the implications of donor insemination on their relationship as a couple and as a family.

Donor Insemination Couples

Couples arrive at DI for very different reasons and with very different medical histories. Some men knew about their infertility from childhood; others suspected it; most others were shocked and devastated to learn of their problem. This section briefly looks at the different groups of couples who consider donor insemination, as well as the ways in which male infertility is diagnosed and treated.

Candidates for Donor Insemination

Almost all couples who turn to donor insemination do so because of male factor infertility; the only exception is when the choice is made because the man is a carrier of a genetic disorder.

Infertility has various causes. For most couples considering DI, male infertility is idiopathic; the nature of the problem can be identified, but its cause is unknown. Infertility can be a side effect of radiation or chemotherapy for cancer treatment; it can be congenital; it can result from a childhood disease or accident; it can be caused by a sexually transmitted disease or an infection; or it can be due to having had a vasectomy.

Those who have family histories of genetic disorders are a small but nevertheless important group of DI couples. If the gene in question can be detected by amniocentesis, it is unlikely the couple will choose DI, unless their religious beliefs preclude abortion. If the gene is not detectable until after birth, many couples elect not to take the risk of passing it on. If the problem gene is autosomal dominant, as in the case of Huntington's disease, any offspring of the father would have a 50 percent chance of inheriting the syndrome. If the disorder is one that is autosomal recessive, such as Tay-Sachs disease or cystic fibrosis and the woman is also a carrier, their offspring have a 25 percent chance of inheriting the disease. Afraid to attempt pregnancy with such odds, a number of these couples turn to donor insemination. Many approach DI reluctantly, feeling cheated out of a biological child but not suffering from the feelings of shame that burden infertile men.

Couples who suffer from male factor infertility of unknown origin comprise the largest group. They, like most other couples, approached parenthood assuming fertility, unaware that the man had a low sperm count, poor motility, or abnormal morphology. In the course of a workup, the diagnosis was made. Many of these couples go through years of testing and treatment, often including the ARTs, before turning to donor insemination.

Infertile men often feel defective, and this sense of defectiveness may be especially powerful for those who together with their wives have undergone extensive testing and treatment without having a successful outcome. Perhaps even more so than other infertile men, they feel helpless, frustrated by their inability to get answers, and even more frustrated by their inability to be successfully treated.

Another group of infertile men—and one that is growing in numbers—are those who have been successfully treated for cancer. These men have a multitude of conflicting feelings. They are grateful to be alive, but once their survival is reasonably assured, the long-term implications of infertility may feel overpowering.

Some men who have had cancer were instructed to bank sperm prior to undergoing radiation or chemotherapy, in order to preserve fertility. Those who have done so have varying degrees of success with their samples. Sometimes in vitro fertilization is used in combination with the frozen sperm of cancer survivors, even in situations with no identified female problem. IVF maximizes their chances of pregnancy and is an efficient way to use frozen sperm. Due to limited samples and the fact that freezing sperm can damage its overall quality, many of these couples will still not achieve pregnancy and may turn to donor insemination.

Congenital problems are another cause of infertility. Examples of congenital problems are absence of the vas deferens (the tubes that carry the semen from the testicles to where it is ejaculated); Klinefelter's syndrome, in which a man is born with an extra X chromosome (in his XY complement, rendering him sterile); or an undescended testicle that was not surgically corrected at a young age. These conditions are not correctable in adults. Men with congenital conditions resulting in infertility have probably lived most of their life with that knowledge. Now, as adults who are prepared to become fathers, these men may find that new feelings of sadness and anger arise.

An illness such as mumps, occurring postpuberty, or trauma to the testicles resulting from injury can also cause infertility in adult males. Similarly, infections—often but not always gonorrhea—can cause blockages in the epididymis or in the ejaculatory ducts. Although men in this group at least have the satisfaction of knowing why they are infertile, it probably does not reduce their pain.

A final group of men who are infertile are those who have had vasectomies, believing they did not want children. Others had vasectomies in an earlier marriage after having all the children they thought they wanted. Although vasectomies can be reversed, the success of the surgery is linked to time; those who had the procedure done many years ago—more than ten—are less likely to have a successful reversal. Unlike those infertile men who feel damaged or defective, men who have had vasectomies tend to be tormented by guilt, self-blame, and regret. They look back upon past decisions—ones often made with great care—and wonder how they could have been so shortsighted.

Diagnosing Male Infertility

Teenage boys learn that only one sperm is needed for conception, yet it is also true that at least 20 million are usually needed to be stored in the woman's reproductive tract. When the egg is ripe they are slowly released. In addition, it is not only the numbers that matter. The percentage of motile sperm moving at the right speed and in the right direction should be 40 to 50 percent normal, and the morphology (appearance) should be at least 60 percent normal.

Medical knowledge about male infertility is constantly shifting. At one time the count was thought to be the most important statistic. More recently, motility has been thought to be even more important, and even more recently, greater emphasis is being placed on morphology. There are, in addition, other factors that affect sperm and can cause infertility, such as antibody problems, infections, and varicoceles (varicose veins in the scrotum).

Male infertility appears to be on a continuum. Although there are some men who have no sperm (azoospermia) and are therefore sterile, most men suffering from infertility do have some sperm (oligospermia). The closer the man's numbers are to the ideal parameters, the greater is the likelihood of an eventual pregnancy. As long as some live sperm are present in the ejaculate, a pregnancy is always possible.

Until IVF, couples with male factor infertility who never had a pregnancy had no way of knowing whether the sperm were capable of fertilizing the egg, even if one should reach its destination. The only diagnostic test that gave any indication about whether fertilization was possible was the hamster egg penetration test: a sperm sample from the husband is obtained, several ripe eggs are extracted from a female hamster (whose eggs are remarkably similar to human ova), and insemination is attempted under laboratory surveillance. Although the test can predict the likelihood of fertilization, it is often inaccurate; many men who have 'failed' this test have subsequently impregnated their wives without any intervention.

In vitro fertilization, though much more expensive, time-consuming, and invasive than a hamster egg test, is understandably a far better diagnostic tool. Assuming that several good eggs are retrieved, a couple will learn whether fertilization can occur. Although it is still not possible to know with certainty what happens in the fallopian tube if fertilization of egg and sperm does not occur in the laboratory, physicians assume that it probably does not occur in the body. (There are, however, many ART programs that offer GIFT as a treatment for mild to moderate male factor, believing that since the fallopian tube is a better incubator than a petri dish, that fertilization may be more likely with GIFT.)

Treatment for Male Infertility

Although male infertility can almost always be diagnosed by a semen analysis and its causes sometimes identified as well, it is difficult to cure. Medical advances in this area have been few, and prognosis is generally worse than for female problems. Treatment for male factor involving count, motility, or morphology can be attempted through the use of medication for hormonal problems or through surgery for problems such as a varicocele or a blockage of the epididymis. Nevertheless, both medication and surgery frequently fail to cure the problem.

Artificial insemination procedures attempt to bypass problems of count, motility, or morphology by depositing sperm closer to the egg—closer than when it is ejaculated during sexual intercourse. Because semen carries prostaglandins, chemicals, that cause severe cramping, sperm must be washed to rid them of the prostaglandins as well as any bacteria present that would impede fertilization. Sperm washing concentrates the sperm so that only the most motile, normal ones are used for insemination, thus bypassing problems of low volume, poor motility, or abnormal morphology. Sometimes this treatment works, and the woman becomes pregnant, but it may take several cycles, and the couple is never sure how long to keep trying. (The less severe the male factor, the greater the chances are of pregnancy occurring.) It is common to combine IUI with superovulation therapy, in which case not only are the sperm getting a head start, but they also have more possibilities for fertilization.

In vitro fertilization was designed to overcome female infertility problems that involve blockage of the fallopian tubes, but it has been an effective treatment for couples with male infertility as well. IVF is a means of bypassing a low sperm count or poor motility or morphology. When sperm do not have to travel (they are placed directly in a petri dish with ova extracted from the woman), the numbers of normal sperm and the speed and direction in which they move are not as important as when they are required to make a long journey. Thus, a significant portion of male factor couples who attempt IVF are able to achieve fertilization (and hopefully a pregnancy as well).

Couples who do not achieve fertilization, assuming the woman has produced at least a few good-quality eggs, often have more difficulty coping with the news than do couples who have negative pregnancy tests, for they know very well that unless they can produce embryos, they have no chance of pregnancy—ever. Sometimes, however, couples who do not achieve fertilization in their first IVF cycle attempt another one in which fertilization does occur or even conceive without medical intervention.

Hence, IVF for male infertility does not always offer couples greater clarity. Some undergo a cycle in which a small percentage of the eggs fertilize—perhaps one or two out of a dozen or more. Other couples whose IVF cycle did not result in any embryos may have only had two or three eggs to inseminate, and their quality may not have been ideal. Hence, the cycle was not truly an accurate test of fertilizability. In these situations the decision about whether to continue with IVF or move on to a second choice is difficult to make.

Until recently, couples who had poor fertilization with IVF, or none at all, usually concluded that they needed to move on. However, micromanipulation techniques are now available in certain ART clinics and are enticing to some couples. Micromanipulation is recommended when the numbers of viable sperm as measured by a semen analysis are too low even for IVF or when attempts at IVF do not yield fertilization. This technique (described in Chapter 2) is a long shot; so far fertilization rates in most clinics doing microinsemination are only about 20 to 30 percent per egg, although a recent report indicated that one technique—intracytoplasmic sperm injection—yielded fertilization in 54% of the eggs that were injected, resulting in a 31% pregnancy rate per treatment cycle. Microinsemination is open to few couples because of its lack of availability and high cost.

Thus the treatment of male infertility is indeed difficult and often confusing. IVF is an effective tool but it is not without its limitations: it reduces confusion for some couples but increases it for others. Repeated attempts at IVF or microinsemination that result in failed fertilization or poor fertilization rates are upsetting and frustrating for a couple. At the same time, however, couples with failed fertilization know they have had the benefit of the ultimate diagnostic test. Unlike those couples who never try IVF and go from month to month wondering if fertilization can occur, they know they have made their best effort to have a bio-genetic child, and they are ready to consider alternatives. Many such couples turn to donor insemination.

Deciding on Donor Insemination

Although many physicians continue to present DI as a 'treatment' for male infertility, the medical profession has come a long way in recent years towards acknowledging that donor insemination is not a simple medical procedure but rather it is a complex emotional, social, and ethical decision that has long-term ramifications for a family. In response to this growing appreciation for the complexities of DI, the AFS has recommended that referral for counseling and evaluation may be very useful to some couples before proceeding with this choice. Unfortunately many couples face decisions about DI alone, with little guidance. And because male infertility is so upsetting, often engendering feelings of embarrassment and shame, it can be difficult for couples to face the issues at hand.

Considering donor insemination is a painful process; it raises intense feelings of loss, confronting couples with their mortality and with their longing for genetic continuity. Many realize that one of their reasons for wanting a genetic child is to continue their genetic line—to live on in their children. Couples embarking on this path must think about what it means to be a parent and how parenting a child who is genetically connected to them may be different from parenting a child who is genetically connected to only one of them. They must also think about attachments and how they develop. They must examine how the addition of a third party, known or unknown, will affect their feelings about themselves and about their relationship. Because donor insemination involves intense feelings and profoundly complicated decisions, a couple's relationship is tested. They must be able to express their feelings to one another, not only about the ways in which infertility has affected them individually but also about the long-term implications of donor insemination.

A 1986 study done in Canada of 120 DI couples supports the notion that the use of donor insemination generates intense and troublesome feelings both within and between spouses—feelings that need to be resolved for everyone's well-being. The researchers state that common reactions for men are loss of self-esteem, emotional withdrawal, and temporary impotence. Anger, guilt, and a wish to make reparations are part of the woman's experience. The researchers emphasize that if these conflicts are not resolved, they can lead to more serious ones.[1]

Considerations Concerning Alternative Paths to Parenthood

The first issue a couple with male infertility must consider when they decide to end treatment is whether they wish to pursue an alternative path to parenthood. Some remain child free. They decide that if they are unable to have a child who is genetically connected to both of them, they would rather not parent at all. For these couples, this alternative is more acceptable than the other two paths open to them: adoption or donor insemination.

In considering alternatives, some couples are clear from the outset that donor insemination is unacceptable for ethical or social reasons. Others are just as clear that if the child cannot be totally biologically theirs, at least he or she can be half biologically theirs. Still others—and this is a large group of couples—approach the end of treatment knowing they want to become parents yet uncertain as to which of those two alternatives will work better for them.

Biogenetic Equality. Biological and genetic equality is an important consideration for many couples. Some fear that the inequality of DI may eventually threaten their marriage. They worry that if a crisis developed with their child, the father would distance himself. They wonder whether he would always feel unauthentic or second class. These couples prefer the relational equality that adoption offers; neither parent is genetically or biologically connected to their child. In adoption, both people ultimately suffer the losses of infertility, and both people begin the parenting venture on equal footing.

Couples leaning toward donor insemination generally feel more comfortable knowing half of the genetic origins of their offspring. They believe their child will feel more familiar to them since he or she is likely to resemble the mother—and members of her family—in physical traits or in personality. They believe that the child will feel equally theirs and that the genetic inequality will not matter.

The Experience of Pregnancy and Childbirth. Of all the potential losses involved in the experience of infertility, the pregnancy-childbirth experience is frequently a major one for most women. Donor insemination, unlike adoption, offers women the experience of gestating and giving birth to their baby. It also offers the couple the opportunity to share a pregnancy. Many women point to this reason as the major force behind their desire to create their family through donor insemination.

Prenatal Care. Couples who opt for donor insemination over adoption know that they will have control over their child's prenatal care, an issue about which most adoptive parents worry. Although adoption agencies obtain as much information as they can about a birthmother's pregnancy, they can never be completely sure that the information is accurate. In some cases, they receive very little information, and many parents who build their families through adoption, begin parenthood wondering whether anything in the prenatal environment was problematic and could be the potential cause of problems later in life.

Social Acceptability and Support. Some couples feel adoption is more socially acceptable than donor insemination. The process of adoption is well known, common, and open, and it offers a large, identifiable peer group with whom couples can relate. Although adopting a child can feel like embarking into unknown territory, adoptive parents are not pioneers. There are many resources open to adoptive couples, including numerous books on the process of adopting and on raising adopted children, support groups for adoptive parents, play groups for adoptive mothers and their children, and family service agencies and therapists who specialize in working with adoptive families.

Compared to adoption, resources for DI families are scant. It is also unlikely, unless they decide to be quite open, that DI couples will find other donor parents willing to share their experiences. Hence a couple may feel that deciding on donor insemination will lead to future isolation.

Privacy and Legitimacy. Some couples choose DI for the privacy it can offer. For them, the adoption of a child becomes a public statement about their infertility, a statement they may not wish to make. Couples who opt for DI may view adoptive couples as standing out to friends and relatives who were privy to the adoption.

Many couples who choose donor insemination over adoption also express fears that if they adopted they might feel different from other parents by virtue of not having given birth to a biological child. Women fear they might feel unauthentic—not the legitimate parents—if they adopt. They count on the fact that the experience of pregnancy and childbirth will make them feel like legitimate parents.

The Likelihood of Success. Some couples choose adoption over donor insemination because it seems more certain. Donor insemination does not always work, especially if there is a female problem in addition to a male factor, the situation in approximately one-third of the cases. Many couples, after years of trials and tribulations in the world of infertility, are hesitant to get back on the emotional roller coaster and are reluctant to continue the uncertainty of time-consuming, invasive treatment. They are ready to put treatment behind them and move on. Adoption generally affords them the security of knowing they will become parents. (Certain kinds of adoptions, however—independent, private, or legal risk adoptions—do not provide much security; there is a chance that the adoption's can fall through.)

On the other hand, many couples are convinced of the woman's fertility and believe DI to be an easier and quicker route to parenthood. Others who choose donor insemination are not worried about the risks; after years of uncertainty, they feel hardened to disappointment and are not convinced that any route to parenthood is a sure bet. Having been disappointed many times, no matter which alternative they select, they select it with skepticism.

Financial Cost. Some DI couples who might prefer adoption choose DI because it is less costly; they cannot afford a private agency adoption and do not wish to wait years for the placement of a child from a public agency. Adoption costs at private agencies currently run between $15,000 and $30,000. The price of a vial of sperm is usually between $150 and $300, plus the fee for the insemination. Frequently these costs are covered by medical insurance, but even when they are not, DI is still a much smaller financial investment.

Loss of Genetic Continuity

Another important issue facing couples considering DI is the loss of genetic continuity. Infertility forces people to think about the importance of bloodlines and of producing bio-genetic offspring who will inherit their traits. The value that each person assigns to these concepts is an important determinant in how much effort a couple will expend in order to conceive a biological child. No matter how extensively a couple pursues treatment, the inability to produce a biogenetic child is always a major loss.

For years scientists, sociologists, and psychologists have debated the 'nature/nurture' question. Although no one has come up with the exact equation—how much of us is determined by genes and how much is determined by environment—the balance seems to be shifting in the direction of nature. No one disputes that environment is extremely important in helping us reach our potential. What is new, however, are findings that traits, once thought to be solely acquired as a result of upbringing, are now understood to have strong genetic components, and this knowledge may make some couples even more determined to have children who are genetically connected to them.

Most couples fantasize at some point long before attempting pregnancy what their children will be like: how they will look, what talents they will possess, and the kind of personality they will have. Although children almost always turn out different from these fantasies, most have some qualities of each parent that are recognizable. Couples who are confronting male infertility and contemplating donor insemination must face their feelings of sadness about not being able to see the husband's traits reflected in their children. They must recognize that no matter how carefully they select a donor who appears to be *just like* the husband, there is no way such a match to the husband can be made.

For some people genetic continuity is not very important. Those who believe in a "humankind gene pool" recognize that no one person has a monopoly on any specific gene. Since each person is a random combination of the parents' genes, there is never any certainty that a particular child will possess curly hair or musical aptitude or any other desired (or undesired) trait of their parents.

On the other hand, there are individuals who believe in a "unique gene pool." Recognizing that there is no one else in the world who is exactly like them, they place a great deal of importance on the unique combination of genes that they received from their parents. Couples who subscribe to this philosophy may feel the inability to pass on their genes as more of a major loss than those who identify more with the humankind gene pool philosophy.

Couples who feel rooted in their family tree, and for whom bloodlines are important, may view donor insemination as severing their ancestral ties. Thus it is common for infertile men to feel as if they will be greatly disappointing their families should they choose donor insemination. They may worry that if their family knew about DI, the grandchild would not be loved or accepted in the way a biological grandchild would be. There is reason for such concerns. Adopted children are sometimes left off family trees or out of a grandparents' will.

Concerns About Attachment

When a couple struggles with DI, the man often wonders whether he could love "another man's child." This uncertainty or doubt may underlie the objections he raises. Attachment for women is usually less of a mystery because most girls grow up playing house or playing with dolls, and they frequently babysit as teenagers. They thus enter adulthood with the understanding that people easily become attached to babies and small children as a result of nurturing them. Since most men had different experiences growing up, they may assume that the reason parents love their children is that they come from their genes. Thus, some men initially reject the idea of donor insemination out of fear they will not be able to love a child they did not create.

Men do not necessarily understand this initial resistance, but over time many are able to acknowledge it. Once these fears are on the table, they can be explored. Couples can talk with one another about their fantasies of parenthood and what they hope for their children. They can think about the children they know and the extent to which they are like or different from their parents. Focusing on parenthood in this way can help with resolution.

Couples who are facing the possibility of adoption or donor gametes frequently find themselves considering whether they could love a particular child they know or whom they observe. Couples may think more about their friends' children and ask themselves whether they would want to have Joey for their child, or Julie, and on down the list. They think about whether they could love the child they see having a temper tantrum in the supermarket or the one whose nose is always running. Women who believe strongly that they could love a child who did not come from them still wonder if they could love *any* child, especially one who is unappealing on the surface. Men, who probably have less faith to begin with about their ability to love a child who did not come from them, may find themselves acutely observing children of all ages, in all situations, in an effort to confirm or deny their feelings.

Adulterous Feelings

A final issue that couples must consider before embarking on donor insemination involves their feelings about having another man's semen placed inside the woman. For some couples this process engenders thoughts and feelings about adultery, as the following example illustrates.

A couple who had been treated for male infertility for three years had just finished their second and last IVF cycle in which they did not get fertilization. Their previous treatment included several IUIs over two years. They made an appointment with the psychologist to discuss donor insemination. The husband stated that he was ready to move on to DI; he had dealt with his sadness over not being able to produce a biological offspring and wanted to be a father more than he wanted to be a biological father. His wife was far more hesitant, telling the psychologist timidly, "I've never told anyone this, but my husband is the only man I have ever had sex with. I'm afraid that having another man's sperm inside me would make me feel like I was sleeping with someone else."

Men similarly may express feelings of hesitancy about DI due to fears that if their wife conceives, they will feel as if she is carrying another man's child. Couples who ultimately choose this alternative means of family building must be able to separate the act of lovemaking from the act of procreation. Long before couples decide on DI or on any other alternative, most have given up the notion that sexuality and family building are connected. Yet donor insemination represents the need for an even greater emotional separation between the two experiences.

Choosing DI means trusting that once a pregnancy is achieved, both members of the couple will begin to feel that it is *their* child. This acceptance does not mean that couples should pretend they conceived in the normal way, at least not to themselves. Rather, they must acknowledge the special means of conception through which they formed their family. Couples who have allowed themselves to feel the range and depth of emotions that stem from their loss are in a strong position to face the decision-making process inherent in donor insemination. Though the feelings of loss probably never disappear completely, the hope is that ultimately they will be replaced by a sense of gratitude to an unknown (or known) man who enabled them to become parents.

Ethical and Psychological Considerations

Creating children through third parties raises profound psychological and ethical issues, regardless of whether the third party is a sperm donor, an egg donor, a traditional surrogate, or a gestational carrier. In some respects, all methods of third-party reproduction are similar and share common psychosocial and ethical issues; in other respects, each of them is unique. Here we address two of these issues as they relate to donor insemination: the use of known versus unknown donors and secrecy versus openness.

Known versus Unknown Donor

One of the first decisions DI couples must make is whether to use a known or an unknown donor. Although the population of couples who opt for a known donor is growing in numbers, most couples do not consider asking someone they know. Thus, the vast majority of DI couples use anonymous sperm from a sperm bank, perhaps due to the fact that secrecy and shame have always been an inherent component of male infertility, and rarely has anyone—including physicians—questioned that aspect of the process. A recent survey compared eighty-two programs that offer gamete donation. Not surprisingly, the author found that although the majority of these programs allowed known ovum donation, the majority did not allow known sperm donation.[2]

In choosing to use a donor, known or anonymous, there are many questions to consider. The first is an underlying ethical one: *Is it morally right to bring a child into the world with an unknown genetic parent?* Historically this question has been overlooked. Perhaps one reason is that nurture was once thought to play a far greater role than nature in human development. People who felt that a person's genetic makeup was unimportant in his or her development did not see a need for an individual to know its genetic parent(s). For if nature is not very relevant, except for physical attributes, it should be almost meaningless to an individual that he or she has no access to a genetic parent. If, on the other hand, nature is believed to be a primary force in shaping human beings, then it becomes less clear about whether it is ethical to create a child with an unknown genetic father. The shifting emphasis of the nature versus nurture debate, once more heavily weighted on the side of nurture, is making all parties to DI rethink what it means to be born with little knowledge about or access to one's genetic parents.

We can speculate that another reason that this ethical consideration has historically been overlooked has to do with fears of jeopardizing or compromising the role of the social father. If the importance of the genetic father is acknowledged, some might fear that the importance of the social or rearing father would be minimized. Efforts have been made to cover up DI—to pretend that the social and the genetic father are the same person. If the cultural ethic changes, and most people feel that a child should not be brought into the world with unknown origins, then social fathers may fear their relationship with their child would be threatened.

Decisions regarding social policy in the use of donor gametes have been discussed by Elias and Annas, a physician-geneticist and attorney-ethicist, respectively. They refer to donor insemination as a contractual agreement between parties and as the accepted paradigm for other methods of noncoital reproduction. They argue that donor insemination places "the private contractual agreement among the participants regarding parental rights and responsibilities above the 'best interest of the child,' and . . . raises a series of societal issues that remain unresolved." The authors go on to say:

> Assuming that deciding about parenthood by contract is socially accepted as currently practiced, we ignore the relevance of legitimacy, lineage, and individual identity tied up in kinship, and thus bypass fundamental questions about the definition of fatherhood and its role in the family and the life of the child.[3]

They then argue the other point of view, suggesting that since issues of legitimacy are no longer important social concerns in the United States and hereditary titles are not bestowed by lineage, questions about genetic parenthood may be irrelevant. It is noteworthy—and testimony to the fact that these ethical issues are extremely complicated—that even these prominent figures seem uncertain about whether the intentional creation of a child with unknown genetic origins should be acceptable.

Reasons for Chosing Known Sperm Donation. Couples who choose known sperm donation are a minority. Nevertheless, they most likely arrived at their decision after a lengthy process and have clear reasons for their decision. The following ones are important to 'known' donor couples

Avoindance of Genealogical Bewilderment. We know a great deal about the importance of genetic ties from the field of adoption as more and more adoptees speak out on the need to know where they came from. The concept of genealogical bewilderment refers to a sense of not knowing who one is or to whom one belongs. Many adoptees describe feeling unrooted and biologically disconnected.

Because of this genetic void, they feel a piece of themselves—of their identity—is missing. This genealogical bewilderment frequently propels adoptees to search for birthparents so that they can fill in the void and develop a stronger sense of self.

Professionals, in recognizing the role that genetics plays in the unfolding of a person's life, are attempting to provide adoptive couples with as much information as they can gather about their child's birthparents—information about their medical, physical, social, and emotional histories. In many situations, however, information is lacking about the birthfather; he is unknown or unavailable, or the birthmother refuses to identify him. There are those who argue that if it is acceptable to couples to adopt a child under these circumstances, then it must be acceptable to create a child using sperm from an anonymous donor.

The key ethical issue, however, is the idea of intentionally creating a child with unknown parentage. In the case of adoption, children are not created in order to be adopted. For various reasons, the birthparents are unable to provide for their children and look to adoption. This unintended situation is different from a deliberate attempt to create a child from donor gametes.

Some couples who choose known donors do so primarily because they believe that it is unfair to create a child who may suffer from genealogical bewilderment. They feel that it is emotionally healthier for a child to grow up knowing who the genetic parents are so that her or his identity will be much more solid. Even if the donor is not someone who is in the child's day-to-day life or is geographically close, the child will still be able to meet him someday.

Control Over the Source of the Gametes. Choosing a known donor provides the couple some control over the gene pool of their offspring. Infertility has taken away their sense of control in regard to reproduction, and using a known donor will help them reclaim some of it. Although no parents ever have control over their child's particular genetic makeup, couples who select a known donor feel more secure that their child will not seem like a random or unfamiliar person.

Many couples who choose known donation opt for a relative, frequently the husband's brother. Preserving the family genes is important to them, as is maintaining a sense of control over their source. Genetically siblings are very similar, because they come from the same gene pools, allowing family bloodlines to be preserved.

A potential problem in using a sibling (and to a lesser extent, any other known donor) is that it stirs up issues of competition. Children growing up in the same family develop feelings of competition about all kinds of issues—power, competence, status in the family, and others—and these feelings do not necessarily cease when siblings reach adulthood. When an infertile man accepts sperm from his fertile brother, emotionally he may feel that he is in a "one-down position." Those feelings may rekindle earlier feelings relating to the power dynamic between the two of them.

A case example illustrates this point regarding sibling competition. A male infertility patient who set up an appointment with a clinical social worker to discuss donor insemination mentioned that he had three brothers. His proposal was to ask each of them to donate sperm and have the physician mix them together prior to the insemination. Thus, no one would know which brother was the genetic father to the child. The social worker saw the proposal as a red flag indicating that he was not emotionally prepared to accept his brother's sperm.

Further discussion revealed that the inability to reproduce was a grave loss for this man, and he believed that his parents would be devastated if he were to tell them about his infertility. In using his brother's sperm, he felt satisfied that he would not be letting his parents down—one brother's genes were as good as the others—and he would therefore not feel guilty about keeping it secret from them. As the interview continued, it also became clear that he had strong competitive feelings toward all of his siblings. Although he had hoped to neutralize these feelings by mixing sperm from all three brothers, the husband realized that this action would increase his feelings of competition rather than diminish them and that he would always wonder which brother was the "real man." The couple decided to use an anonymous donor.

One known-donor situation that sometimes arises is troubling to many mental health professionals and physicians: cross-generational donation of parent to child, or vice versa. Crossgenerational donation raises extensive ethical and psychological issues and is opposed by many professionals who support known sperm donation from brothers or friends. In the case of a son donating to his father, many feel strongly that because of the nature of the parent-child relationship, a child is not truly free in the way others are to say no to a parent's request. In the case of a father donating to a son, some professionals feel more supportive, because the concept of parents' giving to children is already built into the parent-child relationship.

Access to Medical Information. Using a known donor allows the family to have access to the donor's medical history. As the origins of more illnesses are being probed, genetic components increasingly are understood to play a large role. If the donor is part of the couple's life, this history can be updated periodically as more medical information about him and his immediate family unfolds. Couples who use anonymous donors do not have an unfolding medical history available, and their offspring must live with half a medical void.

Psychological and Legal Counseling. Because of the many questions and concerns involved in using known donors, couples and their donors need to have comprehensive counseling from a mental health professional before embarking on this venture. The issues necessary to raise are the ethical and psychological ones that we have just outlined and the ones that we will cover in the next section. It is generally wise for the counselor to meet first with the donor, before she or he has any knowledge about or becomes acquainted with the prospective couple. The counselor can then assume an objective stance and help the prospective donor decide if donating is in his best interest. If the counselor has met with the couple prior to meeting with the donor and has come to know them and feels invested in helping them, then it is much more difficult to be objective.

Couples who are using a known donor should seek legal counsel from an attorney who is well versed in reproductive law. The law in this field is continually changing, however, and varies from state to state. All parties should familiarize themselves with the statutes that apply before entering into an agreement. Both the donor and the parents will want to be protected from future suits or legal entanglements, no matter how close or trusting a relationship they have. The donor needs to know he will not be required to provide any means of care or support for the child, and the parents need to know they will be protected from any claims on their child, legal or otherwise, from the donor. Such legal contracts may or may not be binding, however, and do not assure couples that future lawsuits will not arise. Nevertheless, the act of consulting with an attorney will afford the couple another opportunity to think through many of the crucial issues involved in known sperm donation.

Choosing Anonymous Sperm Donation. Couples who choose anonymous donation are part of the vast majority of couples who form their families via donor insemination. Although there is societal pressure—and frequently pressure from physicians as well—to use an anonymous donor, most anonymous donor couples feel they are making a rational decision and one that is in their child's best interest.

Belonging and Authenticity. Those who choose anonymous donation do so because they feel that in a known situation the offspring (as well as themselves) might be confused about to whom he or she belongs. They are concerned about social or relational bewilderment; that is, the child might be confused to have "two fathers." The closer the relationship is, the greater the likelihood of social bewilderment.

The phenomenon of social or relational bewilderment can be complicated when relatives agree to be donors. When there is an already established familial relationship—for example, the father's brother is the child's uncle—the fact that he is also the genetic father can be confusing to all. Another point of confusion is that if the donor has children, those children, are social cousins and genetic half siblings to the donor offspring. Couples must carefully sort through the issues of belonging and legitimacy, as well as all the feelings they engender, and discuss these issues with their donor before embarking on a course of action that could wreck emotional and social havoc on the family.

DI couples—especially husbands—have concerns that if the genetic father were known, the social father might feel cast aside. It is extremely important that the husband feel he is the authentic father of his child and that he is entitled to assume that role. Whatever choice—known or anonymous—DI parents make, they must be able to feel strongly that their child belongs to them. Couples opting for anonymous donation see this choice as offering them that opportunity. They fear that if the donor were known, particularly if he is someone who interacts frequently with the couple, the husband may not feel like the real father.

Lack of a Known Donor Option. Not all couples who prefer to use a known donor have this choice. They may not have a friend, relative, or aquaintance whom they feel comfortable asking, or they may have asked someone who refused. People who have been turned down by the donor of their choice have two remaining options: to turn to anonymous donation or advertise for a known donor. Advertising for a genetic father for one's child is unusual but does occur. The February 1993 issue of *Boston Magazine* contained an advertisement in the personal section for a sperm donor. The ad, placed by a single woman (it might just as well have been placed by a couple), was lengthy and offered a detailed description of her motivations for having a child, as well as her reasons for wanting to identify the donor. Toward the end of the advertisement she wrote: "Why such an unconventional route? Concern re: child's identity formation. While anonymous donation is ideal for some, I want to spare my children the burden of mystery regarding paternal identity."

Couples who feel that it *is* moral to bring a child into the world with unknown parentage probably subscribe to the humankind gene pool philosophy or are closer to it on the spectrum. They reason that if no one's genes are unique and everyone is part of humanity, then it should not matter who supplies the genetic material used to create a child. The real parents are those who nurture and raise the child.

Whether it is morally right to bring a child into the world with unknown parentage is a question that each person must ponder. Currently our society sanctions anonymous donation and is more equivocal about known gamete donation. As society evolves, however, public opinion changes, and what is thought by the majority to be in a child's best interest today may be regarded differently tomorrow.

Secrecy versus Openness

The vast majority of couples in the United States who decide to form their family through donor insemination do so via an anonymous sperm bank. Although some sperm banks are slowly changing their policies regarding sharing donor information with recipient couples, most banks assure their donors of permanent confidentiality and anonymity. Because secrecy has also been built into the practice of donor insemination, couples choosing to form their family through DI are faced with a dilemma: Should they tell their offspring the truth about his or her genetic origins or keep it a secret?

For many DI couples, the decision about whether to tell is the most complicated, perplexing, and difficult decision they face. In making the decision, they must grapple with what is best for their child—someone who does not yet exist.

Although the climate seems to be slowly changing, the majority of couples in the United States and in other countries as well, decide to keep DI a secret from their child. A recent article, summarized seven studies that addressed this question: three were done in America, two in Australia, one in France, and one in Canada. Couples were asked whether they planned to tell their child about donor insemination. Percentages ranged from one study in which 86 percent said they would not tell, while 14 percent said they would, to another study in which 61 percent said they would not tell while 39 percent said they would.[4]

As we have discussed, in the past physicians introduced the idea of DI to couples by presenting it as a treatment option, strongly advising them to keep the procedure a secret. Many suggested the couple go home after the insemination and have intercourse, so they would never know for sure whether it was the donor or the father whose sperm penetrated the egg, and they could always live with the illusion that it was the latter's. (Some couples request mixing both men's sperm.) Physicians implied, or stated outright, that secrecy was the only reasonable option—the choice of informed, well-adjusted, and reasonable couples; revealing the secret would cause the child to be stigmatized—rejected by friends and family. Furthermore, telling the child about how he or she was conceived would do psychological harm.

Patricia Mahlstedt and Dorothy Greenfeld, prominent clinicians and researchers in the field of infertility, write that physicians typically have responded to couple's concerns about DI by assuring them that "donor conception will be the same as having your own, and that once conception occurs, you will forget how it happened."[5] These platitudes, meant to be reassuring, convey the message to DI couples that there is something terribly wrong with them if they have uncomfortable feelings or nagging questions about DI. This message is damaging; donor insemination is not the same as having a child who is the genetic product of both parents, and couples never forget how their child was conceived, regardless of whether they ever speak about it.

The trend toward more openness in adoption has heralded a similar but probably slower trend in the world of donor insemination. Although more and more clinicians specializing in mental health and infertility are advocating openness for DI couples, the evidence though compelling, is inconclusive about whether it is in a child's best interest and, if so, under what conditions.

The decision about whether to keep DI a secret from the child brings up an ethical dilemma: *Does an individual have a right to know the truth about his or her genetic origins?* and its corollary, *Is it in the best interests of the child, or of the family to lie about this fundamental fact of one's existence?*

Elizabeth Noble, a nationally recognized childbirth educator and author of several books, is an outspoken critic of secrecy in DI and voices both emotional and ethical objections. She quotes several obstetricians (writing in the nineteen seventies) who strongly believe that couples should tell no one—not even friends or relatives. These physicians feel that if couples are unable to keep the fact of DI confidential, they are not ready to do it. One physician even offers a plan of undoing—deception—to those who have previously discussed donor insemination with others. Noble attempts to correct what she considers false assumptions about what is in a DI child's best interest:

> All persons have a moral right to information that concerns themselves and the circumstances of their birth. The truth does not belong to the parents to withhold—*it is the child's birthright*. Parents must develop the wisdom and courage to squarely face the whole issue. It is their responsibility to tell the truth, no matter how difficult or painful that task may be.[6]

Arguments for Secrecy. Virtually all parents—certainly those who go to great lengths to have children—make parenting decisions that are based on what they believe is in their child's best interest. Good parents, however, as well as experts in the field of child raising, frequently disagree about what is in a child's best interest. In discussing secrecy versus openness in donor insemination, it is important to keep this fact in mind: that whatever a couple chooses to do, they are doing what they believe is best for their child.

A major reason couples elect to be secretive about DI is because they believe that their children may suffer from genealogical bewilderment if they were to learn of their DI origins. The Klock and Maier study supports this belief. The researchers investigated the attitudes of thirty-five DI parents toward openness and secrecy and found that the most common reason given for not telling the child was that it would unnecessarily complicate his or her life.[7]

Another important reason that many couples opt for secrecy is that they fear a DI child would never be completely accepted by relatives. To some individuals and in some cultures, lineage is crucial, and children known to be conceived by DI would always have lower status than if they were genetic heirs. Prospective DI parents do not want their children to be subject to any form of discrimination within their family, realizing how painful that would be for their children and themselves.

Additionally, society still stigmatizes donor offspring. Keeping DI a secret means that no one will be able to use the information in a way that could inflict hurt upon the child. Once parents tell their child, the information belongs to him or her. He or she may decide to tell no one or make an announcement in grade school on a day when the class is planting its spring garden. Classmates may go home and tell their parents that "Jessica's daddy did not have enough sperm, and her mommy had to go to the doctor to get some seeds from a donor." Depending on how the parents react, Jessica may or may not be the recipient of a hurtful comment on a future occasion. The point is that telling the child about how he or she was conceived leaves open the possibility of being stigmatized. Parents naturally feel protective of their children, and many see the potential hurt that openness could cause as an argument in favor of secrecy.

A related argument for secrecy is that it allows the parents, rather than the child, to be in control of this private aspect of their lives. Fertile couples do not go around announcing to the world how and under what circumstances their children were conceived. Since sexuality and reproduction are considered private matters, parents who opt for secrecy believe that they are entitled to the same privilege.

Many couples offer as a further reason for secrecy the fact that since there is no way to access records, their child could never learn who the genetic father is. This permanent void might contribute to an even greater sense of frustration and confusion about identity. These couples feel that it is far better psychologically for a child to grow up believing that his genetic and rearing father is the same person than to suffer from a fruitless psychological quest.

Finally, parents may worry that their child might reject her father should she learn the truth. This fear of rejection, however, may be based on an underlying belief or bias that love between parents and their children comes primarily from genetic ties rather than from the daily nurturing and gradual unfolding of their relationship. Couples who have these fears should discuss them together and consider outside counseling. Talking to adoptive couples about their relationships with their children can help potential DI couples sort through their feelings, since donor insemination is "half an adoption."

Arguments for Openness. A major reason given for being open with donor offspring about their origins has to do with the potentially negative effects of keeping a secret. Increasing numbers of professionals—many of them family therapists—are speaking and writing about family secrets. Most of their conclusions are based on anecdotal evidence from families who are in trouble and who sought professional help. The secret, whatever it is, is frequently thought to be the basis of much of the difficulty. The problem with this sort of research is that it can only be imperfect or unscientific. Families with well-kept secrets are not studied in the same way, because they are clearly difficult, if not impossible, to locate.

The lack of scientific research, however, does not mean that we should ignore the experiences of those who are speaking up and urging people not to keep family secrets. Their arguments and examples are persuasive to many people, professional as well as lay. Those who are considering whether to be open or secret should find it helpful to hear the experiences of those who speak out.

Mahlstedt and Greenfeld, although recognizing that there may be certain situations, based on cultural or religious traditions, in which secrecy may be necessary, present cogent arguments for being open with donor offspring about the origins of their conception:

> There is a growing body of research documenting the negative effects of family secrets and their unique power in the family. Since there is no psychological theory which supports secrecy in any situation, secrecy about one's beginnings is particularly difficult to justify, as it places a lie at the center of the most basic of relationships—the one between parent and child.[8]

Annette Baran and Reuben Pannor, social workers who have been involved for decades in the field of adoption and more recently donor insemination, are also known for their strong stand against secrecy in donor insemination. Their book, *Lethal Secrets*, created a stir among professionals in the field of infertility, for whom the notions of donor insemination and secrecy had gone hand in hand. Baran and Pannor studied DI—the effects on offspring and on their families—after being involved in a number of situations in which donor families sought help. Their research spanned six years and included 171 subjects: donor offspring, donor couples, sperm donors, single women, and lesbian women.[9]

These authors have chilling stories to tell: of children who learned they were donor offspring after a parent had died and the remaining parent could no longer tolerate the burden of the secret; of families in which the father could never get close to his children, presumably because he feared that if he got too close, the secret might be revealed; of couples who decided to adopt a second child rather than conceive another through donor insemination, because the father's negative feelings about his infertility had begun to surface and they felt overwhelming.

Baran and Pannor share stories that come from donor offspring themselves. These offspring found out the truth accidently or were told as adults because their parents could no longer tolerate keeping the secret. In some cases, a divorce precipitated the telling; one mother felt that if her children knew the truth, they would understand why their father was abandoning them and might not feel so rejected. The authors point out that although initially in all these situations the parents had every intention of keeping DI a secret, in most cases the truth came out, and in a punitive way.

Many offspring interviewed describe the confusion they felt upon learning about their conception and the feelings of anger and betrayal about not having been told the truth all along. For many, learning the truth was an enormous relief; it explained some of the strangeness they experienced in their family. The consensus of most of the donor offspring, however, is that it is not the fact of DI to which they are objecting—they would not exist without it—but rather the secrecy in which it is practiced that creates the problem.[10]

In *Having Your Baby by Donor Insemination*, author Elizabeth Noble refers to Suzanne Ariel, an activist in the adoption reform and donor insemination movement, who is herself a donor offspring. Ariel learned about the origins of her conception when she was thirty-one, shortly after her mother died. Her father, who could no longer keep the secret, told her the truth in the presence of his therapist. She speaks out about the deception involved in the practice of DI: "The lies and deceptions upon which DI families are built, warp and poison family relationships. No healthy family can be built upon such lies and deception; and in the DI family, deception is at the very core of the relationship. It is a cruel hoax to be played on a trusting child."[11] Ariel openly acknowledges the unhappiness she experienced as a child. It is impossible to know, however, the extent to which the family secret contributed to the problems within her family and whether her childhood would have been different had she been told the truth from the outset.

Candace Turner is another donor offspring who devotes much time to speaking out and educating others about what she feels are the evils in the practice of donor insemination. She learned about her DI status when she was thirteen, in the midst of a family fight. Although she cares for and respects her father, she believes that her parents made serious mistakes in how they handled donor insemination in the family. And although family fights are one way that donor offspring learn about their situation, according to Turner, most DI offspring she knows learned of their status after their father died.[12]

Turner, who experienced six years of infertility herself before conceiving her four children, identifies strongly with the plight of infertile couples. She is not against donor insemination as much as she is against the secrecy that typically surrounds it. She urges that all donors be registered and agree to be identified when the offspring is eighteen.

Turner, who is still seeking her genetic father, founded Donors Offspring in 1981, designed to give emotional support and information to those whose lives are touched by DI and to assist with reunions between donors and offspring. The organization keeps a registry of offspring who are seeking their genetic father and donors who are seeking their genetic offspring.

Some couples choose openness because they are uncomfortable with the notion of keeping a secret and fear that someone will guess the truth, catching them off guard. One DI couple came to meet with a psychologist because the mother, although having agreed initially to keep DI a secret, wanted to change their agreement; she was tired of having to be on guard. The father was hurt and appalled not only by her strong feelings but also by what he felt to be a betrayal of trust. His wife's change of heart had been precipitated by various conversations with friends. On numerous occasions people would ask questions that made her feel uncomfortable and forced her to lie, such as "Where did Jimmy get his curly hair from?" or "Was his father that big when he was two?" One woman who knew the couple had gone through infertility treatment asked, "How *did* you ever get Jimmy?" Although others who do not know the truth rarely guess, the point is that the fear of someone guessing is the real threat. Being open means that they no longer have to live with this fear.

Being open allows family members to be close to one another without having to erect emotional boundaries. Keeping a secret means that there must be some distance between those who hold the secret and those who are not supposed to find it out. The closer one person gets to another—whether husband to wife, or parent to child—the more likely it is that she or he will see something that has not been previously revealed. Being open means that father and child and husband and wife need have no barriers between them.

Family therapists claim that even when secrets do not come out in the open, their existence creates an atmosphere of mistrust. Children pick up on nonverbal cues and sense that something is odd within the family. The exact nature or the source of the problem may not be known, yet children surmise that something or some piece of information is being withheld from them, and they are not supposed to ask. Secrecy also breeds shame, and children who grow up in such families may feel that there is something fundamentally bad about themselves.

The negative effects of keeping a secret and the emotional burden of it may be felt long past childhood, and parents can be anguished for years about whether to reveal the truth to their adult children. A case example makes this point well. A woman in her mid-fifties was seriously considering telling her two DI children, now in their twenties, the truth about their origins. She had been divorced from her husband since the children were very little, and over the years, although he moved hundreds of miles away, she had done her best to help them maintain a relationship. Her ex-husband, however, barely kept in touch with the children, and years would go by without contact. Her daughter, currently in graduate school, had struggled for years with feelings of rejection from her father. She could not understand why he abandoned her and kept blaming herself for their lack of a relationship. Her mother believed that her daughter's low self-esteem was attributable, at least in part, to this abandonment.

The mother sought out a psychologist familiar with these issues because she needed help with her dilemma. Although years ago she had vowed to keep the secret, she was no longer dealing with an abstract idea but rather with a person whose mental health was at stake. She believed that if her daughter knew the truth about DI, she would not experience her father's abandonment of her so personally. The mother hoped her daughter would understand that her father's actions were most likely connected to his unresolved feelings about infertility and that she would then be able to move on in her own life, free from her unresolved feelings toward her father. The mother had no illusions that her daughter's problems would be solved merely by revealing the secret. She understood that telling the truth would result in another emotional dilemma for her daughter, yet her hope was that ultimately the positive effects of telling would far outweigh the negative ones. The psychologist, who could not know what course of action would be best, helped her client explore the ramifications of telling versus not telling. She also agreed to meet with the mother and her children in the future, should she decide to tell, and should the latter desire a meeting.

Advocates of openness hold that it allows trust to develop between parent and child. If there is a secret, and the secret is revealed under unfortunate circumstances or is sensed and guessed by the offspring, the bond of trust is harmed, and it is extremely difficult to repair; when children have been deceived once, they fear they cannot trust their parents again. George Annas, an attorney and ethicist, agrees with this notion:

> It seems to me a similar argument can be made for consistently lying to the child—i.e., that it is a violation of parental-child confidence. There is evidence that AID [artificial insemination by donor] children do learn the truth. . . . If AID is seen as a loving act for the child's benefit, there seems no reason to taint the procedure with a lie that could prove extremely destructive to the child.[13]

Another advantage to being open is that should a medical emergency arise in which locating the genetic father could mean life or death, the child does not have to deal with the emotional trauma, in addition to the medical trauma, that would surface upon learning the origins of his or her conception. Such circumstances are rare, yet many couples have decided to be open just in case they arise. Although they realize that the odds of such an occurrence are remote, they do not want even the possibility of such a traumatic event to be made even more traumatic because the secret might be at the root of the solution.

A more likely occurrence than the child's developing a life-or-death medical condition is that the husband/father (because he is older and illness happens more frequently as people age) will develop a medical condition that could possibly be hereditary. A DI offspring whose father has a serious heart attack at a young age may worry about a similar fate unless he or she knows that the genetic father is a different man. Furthermore, physicians routinely take family medical histories in order to ascertain whether the individual is at risk for any health problems. A DI offspring who does not know the truth will give inaccurate medical information all his life and possibly may receive unnecessary precautionary treatment.

Another reason given for openness relates to the changing nature of the legal system. Although the practice of donor insemination is commonly done via anonymous sperm banks in which both donor and recipients are protected from any knowledge of or claims by the other, there is no guarantee that this situation will always prevail. Some countries handle donor insemination legally and psychologically differently from the United States. Australia, for example, mandated in the 1980s that all donors be registered and identifiable to the offspring at age eighteen, should the offspring desire to seek them out. And although DI couples cannot be mandated to tell their children about their genetic origins, it is probably a fair assumption that Australian couples seeking donor insemination are more likely to be open with their DI children than are couples in the United States. Sweden passed a similar law in 1985, allowing donor offspring to learn the identity of their genetic parent when they reach eighteen.

As our understanding of the psychosocial aspects of infertility increases, we can assume it will have an impact on the legal system. Thus, couples opting for DI today cannot be completely assured that a mandate requiring sperm banks to open their records will not occur in their child's lifetime. Given this possibility, many couples are choosing to tell their child about donor insemination rather than face even the remote chance of a request several years hence by the sperm donor wanting to meet his genetic offspring.

Although reasonable, professional, well-respected people differ in their views about openness versus secrecy, there is one point on which virtually everyone agrees: if a couple is not planning to tell the child or is undecided, it is better to tell no one. (The one exception is that it is always wise to explore the complicated issues of DI with a counselor, member of the clergy, or medical person who is well versed in the emotional issues of infertility, as well as the psychosocial issues involved in using donor gametes.) Despite people's best intentions, secrets have been known to spill out inadvertently, resulting in feelings of betrayal, anger, and deep hurt.

In an ideal world, questions about openness versus secrecy would probably not exist. Children would be loved and valued no matter how they arrived in this world. Infertility would be physically and emotionally painful, but there would not be stigmas attached to the condition, and couples would not feel shame as a result of those stigmas.

We have not yet achieved an ideal world, and DI couples are

thus forced to make less than ideal choices—choices that will affect their family over its lifetime. Mahlstedt and Greenfeld have wise words for couples who are embarking on this course:

> Couples must be helped to acknowledge that the means of coping with donor conception will have an impact, whether it is openness or secrecy. . . . Couples should keep in mind that both of these choices are difficult, and both have effects on the couple and on the child. Whatever the choice, a mutually workable decision about whether or not to tell the child as well as the ways they will discuss that choice over their lifetime should be discussed prior to the procedure.[14]

Personality Variables Affecting the Secrecy-Openness Decision. Couples considering whether to keep DI a secret must also think about how much of a burden the secret would be for them. Consider a continuum. On one end are people who tend to be very private. More often than not, they are quiet, perhaps introverted. They are not necessarily antisocial; in fact, they may have several friends and relatives who are important to them, but they tend to keep their personal affairs and feelings to themselves or may reveal them to only one or two people. On the other end of the continuum are people who are naturally more open. They talk to others about their feelings, their personal affairs, and the circumstances of their lives. They hide very little from friends or family members and have few, if any, qualms about revealing themselves. Secrets make them feel uncomfortable.

People who are naturally private or more closed about their personal life would probably have an easier time keeping DI a secret than those who are more naturally open. The latter may feel that the secret envelops them. Even those who do not believe that individuals have a right to know the truth about their genetic heritage or that it is in their best interest to know might still have difficulty keeping donor insemination a secret if they are people who would place themselves on the open end of the continuum.

Although ethical and psychological reasons ought to be primary considerations in making decisions regarding known versus unknown donors and openness versus secrecy, personality variables need consideration as well. Prospective parents must think about their own personalities—in particular, how private they tend to be or not be—and not make any decisions that feel dissonant with who they are. Baran and Pannor found that most of the donor parents they interviewed were generally open people who do not lie well. Keeping the secret had been a tremendous burden because it forced them to behave differently from their natural inclinations. Having been instructed by their physicians never to tell, they unquestioningly obeyed and paid a heavy emotional price.[15]

Donor couples can sometimes feel as if there is a 'scarlet D' on their chest that the entire world is viewing. Since the secret can feel transparent, in order to be comfortable keeping the secret, husbands and wives must feel that they can respond to others' comments and questions about whom their child resembles without feeling as if they are lying. They must think ahead of time about how they are likely to feel when friends or even strangers comment that "Joey doesn't look at all like his father" or that "he looks just like his father"! Those who know that a couple has gone through infertility treatments, even if they do not know the exact nature of the problem, are likely to ask which treatment worked or what the couple had to do to conceive Joey. Couples who intend to keep DI a secret must plan ahead of time how they will respond.

When and How to Share Information

Although donor insemination has been performed for about a century, the concept of openness is quite new. As clinicians, we have gone through an evolution in our own thinking. When we began working in this field approximately a decade and a half ago, we, like most others, assumed donor insemination was and should be done anonymously. We assumed that offspring had no need to be told and therefore should not be. Although we recognize that certain circumstances relating to ethnicity, culture, or religion may preclude relatives and friends from accepting a DI child, indicating that secrecy may be in that family's best interest, we have been persuaded by the thinking, writing, and research of others, as well as by our own experiences, and have come to endorse the concept of openness, at least as an ideal from which to begin the decision-making process.

Although this book is not about parenting after infertility, many couples attempting to decide about openness versus secrecy in using donor gametes think about how they would explain the process to their children, when they would tell them, and how they might get across the idea that the information, though not a secret, is private and should be shared discriminately. Couples deciding to be open need a game plan—a rough idea about how they might handle the telling—in order to feel more comfortable with their decision. Feeling comfortable with DI is essential before embarking on the process.

Although donor insemination is different from adoption, the knowledge gained from that field—especially about the psychological effects of being adopted, about genetic bewilderment, and about people's need to know about their origins—can serve as a guide in talking to DI children about their origins. The goal in giving the information, whenever it is presented, is to impart it in a way that helps to foster a healthy self-concept and a sense of oneself as normal.

We have seen that there are differences in people regarding the extent to which they consider their genetic makeup unique or as part of a humankind gene pool. These different attitudes toward genes undoubtedly play a role in whether adoptees wish someday to seek out the source of their genes. Although there is no way of predicting which adopted babies will grow into adults who wish to search for birthparents, those who feel in tune with the unique gene pool philosophy are likely to be the ones who are most interested in doing do. Contrary to the fears of some adoptive parents, there appears to be no evidence that adoptees who are unhappy in their families are the ones who most wish to find their birthparents. Anecdotal evidence indicates the opposite: that those who grew up in loving families, in which adoption was spoken about openly and in which they had permission to be curious, may be the most likely to seek out birthparents, for they do not fear rejection from their family.

Family building through donor insemination is like a half-adoption; instead of 100 percent on one's genetic material coming from unknown origins, 50 percent comes from an unknown person. For many donor offspring, however, 50 percent known is not enough to erase their genetic bewilderment. For this reason, couples who elect to do donor insemination, especially if they plan to be open with their child, need to obtain as much information as they can about their sperm donor, even if it is nonidentifying information. Even couples who are choosing to keep DI a secret from their child cannot predict with certainty that a situation that might cause them to change their minds, such as a medical emergency, will never arise. Obtaining information about the donor and keeping it will ensure that if the child ever needs or wants that information, it will be available.

Although professionals disagree to some extent about what is the best age to explain donor insemination to children, virtually all agree that adolescence is not the time to tell. This is the time when teenagers struggle on many levels with identity issues. They need to feel that they fit in and are not different from peers. It is also a time of many physical and emotional changes. Introducing DI during the adolescent years could precipitate an emotional trauma.

Baran and Pannor note that although the usual recommendation about when to tell children they were adopted is between the ages of five and seven, they recommend waiting until age nine or ten years for donor offspring. Adoption, they say, is a fairly easy concept to understand. DI is much more technical and beyond a young child's ability to comprehend. Nevertheless, Baran and Pannor emphasize the importance of creating an open family atmosphere to pave the way for the eventual unfolding of the DI story:

> Growing up in a climate of openness contributes to healthy familial attitudes and relationships. If the parents no longer live with sealed lips and the outlook of a lifetime of secrecy, they are better able to proceed with the telling of the truth at an appropriate time. In this way, they provide the child with a sound emotional climate from the outset.[16]

Children will probably learn some facts related to reproduction in school. What they learn and what they can absorb will depend on their cognitive development. They may ask questions of their parents. It is important to tell the truth about how babies are born without lying about the circumstances of their conception. When children are old enough to understand about conception and reproduction, they are old enough to learn about DI, which is why Baran and Pannor recommend telling no earlier than age nine or ten. When there are younger siblings, parents may decide to tell them at an earlier age, so that they, and not the older child, introduce the information for the first time.

Baran and Pannor state that the initial explanation of donor insemination should affirm three important facts: (1) the father was infertile (or had an inheritable genetic disease), (2) the existence of a donor (genetic) father who is a human being and wanted to provide the sperm, and (3) the child was deeply wanted and is deeply loved. In addition, it is essential that the child be left with a feeling that he or she is normal, having been conceived in the same way as everyone else—through the joining of sperm and egg.[17]

As children grow, they will understand and process their knowledge of their DI origins at an increasingly sophisticated level. Parents need to stay attuned to their children, to sense when they have feelings or questions they may not be able to verbalize and to help them give voice to those concerns. For children conceived from anonymous sperm, with little information available about the donor, Baran and Pannor suggest that patients share whatever they do know while expressing sincere regrets that they do not have more information. Parents can then mention the unique qualities and characteristics their child possesses and acknowledge that he or she probably acquired them from the donor.[18]

Other professionals who advocate openness believe that even small children can be told about donor insemination in a way that makes sense to them. A group of social workers in Australia, the New South Wales Infertility Social Workers Group, wrote a book geared for children between the ages of four and eight. It includes simple illustrations of male and female anatomy, as well as diagrams of sperm attempting to fertilize an egg. It offers a simple but truthful explanation of sexual intercourse, conception, and childbirth and then discusses infertility by introducing a couple who is very sad because they cannot have children. The book explains simple facts about male infertility and the process of donor insemination in a careful way that emphasizes how much the child was wanted and how grateful the parents are to have him or her.[19]

Elaine Gordon, a psychologist, has written another book that can be helpful for parents who want to explain DI to their child. *Mommy Did I Grow in Your Tummy?* also geared to very young children, explains all the new reproductive options and alternatives, including surrogacy, in vitro fertilization, egg donation, donor insemination, and adoption. This book can help a Dl child understand how she was conceived and that there are several alternative family-building options, all of which result in normal, healthy babies and families.[20]

Parents who are planning to tell their children about donor insemination should plan to tell close relatives and friends before talking with their child, or very soon afterwards. Once the child has information about Dl, however, the information belongs to her or him. If parents end a discussion about Dl by suggesting that she not tell anyone, the positive effects of revealing the truth can be undone. It is possible in the same discussion to mention the notion of privacy—"there are facts and feelings about ourselves that we share with people we feel close to but not necessarily with everyone"— thereby encouraging the child to share the Dl story primarily with relatives or close friends, if she or he chooses to do so.

One of the difficulties in being open relates to the societal stigma attached to Dl. Thus, there is always a possibility that someone's negative reaction will come back to the child, causing hurt and confusion. Parents must stay tuned for signs that their child may be feeling upset about donor insemination—feelings that may have been triggered by his or her own thoughts or by another person's insensitive comment.

Probably the most important guideline that anyone can offer to Dl parents, one that may help in decision making, is that being open is a process that happens over time, it is not a one-time event. If parents did not explain it exactly as they had hoped to the first time, there will always be more opportunities. As children develop, Dl will take on new meanings. It is important that Dl offspring should have permission and encouragement from their parents to express the range of feelings, questions, and concerns they have about the way they came into the world.

At various points along the way, especially during adolescence, Dl children may get angry with their parents for choosing donor insemination as well as frustrated if they want information about their donor father and are unable to obtain it. These outbursts will be particularly painful for Dl parents who went through the horrors of infertility that eventually culminated in the birth of their beloved child and who struggled long and hard in deciding against secrecy. Outbursts, however, are a normal part of growing up, and on a positive note, they can indicate the child feels secure enough to know that no matter how intense these feelings, he or she will always be accepted and loved. Parents must have faith that just as they were able to move beyond their anger and frustration about infertility, their children too will move beyond theirs.

The Selection and Practice of Anonymous Sperm Donation

The experience of donor insemination and the climate in which it is performed have changed remarkably since AIDS (acquired immunodeficiency syndrome) has become a health crisis. Before the AIDS epidemic, most donor insemination was performed using fresh semen from a donor who had been selected by the local physician or infertility clinic. The clinic would arrange for the donor to deliver his sample prior to the woman's appearing for the insemination procedure. Although everything was done anonymously, at least one person on staff knew the donor personally. Couples were frequently told that their donor was handsome, or that he was a medical student, or a wonderful athlete, or they were offered some other piece of information that was positive and enabled the couple to feel a connection to their donor.

In 1986, in light of the increase in numbers of people being infected with the AIDS virus, the American Fertility Society revised its guidelines pertaining to the use of anonymous sperm donation. The guidelines strongly recommend that all donation be done with frozen sperm that has been quarantined for at least 180 days, at which point the donor must be retested before the sample was used. Not all physicians made the transition from fresh to frozen semen immediately. Now, however, it is fair to say that responsible physicians recognize the importance of using frozen sperm as a safeguard against disease. This practice, although necessary to protect the health of everyone involved, has led to a reduction in pregnancy rates, because frozen sperm is not as viable as fresh semen. {When donor sperm are used in conjunction with the new reproductive technologies, however, the fact that sperm were frozen does not seem to affect the fertilization rate.}

Emotionally, a drawback to using frozen donor sperm is that the process feels more remote to the recipient couple. The donor becomes truly anonymous; he is not even known to the couple's physician or to the clinic staff. This greater degree of anonymity, however, can be a relief to some couples who know they will not worry about whether their donor was the man sitting next to them in the waiting area.

Couples who elect to use anonymous sperm from a sperm bank make a giant leap of faith. They must be able to trust that their physician is dealing with a reputable and responsible sperm bank that is performing the necessary screening and evaluations on donors. They need to feel confident about the selection process and believe that the donors are physically and emotionally healthy.

The process of banking and freezing sperm is nationally unregulated; no official body regulates and oversees the practices of sperm banks. The American Fertility Society (AFS) has a listing of approximately 100 banks. However, since there is no requirement that a sperm bank register with AFS, it is likely that there are many more than 100—estimates are about 200—in operation. Some programs and clinics operate their own banks, and while they might encourage their patients to choose from among their own donors, most also offer the use of other banks as well. Two states, California and New York, require sperm banks to be licensed in order to operate.

The American Association of Tissue Banks is another organization that encourages membership. In addition to providing guidelines for sperm banks to follow, it also offers an accreditation process, which includes visits to their laboratory and scrutinization of standard operating procedures. Although many banks may comply with their guidelines, few have actually gone through the process to become accredited.

American Fertility Society Guidelines

The AFS is the largest organization of fertility specialists in the country, counting 11,000 members internationally. It is a private, nonprofit professional medical organization primarily involved with education. The AFS includes the Society of Reproductive Endocrinologists, the Society of Reproductive Surgeons, and the Society for Assisted Reproductive Technology under its umbrella. Recently the AFS revised its previous recommendations pertaining to the use of semen donation in *Guidelines for Gamete Donation: 1993.*[21]

According to the guidelines, donors are required to be in good health, free of systemic diseases, and free of genetic abnormalities. A complete family and medical history should be taken in order to rule out the potential for offspring with genetic problems. Donors should not be in a high-risk group for AIDS. In order to screen thoroughly for sexually transmitted diseases, donors should be tested for syphilis and every six months for serum hepatitis B antigen and hepatitis C antibody. Donors should also be tested for cytomegalovirus every six months, and donors who test positive should be used only with positive recipients. Screening for HIV antibodies (human immunodeficiency virus, the virus that causes AIDS) should be performed every six months, and semen obtained at the time should be cryopreserved and used only if retesting after 180 days confirms the antibodies are not present.

Donors should be above legal age but below the age of forty. The guidelines suggest obtaining several samples before undergoing more extensive testing. The criteria for sperm parameters after two or three days of abstinence are motility greater than 60 percent, concentration greater than or equal to 50 million motile sperm per milliliter, and at least 60 percent normal in appearance. These criteria are strict; the numbers are higher than what is required for a man to be fertile. They are necessary in order to offset the negative effects of freezing. Because the criteria are so strict, in many clinics only about one in ten men who apply to be a donor is accepted.

Sperm banks are urged by these guidelines to develop ongoing procedures for monitoring the health of donors. The guidelines do not specify the amount of compensation a donor is allowed to receive for his time and expenses, but they state that monetary compensation should not be the prime reason for the donation. (The standard fee paid to donors seems to be between twenty-five and fifty dollars per ejaculate.) The AFS guidelines also advise limiting the number of pregnancies resulting from a particular donor to ten, which should ensure that the danger of consanguinity from a particular donor—a worry that couples frequently mention—is virtually nonexistent.

The AFS guidelines suggest ways to match the male partner with the donor, advising that clinics ask couples to list the physical characteristics of a donor that are important to them and make reasonable efforts to comply with their wishes. In the event it is not possible to match the couple's criteria, the physician should discuss this with them so as to avoid misunderstandings. (This guideline is obviously unnecessary for clinics that allow couples to select their own donor from the catalogue.)

RESOLVE Inc., the national organization providing advocacy, education, counseling, support, and referral to infertile couples, maintains a list of sperm banks that can be contacted regarding policies and procedures for selecting donors and collecting, freezing, and storing sperm. As of December, 1992, RESOLVE had no specific criteria for being on the list other than filling out the questionnaire. At that time, twenty-four sperm banks were listed.

RESOLVE also has a list of questions about sperm banks, provided to members, urging them to learn the answers before proceeding with a particular bank. RESOLVE suggests that couples inquire about whether the banks keep medical histories on donors, whether they keep track of the number of pregnancies per donor, how long they keep records, and whether the same donor's sperm can be available for a second child. RESOLVE lists criteria for selecting donors and provides a list of diseases for which donors should be screened.

Sperm Banks

Sperm banks, like any other industry, vary in size as well as in the services they provide. Although we did not attempt to obtain a cross-section, we have chosen to discuss three banks that offer especially attractive services. These banks consider the needs of all parties, especially those of the children being created. (We do not wish to give the impression, however, that these three sperm banks are the only ones that are considering the best interest of the child and of DI families.) Couples should feel free to call any of the more than two hundred banks to obtain information about any of their policies or programs.

The larger the bank is, the greater its pool of donors and the more choices available to couples. California Cryobank, one of the largest banks, perhaps the largest, maintains a list of 250 donors, updated monthly. It also offers the largest group of minority donors. Two services that California Cryobank provide are worthy of mention. The first makes lengthy donor profiles available to contracting couples. Donors accepted into the program are required to complete a twenty-seven-page form that asks extensive questions about their personal characteristics, hobbies, interests, and preferences, in addition to genetic and medical information. This information is available to couples for a nominal fee. If they prefer, they can receive free of charge a short form about their donor, which consists of two pages (the first two pages of the long form).

This extensive information about the donor is significant to couples. Through various descriptions, writings, and statements, the donor emerges as a real person rather than as a product. Couples can begin to imagine what he is like and may even feel emotionally connected to him. Some couples have commented that having extensive information about the donor helps them to fill in the void and to feel a positive connection to the donor.

The second service that California Cryobank offers is its Openness Policy. This policy recognizes that unborn children cannot make agreements about their future wishes in regard to the donor and that sperm donors, especially those who are in their late teens and twenties, cannot know how they will feel several years hence about making themselves known to an offspring. Therefore, if at a later date (the bank saves donor records indefinitely) a donor offspring or the parents wish more information about the donor, California Cryobank will obtain it for them. If the offspring wishes to know the identity of the donor in years to come, the bank will act as middleman and ask the donor whether he will agree. If the answer is no, it will not attempt to force a meeting or reveal the identity of the donor.

Xytex, another fairly large commercial sperm bank, requires all donors to write essays, sharing personal information about themselves or their family, including facts about their upbringing, background and personality. Xytex encourages donors to include messages to the unborn offspring about their reasons for becoming a sperm donor, their philosophy of life, and/or their wishes for the offspring. These messages serve the purpose of making the donor become more real to the couple as well as to their child—a person who has a history, a character, and a purpose in life. Xytex also provides a "patriarch program;" it stores cells from the donor, which become his genetic file. These cells can be used later, if additional information is needed about a donor's genetic history.

Larger does not necessarily mean better: small banks may also provide specialized services not offered by other banks. The Sperm Bank of California, in Oakland, is one of two banks (at the time of this writing) that offers a pool of identity-release donors who agree in writing to be identified when the offspring is eighteen, should the latter choose to do so. This fairly small sperm bank, which began in 1982, is a non-profit organization, with approximately thirty active donors, one third of them in the identity-release group. (An additional twenty-five or so donors are on an inactive list, available to couples who already have one donor child and would like a biological sibling for him or her.) The philosophy of the Sperm Bank of California is that the potential child is the key stakeholder in terms of his or her identity—the most affected by the process of donor insemination. In accordance with this philosophy, the Sperm Bank is beginning to conduct research on the psychosocial impact of DI on children conceived this way.

Identity-release donors are carefully screened, according to Barbara Raboy, director of this sperm bank. They must understand thoroughly the implications of their agreement. They are asked about whether they have shared their interest in being a donor with family and friends and what those people's reactions were. They are encouraged to tell their current partner and are urged to think about whether they would tell a future partner and to anticipate how that person might react.

Potential identity-release donors must be comfortable with separating the nurturing aspect of parenthood from the genetic aspect. Raboy explains that she is very "tough" on these candidates, suggesting various future scenarios that could be problematic. In particular, she wants identity-release donors to think about how they would feel should one (or several) of their genetic offspring request a reunion at a later date, particularly if the donor in question has a family of his own. Donors who hesitate or believe that it may be difficult to be sought out in the future are asked to join the anonymous pool. Their hesitation is taken as a no. Donors who do not have a problem with being identified later are also reassured that since their semen must be quarantined for a minimum of six months, they can change their mind during that period.

Donor Counseling

There is clearly a double standard in terms of how male sperm donors have historically been treated and how female donors are being treated in ovum donation programs. In the next chapter we speculate on the reasons for some of these differences. It is worth noting here, however, that none of the three banks we highlighted, as well as others with whom we checked, provide psychological counseling to their anonymous donors. They may do extensive medical and genetic screening but apparently there is little or no mention of potential long-term psychosocial issues.

It is not surprising that counseling about psychosocial issues is not a part of the screening and recruitment process of donors. If donors were encouraged to think about sperm as being part of a biological continuum that ultimately leads to the creation of a person, rather than as a bodily product that is merely going to waste, there might be fewer donors. Baran and Pannor, in doing research for their book, interviewed thirty-seven men who had been semen donors and found that the emotional implications of being a donor may surface much later.[22] The following story illustrates this point.

A psychologist had the opportunity to meet with a thirty-five-year-old physician who had been a sperm donor while in medical school. For years after he graduated, he rarely thought about having been a donor. As his donor offspring were about to enter adolescence, however, he found himself wondering whether he might accidently bump into a young man who looked and was built just like him. The donor himself was the spitting image of his father, a fact that countless people remarked on throughout his life. He had always assumed that if he had sons, they too would carry on this family resemblance. This thought had begun to plague him more frequently, occasionally intruding in his work, and he was contemplating whether to seek counseling. Another reason that this issue probably surfaced, was that he was engaged, and he and his fiancé planned to have children. He wondered about whether he was still fertile and how he would feel if he learned otherwise.

Ken Daniels a researcher in New Zealand, takes a strong stand about the necessity of raising psychosocial issues with prospective donors. A potential donor, he says, needs to think about the fact that he will have offspring whom he will not know. Furthermore, if the donor has children of his own, they will have half-siblings whom they do not know. A donor must think about whether he would tell his children about their unknown genetic siblings. Daniels suggests also that a donor consider whether he will tell his spouse (or future spouse) and how his spouse might react to the information. Preselection counseling should also include thinking about whether he wants to know whether offspring were created as a result of the sperm donation and how the information would affect him over the years. Donors must be made aware of the changing trends in record keeping and the fact that future anonymity cannot be guaranteed. Donors should also consider whether they believe a child should have access to information about his or her genetic parent, or whether that child should even be told that the father who reared him or her was not the genetic father. Donors should consider whether they are concerned about who gets their sperm. Do they have a personal stake in whom they are helping to bear a child? In essence, potential donors must explore both the short- and the long-term issues of providing sperm anonymously and whether it is in their psychological best interest. Daniels states emphatically:

> It is the professional's responsibility to ensure that such consideration occurs. Without consideration of these issues, it is not possible to say that the donor has given "informed" consent. Consent will have been given, but it has not been informed in that the issues associated with and arising from the donation have been considered and understood. To receive appropriate consideration, the psychosocial factors have to be recognized as having a significant and legitimate contribution to make.[23]

Because donating sperm is not the same as donating blood, we hope that sperm banks will begin to offer counseling to potential donors—counseling that addresses the long-term psychosocial issues involved in semen donation. In the interest of helping infertile couples create families, it is important that we not overlook the emotional needs of donors, or they may surface later. They need guidance about whether being a donor is in their best interest, not just for the short term but for the long term as well.

Social Policy Regarding Donor Information and Record Keeping

There is no legislation unifying the practice of anonymous sperm donation, including the screening and selection of donors, so there is no available model of record keeping ensuring that recipient couples have access to important descriptive information about their donor. The AFS guidelines state that

> It is highly desirable to maintain permanent confidential records of donors, including a genetic workup and other nonidentifying information, and to make the anonymous record available on request to the recipient and/or any resulting offspring.[24]

Thus, the practice of record keeping varies from sperm bank to sperm bank and from physician's office to physician's office. Couples should be encouraged to question their physician about their practice regarding this matter and contact the sperm bank in question about its practice concerning record keeping. The urgency for most couples to conceive a child can preclude their best judgment about questions that are likely to surface in the future, such as medical, genetic, and social information about the donor.

The Purpose of Record Keeping. The attitudes toward all aspects of donor insemination are changing, including the necessity of obtaining and preserving extensive information relative to a donor's social, medical, and genetic history. There are two main reasons why record keeping is important. The first is for the parents, so that they can develop a positive feeling for the donor prior to the insemination and feel that he is familiar to them. A second reason is for the child, so that he or she has access to the donor's medical and social background, perhaps avoiding problems of genealogical bewilderment. The role that heredity plays in the transmission of not only medical concerns but personality and social concerns as well is becoming well recognized in the medical community. An understanding of that aspect of an individual can help to illuminate, and in many instances alleviate, similar problems played out in the subsequent generation.

Although many couples typically approach donor insemination with the conviction that it will be a secret, many change their minds. Once the opportunity to get the information has been passed up, it may be too late to retrieve it later, should the parents or the child desire the information. Couples opting for donor insemination should obtain as much genetic, medical, and psychosocial information as they can from the sperm bank. Those who desire to keep DI a secret can save the information in a safety deposit box or in some other safe place, perhaps with an attorney.

The history and practice of donor insemination in the United States has followed the lines of secrecy and anonymity. Prior to the change in policy from fresh to frozen semen, physicians urged secrecy for the contracting couple and felt a similar urgency to protect donors from ever obtaining any information about offspring created or the parents who were raising the child. Physicians feared they would be unable to attract donors if they could not guarantee they would be untraceable. They also feared that if donors were asked to fill out lengthy questionnaires describing their physical, social, psychological, and medical background, they would not be willing to do so. Thus, couples who opted for anonymous sperm donation in the past received minimal information about important characteristics of their donor.

Donors' Willingness to Provide Information. In November 1984, Australia banned payment for human gametes and mandated counseling as well as obligatory record keeping for gamete donors. Although this book is focusing on the United States, the trends, practices, and laws of other countries do influence thinking and decision making regarding these same policies. There is reason to believe that donors in the United States would also be willing to provide far more information to the sperm banks that contract with them than they have been asked to do previously. A look at some recent studies, one in New Zealand and one in the United States, sheds light on this issue.

Ken Daniels, has conducted several studies that offer insight into not only the characteristics of semen donors but also their willingness to share extensive information—identifying or nonidentifying—with sperm banks and/or couples who use their gametes. Daniels found that about half of the donors involved in six programs believe that a child has the right to nonidentifying information about them. Eleven percent of donors (as opposed to 5 percent of couples) believed the child who knows she or he is a DI off-spring will want to learn the identity of the donor. The study also indicated that at least one-quarter of the donors would still donate even if there was a possibility they could be traced in the future. An additional 30 percent said they were uncertain.[25]

A study published in the United States in 1991 by Patricia Mahlstedt and Kris Probasco yielded similar findings. The purpose of their research was to determine the extent to which donors were willing to provide extensive social, medical, psychological, and genetic nonidentifying information about themselves on their applications and to learn what their attitudes were in regard to sharing this information with recipient families. The researchers studied seventy-nine donors from two programs—one in Texas and one in Louisiana. All were between the ages of nineteen and thirty-nine, with a median age of twenty-four.[27]

The results of the Mahlstedt and Probasco survey undoubtedly surprised many people, from physicians who perform inseminations to sperm banks that recruit donors. Of those in the sample, 90 percent returned the new application form that requested extensive information about physical characteristics, personal characteristics, family history, personal health history, and a statement about themselves. Almost all (96 percent) of the donors responded positively to the question, "How do you feel about descriptive, but nonidentifying information about you being given to the recipient family?" Their answers indicated they felt it was important for donor families to have information about the donor. When donors were asked whether they would donate if anonymity could not be guaranteed, 36 percent said they would. In response to a slightly different question, 37 percent said they felt positively toward openness, suggesting that they would be willing to meet the offspring some day; 38 percent felt uncomfortable with openness, and 14 percent were uncertain. Although these results seem to indicate that fewer men would be willing to donate if they were not guaranteed anonymity, they do not indicate by any means that the donor pool would be depleted.

There are no laws in the United States requiring sperm banks to obtain and preserve records of donors. Many in the field of reproductive medicine, like the researcher-clinicians in the previous study, would like such a policy. Elias and Annas, the physician and attorney referred to previously, argue that the policy of secrecy was created mainly to protect the sperm donor from claims arising from his resulting offspring rather than from a consideration of the offspring's best interest. They make a case for allowing donor offspring to have access to identifiable information about their donor parent and refer to a study of sperm donors that indicates 60 percent of them would still donate even if anonymity were not guaranteed. The authors state:

> Since it may turn out to be an extremely important psychological (and possibly medical or genetic) issue to the child seeking information about his genetic heritage, records should be kept of all births in a way that they can be matched with donors. . . . The donor can effectively waive any right to access to such records, but no one should be able to effectively waive the child's future access to genetic, medical, and perhaps even personal information about the donor. These records could have two "levels": level 1 would be medical and genetic history, but not identifiable; level 2 would contain the donor's actual identity. Access to level 1 information should be guaranteed. Access to level 2 should be possible if the child can demonstrate a "need to know."[28]

Although it seems that the United States is a long way from adopting such a policy, it may be moving in that direction. Couples using anonymous sperm banks must understand that by the time their children reach adulthood, banks that were once anonymous may be mandated to open their records.

The Process of Donor Insemination

Once couples make the decision to pursue a family via donor insemination, they approach the process of getting pregnant with both hope and trepidation. Those who believe that the woman is fertile and that the male factor was the only problem standing in the way of a pregnancy will not be too worried about whether DI will work, at least not in the first few months. Those for whom the woman's fertility may still be in question approach DI far more cautiously.

Selecting a Donor

The process of attempting pregnancy begins with selecting a donor. DI couples wonder where in the world they come from, what kind of men would be willing to donate semen, and why they would want to. Their fantasies run the gamut from those who are down and out, to those whose narcissistic leanings compel them to disseminate their genes. Actually donors seem to fit neither of these categories.

Sperm donors are recruited from a number of locations, graduate and undergraduate colleges being the most common. After a highly selective process due to the stringent criteria, approximately 10 percent who apply are accepted.

The motivations and characteristics of sperm donors have not been researched extensively. Ken Daniels, who did conduct such a study, speculates that not only are donors difficult to find because of the atmosphere of anonymity surrounding DI, but he also suggests that over the years, donors (like their semen) have been regarded as a product rather than as a person and therefore have not generated much interest among researchers. In learning about the motivations of sperm donors, Daniels found that of the thirty-seven donors in his study, 91 percent indicated that the desire to help infertile couples was the main reason or a reason for being a donor; 59 percent indicated it was the sole reason for being a donor.[29]

Selecting a donor is one of the most important decisions a DI couple makes. Couples who are able to regard the donor as a person, with unique characteristics and features, generally seem to be more comfortable with donor insemination. But not all clinic staff are equally informed about the psychosocial issues involved in this alternative, and many unwittingly undermine a couple's sense of control and autonomy as they attempt to create their family through DI. Some clinics believe that the couple should not be involved in the choice of a donor—that it might be too overwhelming, or too painful for them, causing them to confront their infertility again. In these programs, staff—usually nurses—select a donor whom they feel is a good match for a particular couple. How they make this determination is not clear.

Sometimes couples, in their urgency to become pregnant, readily agree to let the clinic pick their donor. Their need to deny the reality of DI may encourage them to see the selection process as part of the medical procedure, thus leaving it in the hands of clinical staff whose judgment, they think, must be more astute than theirs. Others feel at the mercy of their doctor and staff, never questioning policy or procedures for fear the clinic will reject them as patients. Frequently in these situations, couples do fine—until a pregnancy occurs. We have known women, pregnant after DI, who sought counseling. Their lack of any information about the donor prompted them to fill in the blanks with horrid fantasies about the baby they were carrying.

Although there are undoubtedly a few couples who may appreciate not having to make the selection, most feel strongly, sooner or later, that they need to make it. Having someone who barely knows them make this crucial decision feeds into their sense of helplessness. Most clinics allow couples to choose their donor, and most have access to more than one bank. All sperm banks provide at least minimal information (many provide extensive information) to recipient couples about the donor(s) they have selected. The information is published in a catalog that is updated regularly and includes certain characteristics: height, weight, build, eye color, hair color and texture, ethnic background, blood type, number of years of schooling, including the donor's major field of study, and key hobbies or interests. We encourage couples to assert themselves with their physicians if they are uncomfortable with either the selection process or with the sperm bank used and to avoid sperm banks that do not provide much information.

Most couples try to match the husband's physical characteristics with the donor's, though it is also important for couples to obtain other information about the donor—personality, character, interests—in order to get a sense of what he is like, so they can develop a positive feeling about him. It can be reassuring to have information about the donor, especially during pregnancy, when DI couples commonly have second thoughts about the conception.

No child is a carbon copy of anyone, and couples must not approach DI with the illusion that they can find a donor who resembles the husband in the important ways. Rather, couples must recognize that their offspring will most likely be different from the father, due to the genetic influences, but that the husband can play a major role in shaping his child's values, attitudes, and interests.

Becoming and Being Pregnant

A significant percentage of male factor couples know they are dealing with female factors as well. In many cases the woman has already undergone infertility treatment prior to donor insemination. When DI does not work after several tries, additional treatment may be recommended, which may include the use of ART. Other couples who elect to do DI know that they must use it in conjunction with IVF or GIFT, or pregnancy will not be possible.

For many DI couples, pregnancy occurs in the first few months of trying. Most feel fortunate that they are on their way to becoming parents. Sometimes, however, the feelings are more bittersweet, as the wife's fertility stands in marked contrast to the husband's infertility.

When pregnancy does not occur after about three to six months, couples face a dilemma about whether to change donors, continue the female medical workup, or try a while longer with the donor they have selected. Changing donors can be psychologically difficult because couples frequently become attached to him, feeling a kind of loyalty. Nevertheless, many couples do changes donors, hoping that the failure to conceive was due to the wrong mix and was not an indication of an undiagnosed female problem. Sometimes clinics advise couples to change donors if they feel that the samples have not been optimal.

Couples using a known donor face a difficult dilemma. If the donor's sperm count was less than ideal to begin with, they must decide how long they are willing to continue with him before moving to a different option. If the sperm samples are normal, the couple will probably want to continue, assuming that a female problem may be at work. Because couples carefully choose their known donors, it is not easy emotionally or logistically to make a change.

A brief struggle with conception can become a positive experience for some DI couples. Though feeling mostly resolved about their decision, many begin inseminations acutely aware of their ambivalence. When a few months go by without a pregnancy, the majority of these couples become very disappointed, and their ambivalence gives way to a feeling of confidence about their choice—a confidence now tinged with worry.

When several months go by without a pregnancy, the focus shifts to the woman in an attempt to discover what may be wrong, if anything. Sometimes in the process of working her up, the male factor is forgotten as couples once again focus on whether conception is possible rather than on how they will feel about a donor child. Men (and sometimes their partners), though feeling disappointed, may also feel a bit relieved that infertility is now shared.

It is common for problems that were previously diagnosed as minor in the woman to be regarded as more major when conception does not occur after a reasonable time. In other cases, new problems are discovered that may have been overlooked when the emphasis was on the man. Couples in this situation are now faced with a series of decisions about treatment, which may include the use of ART.

When conception does not happen easily, DI couples find themselves back on the emotional roller coaster, experiencing many of the same feelings and fears that they had during their initial infertility experience. They may begin to question whether they made the right decision, especially those who agonized for a long time before deciding. Others see it as a sign that adoption is a better alternative for them or that they are meant to live without children.

Fear of Error. Because the process of becoming pregnant is, to a great extent, in the hands of others, couples must have faith that nothing out of the ordinary will occur. They must have faith in the sperm bank that screens the donors and freezes the sperm, and in the clinic that processes it and performs the insemination. They must believe that their goal of a normal, healthy child is not only possible but probable under these circumstances.

Many couples describe the process of donor insemination as feeling very strange. The starkness of the examining room, in contrast to the warmth of their bedroom, can give rise to images of well-intended but mad scientists and experiments gone wrong. It is common for couples to worry about a mix-up, afraid they will get the wrong sperm. So much must happen between the donor selection process and the actual insemination that it is easy to see how those fears arise.

Although physicians and nurses may dismiss these concerns (if couples are brave enough to bring them up) as irrational, they are not implausible. A few years ago the case of Julia Skolnick was highly publicized in the media. Skolnick's husband had samples of his sperm frozen in March 1985, prior to being treated for cancer. In 1986, she gave birth to a mixed-race daughter. When it was determined beyond question that there was no genetic link between her husband (who subsequently died) and her daughter, she sued both the physician who performed the insemination and the sperm bank that sent her the wrong sample. The case never went to trial but was settled out of court.

Although Julia Skolnick's case was a highly unusual situation, it did rattle the nerves of many who work in sperm banks or clinics where inseminations are performed. It rattled, even more strongly, the nerves of infertile couples who need to put their faith not only in technology but also in the people who work with that technology. No matter how scrupulously careful everyone is, there is always the possibility of human error.

Pregnancy After Donor Insemination. Pregnancy after donor insemination brings with it mixed feelings. Couples who had difficulty conceiving with DI may have moved beyond their fears and concerns more than those who conceived soon after the inseminations began. Pregnancy for DI couples can rekindle old worries, in both husband and wife, about genetic inequality, attachment to the child, and social acceptibility if they are planning to be open about donor insemination. If they are planning to keep donor insemination a secret, they may worry that their child will appear so obviously different that others will discover the truth.

Like all other pregnant couples, expectant DI parents worry whether their child will be healthy and whether their pregnancy will be a good one. Once they feel secure in the pregnancy, they may begin to think more about the donor. They wonder in what ways their child will resemble him.

When Things Go Wrong. Although more often than not, DI couples end up with healthy children, this is not always the case. Women pregnant after donor insemination experience pregnancy loss at the same rate as everyone else—approximately one in five times. When a couple loses a child after many years of infertility, it is especially sad. In addition to the universal feelings of loss they share with all other infertile couples, however, there are a few issues unique to DI couples.

The loss of a donor pregnancy, especially for couples who struggled with religious proscriptions before deciding on DI, can bring up feelings (or fears) that they are being punished—that perhaps they made a wrong decision. Such couples may view the loss as a warning from God not to tamper with nature—or, worse, that they are not meant to be parents.

When a couple experiences a pregnancy loss, family and friends may address their expressions of sympathy primarily to the woman. After all, she is the one who carried the fetus and suffered the pain of the miscarriage. When sympathy is expressed only to women, it is hurtful to men, and especially hurtful to DI husbands. If the couple has been open with others about DI and sympathy is directed to the wife, the husband may feel even more removed from the process. It may confirm his own feelings that he is an unimportant, disposable player.

Some couples, no matter how hard and how long they try, may not conceive. This situation seems especially unfair to those who spent years trying to overcome male infertility and eventually turned to donor insemination after careful counseling and deliberation. Now they must reevaluate their situation and make a third choice: to become parents through adoption or to be child free. Making yet a third choice is emotionally draining. Couples have been disappointed so many times that they may feel unable to choose any option that involves risk. At the same time, those who have not discussed DI with anyone may feel especially isolated. No one will know why they are suffering, nor will they have any idea about the emotional ordeal they have gone through.

Male infertility has been a painful burden throughout history, and remains so; from Biblical days to modern times, men have been shamed for not producing children. Donor insemination, a viable path to parenthood, provides a resolution to childlessness, but it does not offer a cure for the inability to reproduce, and it is not without consequences. Although DI has been available for about one hundred years, and has been used extensively in the last several decades, its social, emotional, and ethical ramifications have not been explored until recently. Couples making this important decision must realize that donor insemination is not a one time event. Rather, it is a life-long process that has profound implications for everyone in the family.

Ovum Donation[*]

The practice of using donated gametes to achieve a pregnancy has long offered couples with male infertility the opportunity to experience pregnancy and to have a child that is half genetically theirs. Although it would stand to reason that couples in which the woman is unable to produce healthy eggs (ova) might seek donated gametes, until recently they have not had this option. Unlike sperm, which can easily and efficiently be obtained (and frozen), it was not until the development of in vitro fertilization that eggs could be removed from a woman's ovaries. The use of Pergonal, an ovulation-enhancing drug that has been in existence for approximately thirty years, used in conjunction with in vitro fertilization, makes it possible to harvest several mature eggs simultaneously.

Once the procedure for maturing and removing several eggs from a woman's ovaries was developed, the road was paved for

*Co-authored with:

Susan Levin; LICSW, BCD, Former Director of Psychological Services, Faulkner Center for Reproductive Medicine, Boston, Ma. Member of the GSOATP, Boston Psychoanalytic Institute and Society.

Jeane U. Springer, LICSW, BCD, Director of Psychological Services, Boston IVF, Brookline, Ma.

Sharon Steinberg, RN. MS, CS Psychiatric-Mental Health Clinical Nurse Specialist. Fertility and Endocrinology Department Harvard Community Health Plan, Boston, Ma.

eggs to be transferred from one woman to another. In 1984, just six years after the birth of the first IVF baby, the first pregnancy through ovum donation (also called oocyte donation) was confirmed.[1] With this event, a longstanding dream of infertile couples and their caregivers became a reality.

Although both sperm donation and egg donation have psychological, ethical, and legal issues in common, there are many differences between them. One important distinction is that ovum donation appears to offer more parity, enabling both parents to have a biological stake in their offspring. The man, through his sperm, and the woman, through gestation, make a biological contribution to the creation of their child.

Ovum donation is less widespread, more costly, and less successful than donor insemination, and it is not yet a common path to parenthood. Although IVF makes it medically possible to obtain eggs, for many reasons there are not vast numbers of eggs available for donation. In addition, since ovum donation relies on complex reproductive technology in order to achieve pregnancy, many couples who choose this option do not become pregnant. (However, the pregnancy rates for ovum donation are somewhat higher than for standard IVF procedures because for the most part only young donors are used, and the woman's age along with semen quality, is a crucial determinant of pregnancy rates.)

Another distinction between sperm and ovum donation is that women never see their eggs; they come from deep inside them. Men, on the other hand, have ejaculated sperm since puberty; it is a part of them with which they are familiar. Thus, the concept of removing eggs from a woman's body is completely foreign to most would-be donors and recipients, yet the concept of removing sperm is familiar to all.

There is not a large body of psychosocial research on sperm donors or the families created through donor insemination. Because ovum donation has existed less than a decade (most programs have only been set up in the last few years), there has been an even more limited amount of psychosocial research—and much less written on its legal and ethical aspects—about this alternative. As a result, ovum donation couples are true pioneers.

Ovum Donation Candidates

A woman might be a candidate for ovum donation for reasons ranging from those that are undisputed to those that are controversial. As our understanding about the causes of infertility and the physiology of oocytes increases, it is possible that even more potential candidates for ovum donation will be identified. As long as a woman has an intact uterus and she is given hormonal supplements in order to make her uterus receptive to the embryo, she should be able to carry a pregnancy to term.

The most obvious group of women seeking ovum donation—and those for whom the procedure was essentially developed—are women with premature ovarian failure (POF); their ovaries are no longer producing eggs, and they have therefore ceased menstruating. A woman is generally considered to be suffering from premature ovarian failure if she is under forty years old. Although a forty-one-year-old woman whose ovulatory function has ceased is young to experience menopause, it is not considered premature.

Some women have POF because of prior radiation treatment or chemotherapy for cancer. Others have POF because their ovaries have been surgically removed due to severe infection, endometriosis, or tumor. In rare instances, a woman is born with a congenital absence of her ovaries. Other causes are genetic (POF tends to run in families), autoimmune diseases such as thyroiditis, and environmental toxins. In many instances, however, there is no identifiable cause, and the woman's ovarian failure is considered to be idiopathic. These women have the added emotional burden of not knowing whom or what to pin the blame on. Whatever the cause—medically or surgically induced or organically caused—once the ovaries have stopped working, as measured by follicle-stimulating hormone levels, there is no treatment available. The current estimate is 1 to 3 percent of women suffer from POF.

A second category of candidates for ovum donation are those women referred to as perimenopausal; they are approaching menopause. Although they continue to ovulate, the quality of their eggs seems to be impaired due to the normal aging process. Many perimenopausal women are identified in the course of an IVF cycle. They undergo ovarian stimulation, but either their cycle is cancelled due to poor stimulation or their egg quality is poor and the eggs do not fertilize. Some professionals in the field of reproductive endocrinology are grappling with the question of whether these aging women are appropriate candidates for this new technology. Many clinics, however, are offering ovum donation as an alternative to IVF couples who have been unable to produce healthy eggs.

A third category, also considered controversial, are couples who have completed several IVF cycles and have not become pregnant. They also tend to be couples in which the woman is older. Although they have managed to have eggs retrieved and fertilized, the embryo quality was considered fair or poor. When physicians review the cycle, they conclude that poor egg quality is the probable reason that pregnancy did not occur. Although it is presumed that poor egg quality accounted for their failure to become pregnant, there is no proof of that and no way to know whether another IVF cycle would result in a pregnancy or whether they might ever conceive on their own.

A fourth category of ovum donor candidates are women who are known carriers of a genetic defect or disease that has a high likelihood of being passed on to their offspring. (If the genetic problem is one that is autosomal dominant, the offspring have a 50 percent chance of inheriting the problem; if it is autosomal recessive but the father carries the same defective gene, the offspring has a one in four chance of inheriting it.) Using donated eggs virtually eliminates the problem (except in the unlikely event that the donor is a carrier of the same defective gene). Couples in which the woman is the carrier of an autosomal dominant genetic disease who do not want to take the risk of passing the undesired trait on to their child—particularly if they would not elect to abort should an amniocentesis be able to detect the problem—may prefer to avoid the situation entirely by using a donated gamete. Similarly, when the problem cannot even be detected by existing screening mechanisms, many couples will opt for ovum donation as an alternative, although sperm donation is much simpler, less costly, and less risky.

The final category of candidates for ovum donation—and many would say that they should not be candidates at all—are postmenopausal women. Generally they are in their late forties or early fifties—some are even older—who wish to experience a pregnancy and raise a child. Aware that the technology of ovum donation can push reproduction beyond its normal limit, these women seek the services of ART centers in order to help them achieve motherhood.

The Medical Process

Ovum donation is achieved by using highly technical procedures in combination with fertility drugs. The procedures involve some medical risk, which is one reason why there are a limited number of ovum donors.

The major medical challenge of ovum donation is to synchronize the harvesting of the eggs from the donor with the receptivity of the recipient's endometrium. Synchronization is important because at this point in time eggs cannot be frozen for later use, and unless the endometrial lining is ready to receive the embryos, pregnancy cannot occur. Although eggs cannot be cryopreserved, embryos can and are if the best efforts at synchronization fail. However, the pregnancy rates using frozen embryos are generally not as good as they are when fresh embryos are transferred, another reason that precise timing is important.

The donor, like any other woman undergoing in vitro fertilization, is put on a strict regimen of fertility drugs so that she will (hopefully) produce multiple oocytes. These oocytes are surgically removed when they are ripe—just prior to when they would be released by the ovaries if she were ovulating on her own. They are inseminated shortly after retrieval with the recipient's husband's sperm. Two (or three, depending on the program) days later, a predetermined number of embryos (usually three of four) are placed into the uterus of the recipient, utilizing the same process of embryo transfer as in a normal IVF cycle. GIFT can also be used in the course of ovum donation and may be recommended as a preferred treatment in some instances.

In order to achieve a normal endometrium, the recipient requires careful administration and monitoring of estrogen and progesterone supplementation. Recipients usually wear estrogen patches and take progesterone by injection if ovarian function has ceased. If ovarian function persists, recipients are frequently given Lupron to suppress ovulation, and a similar pattern of estrogen and progesterone supplementation is then given. Many clinics insist on a trial cycle for recipients prior to stimulating the donor, in order to understand how long it takes for her body to adjust to the hormones and for her endometrium to be ready. The hormones are timed such that when the donor's eggs have been fertilized with the recipient's husband's sperm and the embryos are ready for implantation, her uterus will also be ready. If extra embryos exist, they can be cryopreserved and used by the recipient couple in a subsequent transfer cycle if pregnancy, or a successful delivery, does not occur. If a child is born the embryos can be used in a future cycle if the couple desires another child.

Potential Ovum Donors

Donated oocytes are not readily available. Unlike sperm donation, which takes only a few minutes and involves no physical risk whatsoever to the donor, ovum donation is a lengthy process that is physically uncomfortable and inconvenient and involves possible, though rare, medical risks. In addition, there are emotional risks to consider.

Potential donors fall into four categories: infertile women undergoing IVF, fertile women electing to have a tubal ligation, fertile volunteer donors who are known to their recipients, and fertile women who are donating anonymously. The last two groups of donors are the most common. We will discuss each group.

When a woman is undergoing IVF, it is likely that the hormonal stimulation of her ovaries, especially if she is young, may produce far more eggs, and result in many more embryos, than can be safely placed into her uterus. Although most couples undergoing IVF are involved in programs in which cryopreservation is available, and the vast majority of couples choose this option in order to leave open the possibility of embryo transfer later, some are opposed to freezing their embryos for moral or religious reasons. Couples fearing the long-term side effects of cryopreservation (unproved to date) may also elect not to freeze their embryos. These couples may be asked by their physicians if they are willing to donate their extra eggs to other infertile women.

This first group has not proved to be a reliable source of donated eggs, because practically all couples in ART programs agree to freeze extra embryos, at least in the programs with which we are familiar. In addition to the fact that few eggs are available from

ART patients, many clinicians have concerns about the ethics of asking an infertile woman to donate some of her oocytes to another infertile woman. The major concern is the possibility that the recipient, and not the donor, will become pregnant, and the infertile donor must live with this knowledge. Alternatively, if the clinic in question does not tell infertile donors the recipient couple's outcome, they must live with an unresolved question for the rest of their lives. Another ethical question is raised by the possibility that both give birth, resulting in half-siblings who will have no knowledge of each other.

Couples who have no religious or moral proscriptions against freezing embryos may elect to donate if offered a sizable reduction in the cost of their IVF cycle. This reduction might enable some couples who might not otherwise be able to afford IVF the opportunity to attempt ART treatment. The practice of using IVF patients as donors is occurring in several programs. This donor group is a concern for many practitioners, however, because it raises the issue of financial coercion. For ethical reasons, many clinics will not offer reduced fees in exchange for eggs. In contrast, those who feel it is reasonable to accept an infertile woman's eggs in exchange for a reduction in cost argue that without that reduction, many couples would not be able to afford ART and that it would be more immoral to deprive them of the opportunity.

Another potential source for donated eggs are women undergoing elective tubal ligations. Often these women meet the medical and psychological criteria for egg donors. The incentive for them to donate is a free or reduced rate for the sterilization procedure or payment for the time and extra effort involved. In order to donate oocytes, they must receive hormones to stimulate their follicles and undergo frequent monitoring via blood draws and ultrasounds (just as any donor would) in the month prior to their scheduled tubal ligation. After the oocytes are retrieved, the donor's fallopian tubes are tied.

Women undergoing tubal ligation have not proved to be a good source of donated eggs. It is unclear why this source of potential donors remains largely untapped, but it may be that many women have health plans that cover the cost of their sterilization procedure and the offer of a free tubal ligation has no value for them. Another reason might be that because tubal ligations are a source of revenue for gynecologists who routinely perform this surgery, referral to an ovum donation program would be a financial disincentive. In addition, the communication and ongoing coordination necessary to achieve a working partnership with a local gynecologist may be too difficult to maintain in most infertility clinics.

Friends or relatives—known donors—are a popular source—of donated oocytes. Sisters, in particular, are a preferred choice for many couples who have that option available. Other relatives have also been known donors, and some clinics have even allowed daughters to donate for their mothers. Couples less concerned with preserving some genetic connection with the wife/mother prefer to use friends, acquaintances, or co-workers or to locate their own donor.

The recruitment of anonymous egg donors from the general population has become a popular means by which oocytes are obtained for donation. Anonymous donors are usually recruited through advertisements in local newspapers, magazines, or university newspapers. As ovum donation is becoming more common, ads like the following one are seen with increasing frequency in major cities throughout the United States:

OOCYTE DONATION
Healthy female volunteers aged 34 and under are needed to serve as anonymous oocyte (egg) donors. Donors will be required to take medication, have blood screening, and undergo a minor surgical procedure. Compensation will be made for time and expenses. If interested please call. . . . .

Screening of Egg Donors

Because of the possibility for the transmission of disease from donor to recipient or child, or both, donors must be thoroughly screened. They must also fully understand the medical process involved so they can give informed consent. And, due to the invasive nature of the procedure, the ethical and emotional issues are even more extensive than they are for male donors.

The American Fertility Society (AFS) guidelines state that anonymous donors should be of legal age but no more than thirty-four years old, since younger donors are much more likely to respond well to follicular stimulation and older donors have an increased risk of chromosomal abnormalities—a risk that continues to increase as age advances and they experience declining fertility. If the oocyte donor is over thirty-four years of age, this fact should be discussed with the recipient couple as part of an informed consent discussion pertaining to risk, and the recipient should be offered amniocentesis or chorionic villus sampling should a pregnancy result. Although it is preferable that donors have documented previous fertility, AFS does not suggest that it be a requirement for donation.[2]

AFS guidelines specify that all donors, known and anonymous, need to be clear about the procedures involved in ovum donation, because they include drug therapy for ovarian hyperstimulation, close monitoring, and an invasive procedure for oocyte recovery (ultrasound-guided transvaginal follicular aspiration), all of which carry with them potential risks. Although these risks are extremely small, potential donors must be counseled thoroughly regarding these risks, and they must think carefully about their motives and reasons for wanting to become an egg donor.

One of the major concerns for programs utilizing donated gametes is the transmission of the HIV virus. Sperm banks routinely test all donors for the virus, freeze and quarantine all donated sperm for six months, and then retest the donor for HIV. If a donor tests negative for antibodies to the virus, couples can be almost virtually assured that the semen frozen six months previously is free of infection. Because eggs cannot be frozen, the same precaution against transmittal of HIV cannot be utilized. It is unclear whether HIV can be transmitted through ovum donation, however immunologists tend to agree that follicular fluid is a possible means of transmission. The AFS guidelines suggest that couples entering an oocyte donor program be given the following choice: they can assume the low risk of acquiring HIV and use fresh embryos, which yield a better pregnancy rate, or they can elect to have the donated oocytes fertilized and the resulting embryos frozen for six months, after which point the donor is retested. (These choices assume that the donor initially tested negative for HIV.) If she is negative, the embryos can be safely transferred into her uterus. All applicants for ovum donation who have risk factors for HIV infection, such as intravenous drug use or a sexual partner who uses these drugs or who is HIV infected, are to be screened out immediately.

The AFS guidelines specify that serological testing be routinely performed for syphilis, hepatitis B and C, and HIV I-II. They also state that genetic screening be performed on a potential donor before allowing her to donote oocytes, ruling out the possibility that she will transmit an identifiable genetic disease. In regard to record keeping, the guidelines state that a permanent record designed to preserve confidentially should be made available on request to the recipient and any resulting offspring. The AFS guidelines also recommend psychological counseling for all parties involved in the ovum donation process to ensure they are giving informed consent, are not being coerced to donate, are aware of the potential medical risks, and are aware of the potential psychological risks.

Most programs that offer counseling to donors consider that screening is also part of that process. In other words, the psychological counselor may also serve as gatekeeper, determining whether a potential donor is psychologically appropriate. The screening may consist of psychological interviews, personality assessments, or other psychological batteries. Most programs reject donors who exhibit psychopathology, as measured by their test results or as determined in a face-to-face interview. Donors may also be rejected if they have a history that includes psychological conflict and appear to be consciously or unconsciously donating as a way to make up for an unresolved past event.

In a recent survey published, of eighty-two ovum donor programs, 78 percent stated that they require psychological screening for donors. The survey did not state what percentage of ovum donation programs also offer counseling to recipients.[3] We can speculate from speaking to a number of clinicians who work in other programs, however, that probably most programs that screen donors also require counseling (or screening) for recipients. The purpose of counseling for recipients is to make sure they are giving informed consent, are aware of the medical and the psychological risks involved, and understand the ethical and emotional issues involved in creating families through the process of ovum donation.

Ethical Considerations of Ovum Donation

Ovum donation is an exciting new alternative childbearing option for many infertile people. The technologies that make it possible are continually improving, and more and more couples are taking advantage of this technology. As with all of the other new reproductive options, however, our capacity to reflect on the profound and serious ethical issues they raise is compromised by the rapid proliferation of programs. People are undergoing ovum donation before researchers and ethicists have the opportunity to develop an adequate understanding of the life experiences of families created from this option. It will probably be years before we understand the impact of these technologies on the families who use them.

Many of the ethical issues raised by the technology of ovum donation are shared with sperm donation—for example, questions about the psychological effect on a child of intentionally bringing him or her into the world with unknown parentage, and whether a person has the right to know the truth about his or her genetic heritage.

The Changing Nature of Family

There have been many social changes in the last half of the twentieth century that have challenged the traditional definition of family: the increasing incidence of divorce (approximately 50 percent of all married couples eventually divorce), the increasing number of single women who are choosing to have children, and the increasing number of lesbian couples who are bearing and raising children together. Couples who divorce are not intentionally creating nontraditional families. Yet many single women and all lesbian couples by definition are intentionally creating families without fathers in the home. More and more frequently they are requesting technological assistance or gamete donation in order to have families, and these requests are posing ethical dilemmas for many who are involved in the treatment of infertility. The dilemmas center around the question of whether it is in a child's best interest to be brought into the world under such circumstances.

Ovum donation further challenges our traditional understanding of family because it allows women to bear children after menopause—at an age when many of their peers are becoming grandparents. Although there are additional ethical issues that are posed when older women become mothers, the fact that children will be raised by parents who look (and probably act) much more like grandparents is an objection that many clinicians raise on ethical grounds. They feel it is not fair to children to be raised by parents who may not have the stamina for middle-of-the-night feedings, for scout outings, or for the worrisome adolescent years. When single women or lesbian couples opt for ovum donation, especially if they are older, they are creating families that are even more nontraditional.

The Definition of Mother

Prior to the new reproductive technologies, the definition of *mother* was fairly simple: mothers raised their children. Although adoptions created a distinction between birthmother and rearing mother, those were the only ways that motherhood was defined (except for the role of foster mother). The new reproductive technologies, by enabling eggs to be harvested in one woman and implanted in a second woman, allow us to distinguish between the genetic and the gestational mother, as well as the rearing mother.

In virtually all ovum donation situations, the woman who gestates also raises her child. A recently reported case, however, illustrates an unusual situation in which yet a third woman was involved and reared a child who was created from the egg of one woman and gestated by another woman. A sister was the egg donor, the sister-in-law carried the pregnancy, and the baby was adopted by the relative who was unable to provide either her own oocytes or a funtioning uterus. Sperm were provided by the father. This case illustrates how far we have come in noncoital reproduction and shows that when the various components of motherhood are separated, a person can have three mothers.

Traditionally, motherhood and gestation have been linked together; the notion of genetics seemed incidental. However, over the years we have come to understand the importance of genetics in shaping a person's life. Although no one has the definitive answer about exactly what percentage of the resulting person is attributable to nature and what percentage is attributable to nurture, all agree that both are important in determining the whole adult person. The genetic mother—the ovum donor—is therefore extremely important to the child's identity, regardless of whether she donates anonymously or is known to the parents. Those who question the ethics of intentionally separating the genetic from the gestational aspect of motherhood hold fast to their belief that it is not in a child's best interest to be deliberately brought into the world in such a manner.

Although the various definitions of mother are easily understandable, even to those not involved in the new reproductive technologies, in the legal sense they can be baffling. Many would argue that upon birth, the woman who delivers the child should legally be considered the mother, unless or until she gives up her rights to rear the child. Those who argue this point believe that even in situations in which a gestational carrier is used, she is the mother despite the fact that her gamete was not used in creating the child. Others argue that the genetic mother is the real mother, regardless of whether she carries her baby. Our intention is not to argue the legal issues in this chapter but to attempt to elucidate the role that each woman plays in the life of the offspring, and to emphasize that everyone—professional as well as lay—has an opinion, not only about whether it is in a child's best interest to have two (or three) mothers but about who is the "real" mother in the event of a conflict.

The definition of mother becomes even further complicated when we consider the fact that many lesbian couples are choosing to have children and making the point that they are both mothers to their offspring. One might argue that only one of them is the natural or real mother, but what about the couple who applied to an IVF program requesting that one woman donate her eggs to her partner, who would then gestate the pregnancy? Even King Solomon would be hard-pressed to argue that one of those women is more the mother than the other.

Naturalness versus Artificiality of Donated Oocytes

The new reproductive technologies, more than any of the other infertility treatments, separate procreation from lovemaking and sexuality. Some couples hold fast to a moral conviction that nothing artificial should intrude into their sexual relations. This belief is supported by some religious groups, especially the Catholic church, which believes in the sanctity of the conjugal act and frowns on the creation of children through the use of donor gametes. Ovum donation violates both of those concepts.

Others see the development and use of new methods of contraception or reproduction as not only morally justifiable but enhancing the quality of life. In that sense, they are viewed as natural outgrowths of scientific progress. Carried further, this viewpoint sees liberation from some of the unpredictable aspects of reproduction as a major accomplishment. Consequently, the ability to postpone parenting and to have children beyond the limits of one's biological clock is seen by some as a technological marvel. And the opportunity to trade in one's potentially defective genes for others that are thought to be uncontaminated may also be seen as a major achievement of human beings. These differing views represent a broad spectrum of ethical perspective, and it is important to recognize that couples have varying degrees of comfort levels with the (un)naturalness of the new technologies.

The Right to Bear a Child

> The limits on the childbearing years are now anyone's guess; perhaps they will have more to do with the stamina required for labor and 2 A.M. feedings than with reproductive function.[4]

This quotation raises another ethical question that surfaces with ovum donation—one that plagues most professionals in the field of ART: whether a couple or an individual has a right to have a child. Given that the technology of oocyte donation can extend a woman's childbearing years indefinitely, many professionals and ethicists debate the question of whether something should be done because it can be done. Perhaps ovum donation, more than with other type of ART, clearly shows the desires of prospective parents pitted against the best interests of an unborn child.

Many professionals working in ovum donation programs feel a moral obligation to address the question of what is in the best interests of the potential children they are creating. This question arises for a variety of reasons, but the most common is age. Those who set policy must struggle with whether they will set an age limit beyond which they will not allow couples to cycle. Most programs do have age limits, arrived at after careful deliberation. The IVF

America Program-Boston set the age limit at forty-five by checking actuarial tables. Although no child is ever born with a guarantee that the mother will live to see him or her enter adulthood, the practitioners that established the program wanted to feel reasonably secure that a child born as a result of ovum donation would be raised by his or her mother. Recognizing that the role of the father is equally important, however, practitioners at the IVF America Program-Boston also take his age into consideration. If he is under forty-five and the combined average age of the couple is equal to or less than that the couple will be considered for ovum donation.

Other programs believe that it is not their place to decide how old (or young) someone must be when she becomes a parent. Those programs have a higher age limit for ovum recipients or none at all. In a survey of eighty-two IVF programs that offered ovum donation, twenty-two reported they had no upper age limits. Of the remaining sixty that did have upper limits, the average was fifty-five years.[5]

There are other issues regarding the right to have a child. Frequently physicians and mental health clinicians see individuals or couples whom they feel would make poor parents because they are psychologically unstable or in poor health, or their marriages are shaky. Others believe that if an infertile couple is using their own gametes, then their job is to assist that couple to have a baby. They may justify their position by stating that if the couple were fertile, they would easily be able to have children. They also may argue that many fertile couples make extremely poor parents, yet their right to have a family is not challenged (unless the situation becomes so destructive that the state intervenes and arranges for foster care).

The feelings of practitioners who believe they should not be gatekeepers sometimes change when donor gametes are required to achieve pregnancy. In these situations, not only are they helping couples become parents, but through the use of third parties they are creating children who by definition will be born with psychological complications. Those who believe that ethics should not be involved in medical decisions pertaining to reproduction can more easily justify helping all couples who desire children to achieve their goal.

Another related issue concerns the rights of ovum donors. Clinicians frequently struggle with whether they have an obligation to reassure the provider of the gametes that her eggs will be offered only to couples whom they can be reasonably assured will make good parents. This issue may become more pressing when there is a limited supply of eggs, as is the case for many ovum donor programs.

Risks to Donors

Couples considering high-tech treatment must determine whether they are willing to take the risks—some known and some as yet unknown—inherent in the process. Most couples struggle to a greater or lesser extent with whether the gains outweigh the risks. However, when healthy young fertile women are recruited to be egg donors, especially if they have not completed their families, the question is raised of whether it is ethical to subject them to the possible risks of treatment, including the risk of becoming infertile.

A 1993 study indicated a possible relationship between the use of fertility-enhancing medications and ovarian cancer.[6] The study had serious design flaws and utilized a relatively small sample of women, and many practitioners as well as researchers question its validity. However, it does raise questions about the possibility of dangerous and potentially lethal long-term side effects from fertility drugs, particularly for fertile donors who do not receive reproductive benefits. Other studies looking at links between fertility drugs and cancer have shown no greater incidence in women who have used them. Skeptics argue that since Pergonal has been given in such large quantities only recently that the long-term effects cannot be adequately assessed yet.

All donors assume risks when they agree to donate, and these risks must be clearly explained by a physician and clearly understood by the donor; otherwise, the donor is not capable of informed consent. Donors must have a clear understanding of what the ovarian stimulation protocol involves and of the potential risks of the medications. They must also understand the limited risks associated with egg retrieval.

On the psychological side, donors need to give serious thought to what it will mean to them to give their genetic material to an anonymous (or known) recipient and whether they may suffer long-term emotional consequences as a result of this decision. They must be able to separate the genetic from the gestational aspects of motherhood, understanding the significance they attach to each of these components. If the donors have not completed their families, they must understand that although they are fertile now, they may become infertile later, due to various conditions that might develop over time or to aging. They must think about how they would feel about having genetic children in the world if they become infertile themselves. Young donors need to be assessed to determine if they have the maturity to make an informed consent and are not being coerced by third parties or by the lure of financial compensation.

Another concern related to the risks associated with ovum donation is whether the donor has health insurance that will cover any medical complications that might arise. Although complications are rare, hyperstimulation can occur, and serious hyperstimulation may require hospitalization. If the donor does not have health insurance, provision must be made for unanticipated medical costs.

Risks to the Recipient

Pregnancy, labor, and delivery take a toll on even the healthiest and youngest of bodies and carry the risk of medical complications. As women grow older, this risk is compounded. Once, all pregnant women over forty were considered high risk. Now, many physicians agree that if a woman is over forty (or even over fifty) and is in good health, pregnancy is unlikely to present serious risks.

When oocyte donation is used in an older woman, she must be adequately counseled regarding the risks of pregnancy with advanced maternal age. Included should be discussion of the risks associated with multiple gestation, the incidence of premature delivery, and other neonatal problems.

Financial Compensation of Donors

Egg donation is medically risky, physically invasive, painful, and time-consuming. As a result, payment for anonymous egg donation is considerably higher than the usual $50 to $75 for sperm donation. Braverman reported that payments ranged from a low of $750 to a high of $3,500, the average compensation being $1,548.[7]

Some programs have attempted to break down the time commitment a donor must make into a set number of hours, in order to illustrate the point that, hour by hour, donors are being paid only a small amount of money. Whatever the compensation offered, however, there are those who believe that it is tantalizingly high, inducing women to donate their eggs for the wrong reasons; others feel it is insultingly low, tantamount to exploitation.

Some ethicists view donating gametes in the same way they view donating blood: ovum donors should be encouraged to provide their gametes to infertile couples as a public service, without pay, even for their time and inconvenience. Others believe that donors should be reimbursed for actual expenses, such as lost wages, but no payment be made for her time and certainly not for the actual oocytes retrieved. Still others feel that additional payment for pain, risk, and inconvenience is warranted, considering that an egg donor undergoes hormonal stimulation by injection, blood and ultrasound monitoring, and a surgical procedure. Again, the primary ethical concern about compensating egg donors is that the money will serve as a coercive inducement to donate, obscuring any social or emotional reasons that might indicate that donation is not in a particular woman's best psychological interest.

In pondering the issues of ovum donation, ethicists address the potential for commercialization and competition in the marketplace—that these important life-producing cells will be viewed more as commodities and be seriously affected by the laws of supply and demand. Although many find this argument a gross exaggeration of the realities of infertility treatment, it is also true that more and more couples are choosing ovum donation. It is not out of the question that the increasing demand for donor oocytes, in combination with a limited supply, will cause programs to raise the level of compensation they offer donors.

Two other forms of compensation do not involve the direct exchange of money: the offering of free tubal ligations to fertile women and the offer of substantial reductions in the cost of their IVF cycle to infertile women. Both forms of compensation raise the question of whether subtle coercion is involved. If the offer were eliminated, some couples could never afford to try IVF. On the other hand, donating her oocytes is an act that an infertile woman cannot take lightly, and it is possible that the act of donating would haunt her for years to come, especially if the donor did not become pregnant herself and the recipient did.

Insurance Payment

By the time this book is in print our national health care policy will be going through tremendous scrutiny and upheaval. How the insurance industry will be impacted is anyone's guess. The extent to which infertility services will be covered by third party payers is unclear. However these issues get decided, the ethical questions that underlie them remain. These questions deal with whether society has a moral obligation to pay for treatment of infertility, and, if so, when and in what circumstances?

In terms of ovum donation, these questions may appear to be even more complicated, since human beings, especially post-menopausal women, are tampering with the laws of nature. The question also remains, assuming insurance will cover ovum donation, about whose insurance (the donor's or the recipient's) should cover the cost of the egg procurement. Underlying that question is another: whether, given the possible adverse consequences of egg donation, insurance companies should be expected to pay at all when healthy young women serve as donors. These are important questions that profoundly affect the health care industry and challenge our sense of moral justice as well.

Known Ovum Donation

Donor egg programs offer an exciting new opportunity for both partners to have a biological stake in the creation of their child—one through the genetic connection, the other through a gestational one. When a known donor is used, the couple has control over the source of the gametes as well as a medical history. Additionally, if a relative is the donor, the couple is able to preserve genetic continuity.

Known Egg Donation versus Known Sperm Donation: Key Differences

One of the key differences between sperm and egg donation is that known donors are frequently used for ovum donation, but rarely for sperm donation. In fact, according to Braverman's survey of eighty-two ovum donation programs, the majority of infertility programs that offer treatment with donor gametes use known egg donation, while the majority of programs do not use known sperm donation.[8] Although there may be other explanations for this difference, we will identify two major ones: practicality and gender differences.

Practicality. Eggs are difficult to obtain. Ovum donors are required to go through assisted reproductive technology, whereas sperm donors can produce a sample in just a few minutes through masturbation. The former procedure is invasive, potentially risky, and physically uncomfortable; the latter, easy and under different circumstances, pleasurable. Additionally, with sperm donation, insemination of the woman, though usually performed in a physician's office, can be, and has been, performed at home. Hence, ovum donors are much scarcer than sperm donors.

Another difficulty in obtaining eggs is that, unlike sperm, they cannot be frozen and stored for later use, making logistical arrangements a tedious part of the process. As we explained earlier in this chapter, an egg donor's cycle must be coordinated with the recipient's, which involves careful monitoring. Thus two people—each on her own biological calendar—are involved in the ovum donation process, whereas with sperm donation medical monitoring is only necessary for the woman, and her cycle does not have to be coordinated with anyone else's. Since semen can be thawed in minutes, the only necessary logistical arrangement for sperm donation is that it be shipped to the clinic on time. In other words, because anonymous sperm donation can be done so easily through the use of frozen sperm, this makes it a practical as well as attractive option. Since anonymous ovum donation is not any easier than known ovum donation, expediency does not make it more attractive.

Because the process of retrieving eggs is difficult, and because they cannot be frozen once they are retrieved, most programs do not have a large pool of donors available to donate. There are a few clinics, however, who claim to have a 'catalog' of carefully screened donors, but most clinics have long waiting lists of recipients and few donors. The scarcity of anonymous donors prompts many recipient couples to turn to known ovum donation.

Gender Differences. Although a couple may initially choose a known ovum donor primarily for expediency, there is another reason why known ovum donation is popular: gender differences. As we have seen in Chapter 5, over the years most professionals involved in DI have consciously or unconsciously sought to protect men from the shame unfortunately associated with male infertility. Physicians, mandating secrecy from everyone, including the potential child, have encouraged couples to turn to anonymous donors. Although occasional couples have objected to anonymity and have intentionally sought a known donor, most couples involved in sperm donation have accepted anonymity as integral to the process. Although infertility is painful to women, it is not usually shameful.

There are other reasons why known ovum donors are commonly used. One that is important to many couples is that it allows them to take an active role in building their family. After years of feeling helpless and out of control as a result of infertility, choosing a known donor means that the couple has control over the source of their gametes and probably feels more in control of their lives than they have in a long time. They are familiar with the donor's personality, temperament, and physical attributes and presumably have positive feelings toward her.

Another reason frequently cited for choosing a known donor involves the relationship between genes and health. Medical science continues to uncover more and more data indicating that heredity plays a large role in a person's health history. Although few medical problems appear to result from an unalterable genetic blueprint, individuals are born with hereditary predispositions toward certain diseases or physical problems. Although many conditions are passed on through recessive traits and cannot be anticipated, known donors provide recipient couples with baseline information—as much as they would get if the recipient's gametes were used—about a potential child's likelihood (or not) of developing certain medical conditions.

Known donors are also desirable to many couples because the child will have the option of knowing his or her genetic mother. (see Chapter 5, Donor Insemination, for a more extensive discussion of known vs. unknown donors). Although the extent and nature of their relationship must be negotiated, couples choosing known ovum donation feel relatively confident that their offspring will not suffer from genealogical bewilderment and that their child's identity will be enhanced by the opportunity to know his or her genetic mother.

Known Ovum Donors

When couples decide on a known ovum donor they do so for many reasons. First they must think about a crucial question: Who? The answer is very important for whom they select and the reasons why they select her form the cornerstone around which their family will be built.

The typical known donor is a relative or a friend, although some couples have asked co-workers or acquaintances. The experience of known ovum donation differs according to the nature of the relationship between the donor and recipient.

Relatives. When a couple decides to seek a known ovum donor, many turn to a close relative. Women with sisters often feel they are ideal donors because of their similar genetic makeup. With a sister's oocytes, the continuity of the bloodline is assured, and that assurance is important to many recipient couples. Since many ovum recipients are infertile due to aging, chances are that only a younger sister—probably significantly younger—would be fertile. Some have more than one sister and must decide whom to approach. Their decision may be influenced by many factors, including whether each has proved fertility, whether she has completed her family, physical proximity, overall health, and the relationship that exists between them.

Ovum donor couples who do not have the option of asking a sister or are turned down may turn to another relative—perhaps a cousin or a niece. Depending on the nature of the relationship, however, it can be difficult for recipients to ask such an enormous favor of someone who is not an intimate relative.

Another form of intrafamily donation is highly controversial: ovum donation from daughter to mother, in situations involving a second or third marriage. Although women with adult daughters may view them as ideal donors and the daughters may be willing to donate, many professionals, in particular, mental health clinicians, have strong reservations against this practice. They see it as inherently coercive, given the typical parent-child relationship in which children may always feel in some way indebted to their parents. They believe that children are not psychologically free to say no to a parent in the same way they are free to refuse others. In the reverse situation—a mother donating to her daughter—fewer are opposed, since the nature of the mother-child relationship is such that mothers are the accepted and appropriate caretakers of their children. Hence, they might donate eggs to their daughters without violating the integrity of their relationship. Situations in which a mother is young enough to donate to a daughter who is old enough to have a child are extraordinarily rare, however.

Nonrelatives. Couples may seek a friend or acquaintance if a relative is not available or if they prefer a nonrelative. The latter brings with her the advantages of known genes but not the social and emotional entanglements that could occur in the family if their child has an aunt who is also her genetic mother or a cousin who is her genetic mother.

A nonrelative may be desirable to recipient couples if she bears a physical resemblance to the donor. They feel the child will fit into the family better and will be less likely to be the brunt of questions such as, "Whom does he look like?" Couples who use a nonrelative as an ovum donor when a relative may be available do not care much about preserving genetic continuity. They value the fact that the donor is a known entity and comes from good genetic stock. They feel relieved not having to deal with the social and relational confusion inherent in familial donation.

Couples choosing nonrelatives must identify the attributes that are important to them in a donor and the relationship they want to have with her. Their feelings about these matters may point to someone in particular, or conversely, prompt them to rule someone out.

Some couples prefer to ask a close friend. They feel trusting of her and value the special connection between them. Other recipients are afraid to ask a good friend for fear that ovum donation would jeopardize their relationship if something went wrong or if they did not become pregnant. Thus, asking an acquaintance or a co-worker may feel less risky, since there is less to lose.

Motivations for Becoming a Known Donor

What motivates a relative or a friend to be a donor? This question puzzles many people—both inside and outside the field of reproductive medicine—who could never imagine being involved in this process. Some wonder how people could put themselves through such grueling medical procedures; others, who could not imagine watching their genetic child being raised by someone else, are troubled by the 'known' aspect, though they could imagine donating anonymously. Still others feel that under no circumstances could they ever donate their genetic material to another person, known or unknown.

Let us view the donation of gametes on a continuum, ranging from those who feel that giving away ovum or sperm is the same as giving away blood, to those who feel that giving away their gametes is tantamount to giving away a child. Clearly people have vastly different feelings about and relationships to their own genetic material. Actually, a gamete is equivalent to neither a person nor a pint of blood; it is somewhere in between, but where exactly is a matter of individual interpretation. Because known donors are often women who would not have considered ovum donation on their own had a need not arisen with a relative or friend, they find themselves giving careful thought to the question: what exactly is a gamete?

Most potential donors place themselves toward the "blood" end of the continuum. Those who feel an intense connection to their genes, and feel that an egg is close to a person, probably rule themselves out as donors, although they may not be aware consciously of the reason. Women who agree to donate, especially if they are donating to someone they know, tend to regard the ovum, once it is out of their body—and even more so when it is fertilized with the recipient's husband's sperm—as no longer part of them. For them, the embryo takes on a life of its own, and although they recognize that many traits are genetically transmitted and the resulting offspring may resemble the genetic mother in both physical and emotional ways, they believe the genetic contribution is but a small piece in comparison to the gestational and rearing aspects of motherhood.

Most known donors are motivated primarily by enormous empathy for the recipient. In many cases, especially those involving a

sister, the donor has seen the anguish of the recipient and understands how important motherhood is to her. This understanding,
together with her strong feelings of affection, convince her to donate. In many instances she is also motivated by her own joy and
satisfaction in motherhood.

Sometimes a tragedy—frequently a near brush with death—motivates a relative (usually a sister) to donate her eggs. In these situations, donors have acknowledged that they probably would not
have been able to make this choice if it were not for the tragic event
in their family. One couple applied to a donor egg program requesting that the woman's older sister, who was thirty-two, be her
donor. They explained that the prospective recipient had been
treated for Hodgkin's disease nine years earlier and had lost ovarian function secondary to chemotherapy. The donor had two children of her own.

During the counseling session, the intended donor mentioned
that before her sister became ill, she had not believed in IVF or gamete donation. She thought that infertile people should not use extreme measures to have children but should adopt instead. Her
views changed dramatically when it became clear that her sister
would survive her battle with cancer. She described herself as "spiritually converted" and said that she had developed a strong sense
that there was a shared purpose to their lives and she was meant to
help her sister have a baby.

The two couples were accepted into the program, and the recipient did become pregnant. When the pregnancy was confirmed on
ultrasound, the tears of joy that came from both sisters—and their
husbands as well—confirmed that they all had been spiritually converted. Throughout the process, the sisters became closer, and the
donor was present when her sister gave birth.

The Request or Offer

Asking a friend or relative to donate eggs is not an easy task. Most
recipients approach it with great trepidation, feeling as if they have
everything at stake, never having imagined that they would be asking anyone for something that goes so far beyond familiar favors.
Although recipients are fully prepared for the potential donor to

say no, they are vulnerable and know they will be devastated if she does. At the same time they may worry that she will feel forced to say yes. Often the donor agrees without hesitation. Perhaps she had already been thinking about offering help in some way but did not know or understand how she could help. Some thought the only way was to be a surrogate, an act that went a step beyond what they could imagine doing. Many donors were unaware they could donate eggs without having to gestate the child and are pleased when the process is explained to them. Not only are they able to help someone near and dear to them have a child, but they do not have to worry about becoming attached during pregnancy.

Sometimes donors approach recipients. If they know about the technology of ovum donation they may make the offer to their relative or friend. Others make a general offer of help, not knowing exactly what they can do but being aware that reproductive technology can do wonders. In these situations recipients feel grateful and relieved. The fact that the donor offers before being asked is an indication that she is donating because she wants to, not because she feels unable to refuse the recipient.

Many who are asked to donate eggs, however, say no, for reasons ranging from not having the time, to fear of the procedures or side effects from the medications, to feeling that it would be too difficult to watch a genetic child being raised by someone else. This situation is painful for both people. Many who are asked wish they could say yes but realize that they cannot do so.

The recipient may experience a refusal as a personal rejection, an indication that her relative or friend must not care much about her. But in their longing to have a child, infertile couples may not be able to fully appreciate the feelings that some people have about their genes, as the following case shows.

An infertile couple made an appointment to speak with the psychologist in an ART program about anonymous ovum donation. The woman burst into tears immediately and told the psychologist that she had two younger, fertile sisters who had each completed their families. The three sisters had been very close all their lives and remained in the same geographic area. She had approached each of them about being a donor, feeling certain they would come through for her. Both had refused, for essentially the same reason: because their own children reminded them so much of themselves, they could never donate an egg to their sister, or to anyone else they knew, for it would feel like giving away their child. They feared that as the child grew up, they would have different feelings for him or her than for their other nieces and nephews. Both sisters spoke of how difficult it was to say no. Each separately stated that if the sister needed a kidney, say, or a bone marrow transplant, both of which involve far greater physical risk than donating ovum, they would immediately agree.

The recipient felt betrayed. One of the implicit assumptions in her family was that they would always be there for each other. Her sisters' refusal to donate seemed an indication that the assumption was incorrect and that she was not as important to them as she had believed. With some time and distance, the recipient was able to understand that her sisters' attitudes toward their gametes were different from her own. Appreciating the sincerity of their offer of a kidney helped her to see that her sisters really would do almost anything for her.

Psychological Screening of Donors and Recipients

Couples who choose known ovum donation bring their relative or friend to the ART clinic, and she too becomes a patient. They have already invested considerable emotional energy in the process of selecting her and asking her to donate, yet that is only the beginning. Donors must pass a medical screening before they are accepted, and most programs (77.6 percent, according to Braverman's survey) provide psychological screening as well. The physician and the psychologist, or other mental health clinician, must help all parties determine whether the proposed arrangement makes sense medically and psychologically and whether it seems to be in everyone's best interest, including, and most important, the potential child's.

Most programs that have a mental health professional use a team model approach to patient care with physicians, nurses, mental health providers, and sometimes administrators working collaboratively. The role of the mental health professional in ovum donation programs is to assess the emotional stability of both donor and recipient couples and educates them about the complex psychological, social, ethical, and legal issues involved in this process.

The screening process also provides a forum in which to deal with the many concerns of both recipients and donors. Although approaches vary from clinic to clinic, commonly the mental health provider interviews the donor (and often her partner as well) separately from the recipient couple and usually prior to meeting with the latter. Many programs also conduct conjoint interviews with both couples once each has been seen alone. Although a large percentage of programs use psychological testing as part of the screening process, this practice appears more common in anonymous donor screening.

Donor Concerns. Women who are asked to donate fall into three categories: those who refuse, those who tentatively agree and expect the medical and psychological screening process to help them evaluate whether donating is in their best interest, and those who agree readily though they usually find it helpful to review the important social, emotional, and ethical issues with a trained clinician.

Program counselors frequently begin by interviewing the potential donor first. The clinician's job is to be everyone's advocate—including the unborn child—and to help all parties make a decision in the best interest of everyone. When clinicians meet with recipient couples, it is easy to empathize with them and to want to help them achieve their goal. Thus, if a clinician is already invested in a particular couple, (having met them prior to meeting the donor) he or she may not be able to be objective when screening the known potential donor.

During the screening session, program counselors help a donor understand her concerns or conflicts about the process, and help her determine their significance. Frequently donors find that by voicing their concerns to someone who understands, they can make better sense of them. If her concerns prove serious, the counselor can help the donor decide to say no, and, if she wants, intervene in her behalf.

Most donors are not able to anticipate all the problems that could occur. An important part of the counseling process, therefore, is to raise all the potential complications for the donor to ponder. They are asked to think about, and to respond to, various "what if" questions: What if you decided to have (more) children and discover you are infertile? What if the childlooks just like you or is just like you in some major way? They must think about future relationships: What kind of relationship do you wish to have with the recipient couple? The child? If the recipient couple dies, will you want guardianship of the child? The responses will help everyone assess whether the woman is prepared to donate and if it is in her best interest.

Inability to Separate. Donors may wonder whether they can truly separate the genetic aspects of motherhood from the gestational. When the concern is a nagging worry rather than an occasional thought, it is important for all involved to examine it. The following case is a good example of a donor's having doubts that were strong enough to cause her to have a change of heart.

A forty-year-old married woman who was a candidate for ovum donation brought in her sister who was fourteen years younger. The sister was a divorced woman with a five-year-old daughter. During the initial interview, the psychologist probed her feelings about genetics, bonding, attachment, her relationship with her daughter, and her relationship with her immediate and extended family, along with other relevant issues. The potential donor felt close to her sister and sincerely wanted to help her have a child. During the interview, however, she became aware of the extent to which she felt connected to her own daughter, in part, she thought, because she looked and acted so much like her. She left the session having doubts about whether she could emotionally separate from a child who was created from her egg and feel like an aunt to him or her in the same way that she felt like an aunt to her other nieces and nephews. It was agreed that as long as she continued to have even the slightest of doubts, donation would probably not be in her best interest or anyone else's.

Sometimes a donor is unaware of her doubts, and the counselor must help her to identify them. A psychologist was interviewing a woman who hoped to donate eggs to a close friend. In the course of the interview the psychologist pointed out to the potential donor that the resulting child might very well resemble the donor, in physical characteristics or in traits. The donor, a reasonably intelligent woman, asked, "Since Mary will be carrying the child, doesn't that mean that some of her will enter the baby?" The psychologist began to understand, as a result of exploring the meaning behind her question, that the potential donor needed to view the ovum donation process in such a simplistic way. The donor's wish was to be able to help her friend have a baby; her fear was that she herself would feel connected to the child. By creating an unrealistic fantasy, she hoped to remove herself psychologically from the process. If she had no connection to her eggs once they were removed from her body, she would not have to feel connected to the child.

Feelings About the Recipient's Partner. Donors may have concerns about the couple's relationship or about whether they will be good parents. They may also have mixed feelings about the recipient's spouse. Most known donors have a close and special relationship with the recipient, but that closeness does not necessarily extend to her partner. Negative feelings about spouses are usually troublesome and can give donors pause to think about what they are doing and for whom they are doing it.

An example of this situation is illustrated by a case in which a recipient asked her best friend to donate oocytes to her, but the friend had ambivalent feelings about the recipient's husband and was reluctant to talk directly to her about this issue. She did, however, express them to the clinical social worker, who helped her to sort through her feelings. The donor found that she had to decide who was receiving her eggs: her friend or the couple. If she was donating them solely to her friend, her feelings about the husband were not important. If she was donating them to the couple, however, then she believed they were important. The dilemma was complicated for the donor because she knew that her friend had experienced four pregnancy losses and would be happy to adopt, but her husband was determined to have a biological child and wanted to use known donor gametes. The donor came to the conclusion, after a great deal of counseling, that she was donating to her friend and not to the couple. She put aside any negative feelings she had about the husband in order to help her close friend.

Bonding. Like most other people, donors associate motherhood with gestation. This association allows them to believe that the pregnancy will transform the recipient into the "real" mother and that the process of having their eggs removed will allow donors to let go of any emotional ties to them. Nevertheless, it is common for potential donors to have nagging fears that it might be the genetic connection, after all, that accounts for bonding.

Good Genes. Donors worry about passing on "good genes." They know that the recipient couple has positive feelings toward them, or they would not have been asked to donate in the first place. Donors are aware, however, that genes are randomly distributed, that each egg is genetically different, and that an offspring could inherit less desirable characteristics. They may still feel a strong sense of responsibility, however—even though they have no control—to donate a "perfect" egg. Donors worry about how they, and the couple will feel if the child is born with a serious problem.

Obligations Toward the Child. Donors wonder whether the child will conceptualize the donor as the genetic mother or simply as a donor. The notion of being any kind of mother to someone they are not choosing to parent may seem frightening. Donors wonder whether they will be responsible in any way for the well-being of the offspring or have any obligation—legal, social, or emotional—toward him or her.

Most programs recommend that known donors and recipients seek counsel from an attorney who has experience in this area of law. A contract can spell out the rights and obligations of all parties. The contract may or may not be legally binding if it is challenged in the future by one of the parties, say the donor wanting to claim the child as her own. Because many of the legal issues are tied in with the emotional and social issues, however, the act of meeting with an attorney can help all parties understand what is involved in the process of ovum donation.

Recipient Couple Concerns. Although virtually all recipient couples begin the process of ovum donation with hope and excitement, most are not blinded by such a strong desire to become parents that they minimize potential complications. Counseling sessions allow the couple to express these concerns and to explore the ramifications of the arrangement with a clinician. In addition, as with donor screening, counselors must raise a host of "what if" questions.

Bonding. The experience of gestation has always been closely associated with the role of mothering, a connection that may explain why many infertile women readily embrace ovum donation. Nevertheless, most recipients wonder how they will feel carrying another woman's genetic child and whether they will bond to that child in utero. This question has another facet when they know the donor. They may wonder if, during pregnancy, they will look at the donor and feel that the baby belongs to her.

Still, most women know from experience that attachments can form through nurturing. Because they associate the maternal role with gestation and have faith in their ability to bond with a baby who did not come from their genes, we have found that this concern, though genuine, diminishes over time.

Authenticity. Recipient mothers wonder whether they will feel like the real mother of their child after birth and throughout his or her lifetime. If the donor is someone with whom they are in regular contact, such as a sister or a good friend, they may wonder if during Thanksgiving dinner, for example, they will look at their sister and feel like a fraud. They may wonder what others will think and feel and whether all who know will regard the donor as the true mother. They may wonder also whether their ability to claim the child as theirs will be even more threatened if he, or more likely, she, resembles the donor.

Inability to Separate. Recipients have worries about the donor as well. One concern is that she will not be able to separate emotionally from her egg and that, as pregnancy progresses, the growing fetus will feel like her child and that she will experience feelings of depression, longing, and emptiness, regretting having ever made the offer. Sometimes these worries prove to be real, as in the case previously mentioned in which a twenty-six year old woman, determined to help her forty-year-old sister have a baby, realized through the screening process that she could not regard a child who came from her genes as "just another niece or nephew."

The Desire for a Positive Experience. Almost all recipients want the donation to be a positive experience for their donor. Most are extremely sensitive to their potential donor's feelings, reassuring her frequently that there will be no hard feelings should she change her mind. Recipients frequently tell potential donors that they will always be grateful for even considering being their donor.

The following case is an unfortunate, and unusual, situation in which the recipient did not seem to be at all concerned about her donor's future reaction to the experience. A forty-year-old woman asked her younger sister to be her donor. The sister initially agreed, but in the course of the counseling session, the donor realized that she did not want to be involved in the complicated familial relationship that would occur. As it was, she felt her family was overly involved in each other's lives, and although she felt deeply for her sister, she realized that ovum donation was not right for her.

The recipient, who never liked the fact that counseling was a requirement, called the clinic a few weeks later and told the coordinator she had another sister who was willing to be her donor. After the coordinator requested the second sister's medical records, the recipient queried, "She doesn't have to see that psychologist who will talk her out of it, does she?" This statement alerted the team to what they already suspected: that the recipient was either not willing or not able to understand the potential conflicts or complications in relationships that can arise in known ovum donor situations. Because of her refusal to recognize the psychosocial aspects of the process and the team's belief that unless all parties are open to examining these complications, it should not be offered, the recipient couple was asked to come in for an interview. At that time the reasons why they were being denied the treatment were explained.

This case illustrates the need for mandatory counseling. Had the donor's feelings not been probed, she may have overlooked them herself in her strong desire to help her sister, and possibly also to avoid her sister's wrath. We can speculate about the emotional sequelae that may have resulted, and the long-term consequences on the family as a whole, had the original plan been followed.

Fear of Obligation. Recipients worry that their donor may feel obligated to donate and that she may be afraid to tell them if she has a change of heart. As the screening process unfolds, many things can come up that will cause the donor to feel ambivalent. The donor may be frightened of the medical process, rethink what it means to donate gametes, or be concerned about the confusing familial relationships that will occur.

When a family member is considering ovum donation, especially in the case of sisters, she may experience additional pressure from relatives who want to see the infertile couple become parents.

Sometimes in their enthusiasm to embrace an option that seems like a perfect solution, relatives (frequently the parents of the sisters) may overlook potential complications.

Identity Confusion. Recipients have concerns about their potential child and how she or he may feel in the future about the manner of conception. Recipients wonder whether their offspring will have identity confusion, especially during adolescence when the search for identity is paramount and when teenagers commonly reject their parents. When third parties are involved in reproduction, especially when they are known, recipient parents may fear their children are likely to form a stronger attachment to their genetic parent than to them. If the donor is a close friend or relative who frequently spends time with them, this concern may be especially troublesome.

Conjoint Counseling

Once both parties want to proceed, a joint interview is very useful, many would say necessary. It is a time for each party to share the concerns they discussed in their separate interviews—concerns that might affect the outcome. It is also an opportunity for the clinician to determine how well they listen to each other, communicate, and problem solve—skills that will be necessary in their joint venture.

Shared Expectations. Any discrepancies, however slight, that arose during the individual sessions need to be brought up for joint discussion. This session provides an opportunity to assess the nature of these differences and to determine whether there is or can be agreement. The parties also have to agree about:

- Logistical arrangments during the medical process—rides to the clinic, for example, and injections.
- Whether the donor will be reimbursed for her time or expenses or both.
- What to do if an amniocentesis indicates a problem with the fetus.
- Whether they will consider multifetal reduction if more than two fetuses result.

They must also agree about the nature of the relationship the donor would like to have with the recipients and, more important, the offspring. For example, if a donor expects to have a close relationship with the child—perhaps become the godmother—and the recipient couple does not intend for her to have a major role in the child's life, the arrangement may not be workable unless they can reach a point where their expectations are shared.

Openness versus Secrecy. Another shared expectation relates to telling, or not telling, others. This question is of fundamental importance; it is crucial that all parties have the same understanding about who, what, and when they will tell. It appears that almost all known donor ovum couples choose to be open about sharing that information with other people, including the child. Being open, however, does not mean that privacy must be compromised. Those involved may decide to tell others selectively; who and under what circumstances must be negotiated. If couples wish to keep the process a secret, it is more difficult, and for that reason many clinicians strongly advise against secrecy where the donor is known.

This decision about being open (or not) involves an ethical dilemma: whether a person has the right to know the truth about his or her genetic origins. Chapter 5 contains an extensive discussion of the ethical and psychosocial issues inherent in the openness versus secrecy debate, and these issues pertain to both donor insemination and ovum donation. Here, we briefly review why couples make the choice they do.

Those who choose to be open with their child do so because they feel comfortable with using a third party for purposes of reproduction, and they want to maintain an open, trusting relationship with their child. They feel that when a lie forms the foundation of their relationship, the basis for trust is removed. Additionally, maintaining a secret would be a tremendous burden to themselves and to their donor. Finally, they believe that their child has a right to know about his or her genetic origins for medical and well as psychological reasons.

Known donor ovum couples who decide to keep the donation a secret, and they are probably few in number, fear that the child would be confused to learn that the gestating-rearing mother and the genetic mother were not the same person. They may also fear that their child would become angry and reject the mother if she or he were to learn the truth. Finally, they worry that the child may not be accepted as readily by other people—family members, friends, and acquaintances. Couples who opt for secrecy usually value their privacy and the privacy of their donor.

Sometimes, however, even the most thoughtfully constructed plans may need to be changed if life circumstances take an unexpected turn, as one couple found. They had decided not to tell anyone that a friend had been their donor. They were concerned that since the donor came from a different culture, their families might not accept a grandchild who was not part of their lineage. When their child was two years old, the wife's sister died suddenly of a heart ailment. It was thought that this particular ailment was genetically transmittable, and there was no means by which the presence of the gene could be detected. There was a great deal of concern in the extended family, that not only the mother and her siblings but also the only grandchild could be at medical risk for the heart problem. After seeking counseling with the social worker who initially met with the donor and recipient couple, the parents decided to disclose the donor conception to their families.

Not all couples who found themselves in this troublesome situation would make the same choice. Every couple is different, as are their families and friends. What is in the best interest of one family may not be in the best interest of another. The reasons governing a couple's choice to be open or private are profound and challenging to everyone, from professionals in the field, to the couples who avail themselves of these new technologies.

Dyads Within a Triad: Bonding and Separation

The addition of a third person to the complex technological procedures involved in making a baby, drastically changes the ART dynamic. When there are three people involved, all of whom have an essential role in the creation of the child, it is inevitable that separate relationships occur between each of them. Three two-way relationships emerge: the couple, the donor-recipient, and the donor-husband.

Throughout the ART process, all parties involved in the triad go through various stages in relation to one other. The feelings that each person experiences are multifaceted, and the ties that develop intensify as the cycle progresses. The group begins as a triad, united in their common purpose. Yet as the drama unfolds, dyadic relationships emerge, and each plays a prominent role during a particular stage. Depending on the stage, each person has the capacity to feel central or, conversely, left out of the picture.

The bond that develops between the recipient and the donor is usually intense. Both women are sharing in the preparations for an IVF cycle, but in a sense the roles are reversed: the donor is undergoing hormonal injections and having her blood drawn and her ovaries monitored by ultrasound, while the recipient looks on, perhaps assisting with injections or rides to the clinic. If stimulation does not go well, and it sometimes does not, it brings heartache to all involved.

One woman in her mid-thirties who was donating to her sister became quite despondent when her cycle was cancelled because of poor stimulation. Although the recipient continued to express strong feelings of appreciation to her sister, the latter felt guilty, fearing that she had done something wrong. In this case the program psychologist met with the donor to reassure her that it was not her fault. What was striking, however, was that as disappointed as the recipient was about the outcome of the cycle, the donor appeared to be suffering as well.

As the time for retrieval approaches, the husband-donor dyad comes into the foreground. Questions about the number of eggs that might be retrieved and whether fertilization will go well surface. One recipient shared her feelings about this with the clinical social worker at her ART clinic:

> I felt like the odd woman out in the donor egg process, as my old friend from college was my donor, but this meant that *her* eggs would be fertilized by *my* husband's sperm. They are making the embryo/baby while I wait; then I'll carry *their* embryo that I didn't contribute to conceiving.

If the retrieval has gone well and several eggs are obtained, all three—once again a united force—support one another while they await the results of fertilization. Assuming the news is positive, the couple dyad then emerges as the central pair in the process. The next two weeks crawl by at a snail's pace, as the tension builds.

When the Test Is Negative. When a known donor ovum cycle fails to result in pregnancy, all involved are extremely disappointed, especially if it was the couple's only chance for pregnancy. There is a tendency for each person to examine his or her role in the process, looking for an explanation. Donors commonly blame themselves, assuming their eggs were not good enough. If the cycle was cancelled due to poor stimulation, there is some truth to this assumption, though the donor did nothing to cause the problem. When the cycle went well but the pregnancy test was negative, no one knows what may have gone wrong. Questions may immediately arise about whether to try again.

Recipient couples need a lengthy period of time to grieve when the process does not work. Most put a great deal of hope into the cycle, having believed that the donor eggs were the remedy they needed. Depending on the financial resources of the couple, and the willingness of the donor, they may attempt another cycle, but each person first needs to pull inward for a period of time.

Pregnancy After Known Ovum Donation

Pregnancy after known ovum donation is a fairly recent phenomena because the procedure itself is so new. Thus clinicians in the field do not have extensive experience working with couples who are pregnant after known ovum donation. Nor has the process been described in the literature. Although we are not able to make definitive conclusions, we can, however, draw on our time-limited experience to make some preliminary generalizations about pregnancy after known ovum donation.

Although known donors are genuinely thrilled for the expectant couple when the news is good and are usually ready to get on with their lives, they may experience some mixed feelings. They have been central to this intense drama and may feel left out at this point in the process. They also know that the couple's attention is focused on their pregnancy rather than on their donor.

Once a pregnancy has been confirmed, a process of separation and differentiation occurs among the members of the triad. Each needs to experience and take credit for his or her unique role in the ovum donation process. Recipients commonly have expressed a need to pull back from the donor when they are pregnant, giving themselves some time to bond with the growing fetus inside them. One recipient stated that she wanted to "get in touch with my own contribution to the pregnancy and creation of my child." Another woman expressed her need to pull back "in order to feel involved, not wanting to share the pregnancy with anyone else quite so soon."

Although these tendencies (and needs) are common, they are not exhibited by all recipients. In the following case, the recipient did not feel a need to pull back from the donor; in fact the process brought them even closer.

Ms. B. was a thirty-one-year-old woman who was born with only one ovary, which was surgically removed when she was twenty-four, as a result of a benign but invasive cyst. Her resulting infertility was initially devastating, but in time she and her husband accepted the situation, assuming she would never bear a child and that they would build their family through adoption.

About five years after her surgery, however, she came across an article on ovum donation. Cautiously she investigated infertility programs that offered this service, and eventually Ms. B. decided to ask her only sister, to whom she felt very close, to be her donor. Known ovum donation excited Ms. B. because not only would it allow her to actually become pregnant, but it would enable her to have a child who would carry on the family's genes. The sister, who was married and had three children, ages ten, eight, and six, was overjoyed to help her sister have a child.

Ms. B.'s husband reacted to the idea with apprehension. He was afraid that his wife would become obsessed with the process and would feel devastated if it did not work. Moreover, he felt comfortable with adoption. Ms. B., however, felt strongly about wanting to attempt known ovum donation, and eventually her persistence won him over.

After extensive counseling that included separate interviews with both couples, as well as an interview with everyone together, they were accepted into the program. From the beginning, all four people were a cohesive unit, working together toward a common goal. Although the sisters lived an hour's drive from each other and each lived approximately an hour and a half from the clinic, Ms. B. always drove to the clinic with her sister, and on occasion the two husbands drove with them as well.

Ms. B. did not become pregnant during her first IVF cycle. She was extremely disappointed, but her disappointment was diminished when her sister volunteered to go through another cycle. Additionally, they had four frozen embryos left from the first cycle. Ms. B. decided to try a frozen cycle and, if it did not work, to accept her sister's offer. She resolved that if a second fresh cycle and any remaining embryos did not result in pregnancy, they would end treatment and move on to adoption.

Ms. B. did become pregnant from the frozen embryo transfer cycle. She and her husband were thrilled, as were her sister and brother-in-law. Instead of feeling a need to separate, however, everyone felt that it was truly a family affair that brought them closer together. This closeness continued throughout her uncomplicated pregnancy.

In reflecting back on the pregnancy, Mr. B. stated that he rarely thought about the fact that his wife was not the genetic mother. Rather, he focused his worries on whether the cryopreservation process would affect the fetus. By contrast, Ms. B. was not at all worried about the effects of cryopreservation but did occasionally wonder whether she would feel like a second-class mother to her child, especially in her sister's presence. She wondered whether her sister's genetic connection might overpower her own maternal bond.

To Ms. B.'s delight, her sister and brother-in-law were present during her labor, which ended in the birth of a healthy baby boy by cesarean section. Ms. B. attests that from the moment her son was born, any doubts she had about who the mother was were erased entirely; it was clear to everyone that the baby belonged to her and her husband.

The bonding that occurred among the four adults during the ovum donation process and the subsequent pregnancy and delivery has remained intact. Ms. B.'s sister and brother-in-law adore the baby (now ten months) but do not feel possessive of him. This fact became clear when Ms. B. and her husband received an invitation from the clinic to attend its annual ART family reunion. Ms. B. assumed her sister and brother-in-law would attend as well, since they were part of the team—along with her and her husband—that produced her son. Her sister, replied, however, "This is your baby now; you don't need me. You're the parents."

Ms. B. and her husband are thrilled with their outcome, yet they know that they face many challenges ahead. Mr. B. said that the only time he thinks about the fact that his wife is not their child's genetic mother is when he contemplates how or when they will tell their son the story of his birth. Ms. B. says she thinks about it when people comment that her son has her blue eyes or some other feature; usually she explains why he cannot possibly have *her* features.

The experience of these two couples has been an extremely positive one, perhaps unusually so. Ms. B. and her sister began the process as close, loving siblings, and through ovum donation they became even closer. Although Ms. B. had occasional doubts during her pregnancy about who the child would *belong* to once he was born, it was clear to both who was the mother and who was the aunt. It is not possible to draw any conclusions from just one case history, but it is probably fair to say that the doubts Ms. B. felt on occasion are probably common given the nature of this parenting option. And although the bonding between the two couples was probably more intense than usual, the joy that the recipients experienced as a result of known ovum donation is not unusual at all.

Anonymous Ovum Donation

The medical process for ovum donation is identical whether the donor is known or anonymous; many of the social, psychological, and emotional issues are very different, however.

Some couples who decide to use donated eggs feel certain that they prefer anonymous to known donation; they see this process as less complicated emotionally in the present as well as in the future. Other couples would have preferred a known donor, but no one is available. Thus, for the first group of couples, anonymous donation is a second-choice path to parenthood; for the second group, it is a third choice. This distinction is significant because the latter group comes to anonymous ovum donation with additional losses that may touch old wounds. If such couples do not acknowledge and grieve these losses, they are likely to have difficulty embracing the option of anonymous donation.

Couples who prefer to have a known donor and do not have this option have additional feelings of loss and disappointment and feel out of control in the realm of reproduction. Their best efforts to form their family have been thwarted. Sometimes they attempt to ignore these feelings. Instead, they need to acknowledge and grieve their previous losses before they can choose and move on to anonymous donation, as two examples show.

In the first case, a potential recipient expressed great sadness to the clinical social worker about using an unknown donor. She had a younger sister who had died in a car accident several years earlier. Now, in thinking about ovum donation, the recipient imagined that her sister would have been a wonderful donor and that she would have readily agreed to donate. As she spoke of this loss of her ideal donor, the recipient realized that she had never fully mourned her sister's death. With guidance from the clinician, she understood that she needed to work through this earlier loss and the ways in which it was connected to her infertility trauma before she could proceed resolutely with anonymous ovum donation.

Another potential recipient told a clinical social worker that she was hurt because her sister had refused to donate. This experience of being turned down rekindled earlier feelings of being disappointed by her sister, whom she had always considered selfish. The recipient felt certain that if the situation were reversed, she would gladly give eggs to her sister, because she had always been the one to give in their relationship. Her sister's refusal also caused the recipient to feel even less in control of her reproductive life; not only was she "forced" to use an anonymous donor but also to reveal her infertility, and especially her need for ovum donation. With help, the recipient recognized that this experience meant she must let go of her hope for genetic continuity, as well as her hope that her relationship with her sister would live up to her expectations.

Choosing Anonymous Ovum Donation

Despite the understandable disappointment of couples who would prefer known donors, there are many others who prefer anonymous donation. Some of them may have an appropriate donor but feel that anonymous donation offers them some clear advantages:

1. *Avoidance of Social Bewilderment.* These couples do not want to have an ongoing relationship with the donor. They believe

that if the child's genetic mother were involved in their lives, the child could be confused about who his or her "real" mother was. Furthermore, if the donor were a relative, a sister, for example, they believe the child would face the additional confusion of not knowing whether to relate to her as an aunt or as a mother.

2. *Authenticity*. Couples who have battled long-term infertility are left with a sense of insecurity about parenthood and a lack of entitlement about their right to be parents. Couples choosing anonymity believe this route will enhance their sense of authenticity and allow them to feel like the real parents. They fear that if the donor were part of their lives, the recipient's relationship with her child would be undermined.

3. *Security*. Some couples considering known ovum donation have fears that the genetic mother might try to claim the child as her own and take him or her away. Couples choosing anonymous donation feel protected by the anonymity, seeing it as creating a psychological barrier between them and the donor, enabling them to feel more secure as a family.

4. *Privacy*. Couples frequently choose anonymous donation because it affords them privacy, although some might like to know the source of their gametes. They feel that using a known donor would compromise their privacy and force them to disclose how their child was conceived, thus interfering with the foundation and future of their family. Being private gives them control over the information regarding their child's conception.

The Donors

Couples considering anonymous ovum donation almost immediately question who the donors are. Many wonder why someone would put herself through a grueling procedure for someone she did not know. They may conclude that donors must be psychologically disturbed. Others assume that because compensation is usually involved, donors must be in financial difficulty. The truth is that most programs require donors to go through an extensive psychological and medical evaluation, and those with psychopathology are immediately screened out. In addition, many programs attempt to avoid including donors whose motivations are strictly financial.

Recruitment and Motivation. Most women who apply for ovum donation do so in response to an advertisement in their local newspaper, on a bulletin board (in settings that range from college campuses to supermarkets), or in medical centers. Other prospective donors learn about ovum donation because they had a friend who was a donor, because they know someone who works in an ART program, or because they saw a television program or heard a radio broadcast that piqued their interest.

Regardless of how she arrived at a clinic, however, the typical anonymous donor is a young, appealing woman in good health who has given careful consideration to the process. In many cases, donors are women in transition: students, mothers with young children who are not working outside the home, or women who are between jobs. Most are drawn to ovum donation for reasons of empathy or altruism. Others are drawn to it as a result of having suffered reproductive losses.

Empathy and Altruism. It is common for donors to know someone who is or who has been infertile. If the infertile woman is a close friend or relative, the donor understands her heartache. Many donors have said that were it not for their relationship with their infertile friend (or relative), they would never have thought of donating eggs.

Other potential donors, who may or may not have known an infertile person, are mothers with young children who state unequivocally that motherhood has been the most rewarding experience of their lives. They feel deeply for couples who desire children and are unable to have them and seek the opportunity to help such couples.

Donors who are primarily motivated out of altruism or empathy usually think of their eggs as genetic material, not as a baby. They view their eggs as going to waste every month, and since they do not need them and someone else does, why not donate them? They believe that if they can do something of such importance for someone else, at little cost to themselves, that it is worth doing. Many donors include women who donate their blood regularly and regard egg donation as a comparable act of charity.

Reproductive Losses. Some donors may be attempting to "make up" for past reproductive losses, perhaps an elective abortion, about which they still have ambivalent feelings. One prospective donor had three young children and had completed her family. She had had an abortion when she was seventeen, and although she believed that she made the best decision at the time, she did not take her action lightly. One of her reasons for donating eggs was that she "took away a life, and now wants to give back a life."

Another woman in her early thirties who wanted to be an egg donor had undergone a hysterectomy, but her ovaries remained intact. She was married to a man several years older than she was, with children from a prior marriage, and although they had not ruled out alternatives, she was reasonably certain that they would not have children together. Having lost her fertility, she empathized deeply with women who were unable to have children. Aware that her ovaries were intact, she felt strongly that "rather than let her eggs go to waste," she would donate them to a couple who needed them.

Women who have placed children for adoption sometimes apply to be ovum donors. Depending on the psychological assessment, it may or may not be wise for them to become ovum donors. On the one hand, they have already experienced a loss that is presumably much greater than the loss of an egg. They should know whether they can handle the long-term implications of egg donation. On the other hand, there is always the possibility that this prospective donor, like some women who have undergone elective abortions, is still suffering from feelings of guilt or grief and is hoping that the altruistic act of donating eggs to an infertile couple will make up for the loss of their child.

Adoptees have also applied to become ovum donors. Many programs will not accept them, though, if important medical information is missing. Other programs, however, will consider them as donors if they have access to their medical history. For example, one woman who sought and found both her birth parents and five genetic siblings, applied to become a donor. The program felt comfortable having her as a donor, since she had obtained her entire family medical history. Although adoptees' motivations may differ, ovum donation may be a way to ensure they have established genetic connections in the world.

Some clinicians feel that women with histories of reproductive losses should not be donors; in such instances, ovum donation may be an attempt to undo a traumatic event rather than to grieve it. Other clinicians feel that ovum donation may allow some women an opportunity symbolically to "redo" rather than "undo" an event. In the case of the woman who "wanted to give back a life because she took a life," ovum donation did turn out to be a healing experience, one for which she was very grateful.

Psychological Screening and Counseling. The differences in screening sperm donors and egg donors are striking. Although the medical screening for sperm donors is thorough, the psychological screening is virtually nonexistent. Some feel this dual standard is sexist or paternalistic—that it reflects an inherent assumption that women are not capable of making a good decision without the help of a professional. Others believe that the screening processes for egg donors evolved from concerns raised about the lack of a similar process with their male counterparts. In other words, what is standard practice among sperm banks is far from what many mental health providers consider acceptable and is recognized to be a poor model for ovum donor programs.

Ovum donor programs tend to view the potential donor in one of two ways: as their patient or solely as a provider of gametes. Programs who regard donors as patients are generally concerned about both the medical and psychological well-being of the woman. They are concerned that the donor is well informed about the medical process and risks and that she understands the legal, ethical, social, and psychological implications of "giving away" her genetic material. In addition, such programs are concerned that the potential donor have reasons for donating that will enhance, rather than detract from, her self-esteem.

Clinics that view donors as providers of gametes—much as they view a pharmaceutical company as the provider of medications—are concerned primarily with the end result: whether they are providing patients with good (and viable) gametes. They are not as concerned about the psychological state of the donor. They assume that she can make an appropriate decision about whether ovum donation is in her best interest, and she does not need a mental health professional to help her make that decision. These programs are usually concerned about thorough medical screening, and some may administer routine psychological assessment tests to rule out donors with serious psychopathology or personality problems, but they probably have little personal contact with the potential donor and are not worried about the long-term psychological effects on her or the family.

Most programs view the donor as their patient. In Braverman's survey, 77.6 percent of the eighty-two programs reporting stated that psychological screening was required. Of those programs requiring psychological screening, 78.4 percent used personal interviews as part or all of the screening process. Some of the programs requiring psychological screening used personality assessment tests (43.1 percent), and some used other standard psychological tests (27.5 percent). (These statistics indicate that although most programs requiring screening include a personal interview with the donor, there are some programs that require only the use of standardized testing in their psychological assessment.) Furthermore, most programs (58.6 percent) require partners to be seen as well. Depending on the time allotted to the counseling and screening process, clinicians may see the potential donor anywhere from one to three times.[10]

The purpose of psychological screening and counseling is threefold: to ensure that the woman is psychologically appropriate to be a donor (mature, responsible, and with no underlying psychopathology), to inform her of both the short- and long-term psychological risks of donating ovum, and to be sure the program is protected in the event of future litigation.

In attempting to determine psychological appropriateness, a family and individual history is usually taken, which includes questions about prior substance abuse, mental illness, and reproductive losses. This allows the clinician to form a picture of the potential donor and to understand what social and psychological forces have shaped her life and prompted her to apply for ovum donation. The information gathered, in combination with her motivations and current life situation, helps the clinician determine whether she is suited to undertake ovum donation at this time.

The following case concerns a twenty-five-year-old woman whose status as a donor was put on hold as a result of her psychological interview. Her stated reason for applying to be a donor was that she wanted to be a generous person like her mother, who had died fifteen years earlier and to whom she had been very close. Her image of her mother had become quite idealized in the years following her death. During the interview, some important and reveal-

ing information came out. The donor mentioned that she had difficulty sustaining relationships and that she had sought therapy a
year ago in order to get help with this problem. She did not believe
that she would ever have a good relationship with a man or be able
to have a family of her own. The donor added that her therapist,
who was pregnant and about to deliver, had temporarily terminated treatment until after her maternity leave.

Two important realizations emerged from the session. The first
involved the donor's fantasy that her mother would not only
be pleased by her generosity in donating her eggs but that it
would also be a way to ensure that her mother's (good) genetic
material was passed on, since she did not expect to have children
of her own. The clinician suspected that the donor's emphasis
on her mother's "good genes" reflected her own poor self-image
and her fantasy that by this generous act she might become more
like her mother. The second realization was that she was both
angry at her therapist for leaving her alone for three months and
jealous of her therapist's family situation. Ovum donation was
her unconscious way of saying to her therapist, "I'm just as fertile
as you," and "I don't need you to help me make important decisions." This young woman was open to examining these issues
and was able to see that she was motivated, in part, by unconscious reasons that needed to be explored. She agreed to postpone her decision about ovum donation and to discuss it with her
therapist when she returned to work.

Another important part of the assessment interview is making
sure that donors comprehend exactly what it is they are giving
away. Counselors must try to learn whether a potential donor views
her gametes more as blood or more as a person. Those who consider their eggs similar to a person usually screen themselves out as
donors—if not before, then as a result of the interviews.

Program counselors help prospective donors see the long- as well
as the short-term implications of their donation. The counselor
tries to anticipate potential events that might cause them to have
regrets. One way this task can be accomplished is by asking a series
of "what if" questions, similar to the questions asked of known
donors. For example, if a potential anonymous donor has not completed her family, she must think about the possibility that something might happen in the future that would cause her to be infer-

tile. If that unfortunate situation were to occur, would she regret having donated at a younger age?

Donors must think about the possibility that the offspring might want to find them someday. Laws are continually changing, and it is possible that eventually all programs using donor gametes will be mandated to open their records. Prospective donors must also think about the possibility, though remote, of a medical emergency—that an offspring may need to find a match for an organ transplant, and the donor could be contacted.

Potential donors must consider whether to tell their future partner or future children that they had been an ovum donor—or their existing children, if they are already mothers. They must be made aware that their children will have half-siblings in the world whom they will probably never know. They must imagine themselves in the grocery store or in the local mall spotting a young child who resembles them at that age. Would the prospective donor wonder, for more than a passing moment, about whether it was her child?

An important consideration for all donors, regardless of whether their decision will be affected by it, is the reaction of their family. Recently a few "donor grandparents" have stepped forward to share feelings of sadness and loss about having grandchildren in the world whom they will never know. It is important for potential donors to understand that although they themselves may not feel a particular connection to the genetic material they are passing on, other family members may feel differently.

Potential donors must consider how they feel about revealing personal information. Many clinics ask donors to fill out a lengthy questionnaire that inquires about their social, psychological, physical, and medical history, and this information is offered to recipient couples if a pregnancy occurs. Potential donors must be comfortable with the idea of sharing extensive (though nonidentifying) information about themselves.

Each program has its own policy regarding disclosure of information about recipients to donors, including whether a pregnancy has occurred. Some programs refuse to give a donor any information about who is getting the eggs and refuse to inform the donor if a pregnancy occurs, believing that it is in her best interest not to know. These programs feel strongly that if the donor cannot live with uncertainty, she should not be a donor. Other programs leave the choice about receiving that information to the donor, believing that she knows what is best for her. Our initial impression is that most donors, when given the option, like to be informed; they prefer knowing the truth to living with uncertainty. Those who say they do not want to know may be ambivalent about the ovum donor process. It is important to explore their reasons for not wanting to know in the event that unconscious conflicts are revealed.

Of the eighty-two ovum donor programs that participated in Braverman's ovum donation survey, 60.3 percent stated that they had developed specific psychological criteria to reject ovum donors. Although it can be assumed that the remaining programs (39.7 percent) reject donors they feel are psychologically inappropriate, it is not clear on what basis—presumably a subjective one—they are rejected.[11] The Ovum Donor Task Force of the Psychological Special Interest Group of the American Fertility Society has recently developed guidelines for accepting and rejecting ovum donors. They are available through the American Fertility Society. Legal protection is also a necessary reason for donor screening. Litigation in the area of reproductive technology is rare, and there has been no known lawsuit involving either an egg donor program or recipients or donors who have been involved in these programs. However, other cases involving third parties or advanced technology have received significant attention. As a result of these cases and others less widely publicized, ART programs recognize that something could go wrong that could cause irreparable damage to their reputation. Programs hope to minimize the chance of litigation by thoroughly screening both donors and recipients.

The Donor's Experience. When the medical process is completed, most donors report that they did not find it difficult. Their relative ease is probably due in part to the fact that women who fear needles and other invasive medical procedures either do not apply to be ovum donors or screen themselves out when they learn what the process entails. Some programs report that many of their donors volunteer to recycle, which serves as testimony that the process was not too trying. Other programs, however, have reported an unexpected number of donors who have had difficulty with the medical protocols and who appear to be mildly depressed.

During the screening interview, donors sometimes ask about the recipients, but their questions tend to be general. We have found, however, that as the process begins, donors become more curious about the couple (or couples; some clinics divide one donor's eggs between two recipients) receiving their eggs and frequently ask for more information about them. One donor told the psychologist that before beginning the process it was enough for her to know that the recipients were good people who wanted children very badly. Once egg donation became more real, however, she wanted to know more about who would be raising her genetic children. Certain questions, such as "are they religious people?" and "will they have close relatives who will be involved in their lives?" became especially important. The psychologist handled this situation by asking the donor to list a few questions that concerned her. She explored the meaning of these questions with the donor, and then, after consulting with the recipients, answered each of them. The donor, who was seen in a follow-up appointment after the cycle was over, reported that having the information helped her to stop obsessing about the recipients and to put closure on the process.

Some donors never ask about the recipients. It is enough for them to know that recipients are couples who want children and that the program agreed to treat them. Such donors need to separate the process of donating gametes from the people receiving them. Some may fear that they would become too invested in the outcome if they knew more about the recipients. Others worry that the more information they have, the less anonymous the process is.

During the ovulatory phase of the cycle, when donors are receiving daily injections and must report to the clinic each day to be monitored, they receive a great deal of attention and appreciation from the staff. Most donors enjoy being in the spotlight; they know they are providing an invaluable service to infertile couples and, unless the medications are seriously affecting their moods, usually report to the clinic in good spirits.

When the egg retrieval is completed and the donor's immediate obligation ends, some donors go through an unexpected but understandable depression, which may be due in part to the hormonal changes they are experiencing. Some of the depression may also be due to the loss of their special status as egg donor and the attention that it brings. The abrupt change in a donor's demeanor may be puzzling to staff if they have not prepared themselves for this possibility.

Many clinics ask donors to come in for an exit interview with either the counselor or a nurse after the retrieval is completed. This interview offers the donor an opportunity to say good-bye to the staff and to put closure on her experience. It also offers the program an opportunity to learn about her experience so they can better understand and work with future donors. Finally, the interview can help establish a system by which donors notify the programs of significant medical information in years to come.

The Recipients: Psychological Screening and Counseling

There is a double standard when it comes to psychological assessment of couples undergoing ovum donation versus those undergoing sperm donation. This double standard has historical roots that include differences in gender roles as well as biological differences. These differences between men and women, and how they are regarded by society, form the cornerstone of the double standard.

Role of the Mental Health Clinician. Although ART programs have very different standards for acceptance or rejection of donors, virtually all agree that not everyone is psychologically fit to be a donor. In counseling recipients, however, mental health clinicians, as well as the physicians with whom they work, struggle with a basic question about their role: are they gatekeepers or consultants? If they are gatekeepers, their job includes screening potential recipients in or out of treatment. If they are consultants, their job is strictly to offer information to recipients and to engage in a discussion with them about that information rather than to screen them.

Those who oppose gatekeeping point out that no one screens fertile couples; moreover, *they* are not in a position to judge who will be good parents. Counselors who argue this viewpoint also remind professionals that many couples who appear to have their lives in order and are model citizens make poor parents.

Those who feel that counselors should be gatekeepers point to adoption as the model from which they base their opinion. They feel that the best interest of the unborn child should be everyone's primary consideration and that professionals have an obligation to offer their specialized services only to those who would in all probability make good parents. Furthermore, since eggs are scarce, they believe it is morally wrong to give them to couples who are not emotionally equipped to parent. Some professionals also feel a moral obligation to the donor—to do what they can to ensure that a child created from her donated eggs will be parented well.

Most mental health clinicians appear to take a middle-of-the-road position, adopting liberal screening criteria. Unless a serious problem emerges in the counseling-screening interview or unless the recipients screen themselves out, the couple is approved for the program. However, the definition of "serious" depends on the clinician and the clinic. Standards for acceptance or rejection vary greatly from program to program.

The Purpose of Counseling Recipients. The purpose of the counseling-screening interview is to assess the psychological readiness of the couple to undergo ovum donation and to help the couple anticipate both the short- and long-term social, psychological, and ethical implications of ovum donation. In the event that the counselor functions as gatekeeper, the task is also to determine whether the couple is accepted into the program. If the counselor is solely a clinical consultant, he or she can work more actively with the couple to help them decide whether ovum donation is in their best interest.

In assessing readiness for ovum donation, counselors attempt to understand how well each member of the couple—and the couple as a unit—functioned prior to infertility. They explore how the couple has coped with infertility and how it has affected their lives. Other questions investigate support systems, whether they have mentioned ovum donation to anyone, and how and why they decided to pursue it.

The extent to which the couple has grieved the loss of having a biological child together can be an important barometer of their psychological readiness. The following case concerns a woman who was not ready to accept egg donation. During the screening interview, when the social worker noted that their child might look and act very different from her or her husband—and might be much like the donor—the prospective recipient looked puzzled, then said: "Maybe if I'm lucky enough to conceive, my genes will get mixed in while the baby is in utero." After further investigation, the social worker recommended that they think longer about the process and that they take time to acknowledge the loss of having a genetic child together.

The second reason for screening recipients—to help them anticipate potential problems—can be done in many ways, including asking "what if" questions: What if your child someday wants to seek his or her genetic mother? What if laws change, and donor records can no longer be anonymous, and the donor wants to meet your child? Counselors are also interested in whether the couple plans to be open with others about ovum donation and, most important, whether they plan to tell their child about how he or she was conceived.

Expectations About the Donor. Oocytes are difficult to obtain, and most programs do not have a large supply of donors. Even programs that allow recipients to have some voice about their donor are not able to offer them much choice. Nevertheless, it is useful for counselors to discuss with prospective recipients their expectations about the donor. Such a discussion can help the program counselor determine whether they are being realistic in their expectations, and if not, why not. Asking about the donor can also help the team members be as responsive as possible to the couple's request.

Most recipient couples have few expectations or requirements of a donor. They realize donors are scarce, so they cannot be too particular. Moreover, as we will discuss later, most couples plan to be open about their child's conception, and so the need to match recipients with donors in order to mask the truth is not a factor. When asked about their expectations, most recipients say they hope she is a "nice" or "good" person. Couples who are well educated hope for an intelligent donor, and some couples mention physical features, but they are not a primary focus for most recipients. When physical features are mentioned, they usually concern issues of height or coloring.

Asking individuals and couples about their expectations for a donor helps clinicians determine their preparedness for this parenting alternative. For example, one husband stated to the counselor that he wanted the donor to have a curriculum vitae. He then listed the features and characteristics he wanted the donor to have: high intelligence, physical attractiveness, high energy, and ability to understand and use computers (his wife was a computer operator). Although the clinician was initially put off by his requirements and by his attitude toward the donor (he viewed her more like a job applicant than a person providing gametes), further exploration revealed that the husband had not come to terms with the loss of his wife's genes. He had always admired her physical beauty, as well as her intellectual skills and extroverted personality. Finding a woman as desirable as his wife was his unconscious way of attempting to preserve her genes and to deny the reality of their loss. It was also a way for him to stay in control and to maintain emotional distance from their infertility.

In another case, a prospective recipient, seen in consultation with her husband, stated that she wanted very specific physical characteristics, and they were the opposite of her physical appearance. Investigation revealed that she had always felt inadequate and unattractive, and her feelings of low self-esteem had only worsened as a result of infertility. Her fantasy was that the opposite of her would not only produce a perfect child but that it would also fix something in her. The social worker helped this woman recognize that she needed more psychological attention before proceeding with ovum donation.

A final case offers another example of how the counseling/ screening process can reveal a couple's psychological readiness for ovum donation. The recipient seemed anxious about the physical size of the donor. She feared that if the donor was too big, the baby would be too big, and her uterus might rupture. The prospective recipient continued to focus on ways she imagined the fetus could damage her. The clinician was able to help the woman identify her underlying fear that the child would feel like a stranger—that she might never be able to connect emotionally with him or her. After some additional counseling sessions outside the clinic setting, the couple decided they were more comfortable with adoption.

Openness versus Secrecy. Clinicians observe that a much larger percentage of ovum donor than sperm donor couples appear to be choosing to be open with their offspring (and with others) about how their child was conceived. Although there has not been research exploring why this is so (and if it is truly so), we can speculate about the reasons.

Until ovum donation became a reality less than a decade ago, gestation and motherhood were inseparable. Because the woman who carries and bears a child has always been seen as that child's mother, ovum recipients do not seem especially vulnerable to feeling unauthentic. They assume they will bond with the child they carry. In this way, their experience is very different from the infertile man whose wife conceives with donor sperm: he must wait until after birth to establish a relationship with his child.

Additionally, women tend to be more open in our culture about their personal lives. They are accustomed to sharing problems with friends and family and looking to others for mutual support and advice. There may also be less stigma attached to being an infertile woman than to being an infertile man, perhaps because infertility, at least in the greater society, is assumed to be a woman's problem. Thus, women in general are more open about infertility than are their male counterparts, and so it stands to reason that they would be more open about ovum donation than men are about sperm donation.

There is another reason for what appears to be greater openness among ovum donor couples than among donor insemination couples. In Chapter 5 we noted that there may be sexual overtones for some couples electing to do donor insemination. The woman may feel as if she is having an affair or being adulterous, and her husband may have similar feelings. In ovum donation, sexual overtones seem to be absent. Because the woman is receiving an egg—something her body would normally produce—and because an egg is not associated with lovemaking, as are sperm, she does not feel that she is involved in a moral transgression.

As we noted in Chapter 5, the question of openness vs. secrecy is an extremely fundamental, as well as complicated one, involving profound ethical, legal, and psycho-social issues. Historically, sperm donation was almost always done anonymously; this trend, however, appears to be slowly changing. We encourage those couples considering ovum donation to read Chapter 5, in particular, the section on "Openness versus Secrecy, as a means of guiding them.

Whatever couples decide, it is important that they consider, prior to undergoing ovum donation, whether they will tell their child about the conception. If they decide to be open, they must determine at approximately what age they will tell him or her. Counseling can help couples to sort through those issues and anticipate future scenarios.

It is important to keep in mind that couples want to do what is best for their child. Many who would prefer to be open are afraid that in doing so their child will be stigmatized or may suffer in other respects. Others, who would prefer to forget their child's conception and put all references to it aside, feel obligated to be open because they feel that a family secret would be damaging to their child. Like most other couples exploring and undertaking alternative paths to parenthood, these couples recognize that their own desires and preferences may not be in the best interest of their unborn children.

Finally, in meeting with recipient couples, the clinician must be certain they recognize that ovum donation is a lifelong process. The issues underlying this parenting alternative, as well as with others that involve third parties, are highly complicated and evoke intense feelings. A family created as a result of this technology will undoubtedly have hurdles to face. Thus, there is also another purpose to screening and counseling recipients: to establish a comfortable relationship with a mental health professional. This contact is designed to lay the foundation for psychological support and assistance, should they feel a need for it in the future.

Matching Donors and Recipients

One of the most challenging aspects of ovum donation is the 'matching' process. Depending upon the protocol of a given program, this task may be accomplished by one individual (usually the nurse or coordinator) or by a team. In either event, those involved in this modern form of 'matchmaking' find themselves in an awkward position, feeling as if they are "playing God."

Actually, the word 'match' is somewhat of a misnomer, as that term implies a 'fit', or a 'duplicate.' Since everyone has a unique set of genes, there is no possibility of 'matching' one person to another, although sperm banks, with their vast numbers of donors, create the illusion that it is possible. Thus couples involved in donor insemination are sometimes able to 'fool' themselves into believing they have found a perfect match—a donor who seems just like the husband. When it comes to ovum donation—where eggs are scarce—such illusions are not possible.

Those involved in pairing donors and recipients—an individual or a team—take a variety of factors into consideration. They look at physical appearance, trying to avoid obvious mismatches, such as a five-foot blond recipient and a six-foot dark-haired donor. They also attempt to take some personality characteristics into account, aware that many traits once thought to the product of environment are now seen as inherited. Such knowledge increases the anxiety of the 'matchmakers,' although they are also comforted by their awareness that there is never a guarantee that any trait—desirable or undesirable—will be passed on, as children are often very different from their genetic parents.

Some programs use pictures of donors and recipients to narrow the possibilities and to avoid confusing one person with another. Intuition, however, is probably the most important variable in selecting donor-recipient pairs. Many involved in this process attempt to use their "sixth sense" about who fits well with whom, to guide them in the selection process.

Those involved in this task try not to let personal biases get in their way. Nevertheless, they may feel a special connection to a recipient couple and want to match them with a favorite donor. Conversely, certain prejudices may cause them to be reluctant to pair other women together.

Because matching donors and recipients can feel like a heavy burden, many programs are allowing recipients to participate. One way to do this is to find a tentative match (or perhaps two or three) and allow recipient couples to review information about the donor that includes a family medical history, physical attributes, interests, and talents. The recipients have the right to reject any or all of the donors offered, knowing that this may cause a delay, but that sooner or later there will be other donor profiles to review.

Couples who are involved in the selection process not only feel more in control but have an additional opportunity to think about what it means to accept a donated gamete. They must wrestle with questions such as whether they prefer a donor who has a family history of heart disease or a donor whose brother is alcoholic. The process also means that couples must face the fact that there is no perfect donor, just as they do not come with perfect genes. This knowledge may help them to have realistic expectations of their child.

A few programs allow (even encourage) donor and recipient couples to meet. Many programs have found that these open arrangements are extremly satisfying to everyone. Elaine Gordon, a psychologist who works with several ART programs in southern California, commented that the people who appear to be the most comfortable with ovum donation—both donors and recipients— are the ones who participate in open arrangements. She believes that when ovum donation is open, everyone seems less anxious, and the process goes much more smoothly. As the cycle progresses, they tend to voice fewer complaints and appear comfortable with the protocols. When the process is open, she has found, everyone has a sense of peace as well as pride that what they are doing is right for them. Even when the pregnancy test is negative, recipient couples seem more resolved: their feelings are more sad than angry—the opposite of what they usually are for those who have not wanted to meet their donors.[12]

Pregnancy Through Ovum Donation

Although ovum donation places relatively few physical demands on a recipient, it is immensely stressful from an emotional perspective. Most recipients go through the process with a great deal at stake. For some, the cycle represents their last hope for sharing pregnancy and childbirth, and for those unwilling or unable to consider adoption, it is their last chance of becoming parents together. Because so much is at stake and there is so little they can do about it, recipients are understandably anxious. During the first part of the cycle this anxiety focuses on their donor; recipients become increasingly curious about who she is and how she is doing. Although clinics try to schedule appointments so that donors and recipients will not meet in the waiting room, recipients find themselves looking around and wondering if the woman sitting across the room or the one who was leaving as she was arriving is her donor. Later, following transfer, the recipient's anxiety typically shifts to her own body and to what she can do to maximize her chances for successful implantation and pregnancy.

Many recipients have a negative pregnancy test. This news is especially painful for those who come to ovum donation with a history of reproductive loss such as cancer or premature ovarian failure. These women are even more prone to feel that their bodies are defective and have betrayed them once again. Recipients who did not become pregnant may feel a sense of failure and guilt. They know that substantial effort from several people went into producing and obtaining the eggs, as well as creating the embryos. It was truly a team effort, and recipients may feel that they have not only let down their husband but the donor and staff as well. The overriding feeling, however, is profound sadness and loss. Once again their bodies have let them down, and once again their wombs—and their hearts—are empty.

A positive test beckons very different emotions, and about 40 to 50 percent of ovum donation recipients do become pregnant. For many recipients a positive pregnancy test is confirmation that their body is working properly. The news, however, is also received cautiously; couples who have been through long-term infertility know that there are always additional hurdles ahead—medical and emotional ones.

Because pregnancy after anonymous ovum donation is a recent development, there is little extensive clinical expertise to draw upon. We can only speculate, based on our limited experience, that a pregnancy that begins in this new way brings special challenges for the couple—in particular, the woman. The following case explores some of the issues that arise for women pregnant after anonymous ovum donation.

Ms. T. was a forty-three-year-old woman who had been through three years of infertility treatment that included two cancelled IVF cycles (her ovaries had not responded to Pergonal). The patient and her husband were happily married (both for the second time), and she had teenage stepchildren from that relationship. Her biggest regret was that she had waited so long to attempt pregnancy.

When the idea of ovum donation was first presented to her, Ms. T. was hesitant, not because she was uncomfortable using donor gametes but because her body had failed her for so long she could not imagine that it would actually work. Furthermore, the idea of pursuing one more treatment filled her with dread. Nevertheless, she and her husband decided to try it. Ms. T. would have preferred a known donor, but she did not have one. Thus, she approached ovum donation tentatively, disappointed that she would not be able to pass on her family's genes and skeptical that her body would not work properly.

Ms. T. became pregnant during her first ovum donation cycle and reacted with great delight that her body was functioning as it was meant to. Soon after, she learned there was a possibility that she was carrying three fetuses. This information, although shocking (and worrisome), was thrilling as well; a multiple gestation provided more evidence that her body was working.

Ms. T. miscarried one fetus very early on, shortly after it was seen on ultrasound. This loss was not unanticipated (the ultrasonagrapher had not been able to view a heartbeat) and was to some extent a relief. She then unexpectedly miscarried a second fetus at thirteen weeks. This second miscarriage was devastating and one of the pivotal points in her pregnancy. Ms. T. blamed herself for the loss; the miscarriage reconfirmed her sense that her body was defective. Although she believed the eggs were strong (from a twenty-three-year-old donor), her body seemed old and incompetent. Ms. T. now questioned whether she had gone too far in tampering with nature.

Another pivotal point in Ms. T.'s pregnancy occurred when she and her husband discussed amniocentesis. There was no medical reason to undergo this invasive diagnostic procedure, as the odds of the fetus carrying a genetic defect were the same odds as they were for the donor—very, very low because she was only twenty-three. However, emotionally Ms. T. felt a need for the test. So much had gone wrong already that she could not believe she was carrying a healthy child. At the same time she knew that miscarriage as a result of the procedure, though rare, was a risk, and she could not imagine being able to bear the loss of her surviving fetus. In discussing her ambivalence with the therapist with whom she had been in treatment, she became aware that she had other reasons for wanting an amniocentesis: she was increasingly curious about the donor, realizing that she knew very little about her. Having had this insight, she decided against the procedure, realizing that it would not provide her with what she wanted.

Ms. T.'s curiosity grew and intensified when during her last trimester an ultrasound revealed that the fetus was a male. She now found herself wanting information about the donor's father, for he was one of two genetic grandparents who was the same sex as the child. After some exploration with her therapist, Ms. T. realized that she did have information about her son's maternal grandfather; the clinic had supplied her with several details about the donor's family and medical history. It soon became clear, however, that it was not medical facts or physical information that she really wanted. Rather, she was searching for a way to feel that the child truly belonged to her. Because he came from a foreign egg and because he was a foreign sex, Ms. T. was afraid that she might have difficulty bonding with her son. Her request for more information was her effort to ease this anxiety.

Another pivotal point in her pregnancy occurred when Ms. T. and her husband discussed names for their son. Both wanted to name him after their fathers. Ms. T. quickly gave in to her husband, expressing to her therapist that she felt it was more her husband's child. Because it was genetically his, she felt he was more entitled to having his family's name passed on. When she explored this issue, she realized that the speed with which she relinquished her claim on naming him might be an indication that she would also be quick to step aside and allow her husband's views on child rearing to take precedence over her own.

Ms. T. was able to discuss these insights with her husband, who was very sympathetic. Neither of them wanted to raise their child in an environment in which one of them felt and acted like a second-class parent. They eventually agreed not to name their son after either family. Instead, they chose a name they both liked that was not associated with either of their family histories.

Although Ms. T. had an easy and uneventful pregnancy after the loss of the second fetus, she tired easily in her third trimester and became concerned that she would be too tired to take care of the baby. Although these concerns are not uncommon for many mothers-to-be in their third trimester, Ms. T. was again confronted with her feelings about being too old and too defective. She expressed sentiments that the genetic mother would have done a better job and wished that she too was twenty-three—though she quickly realized that at twenty-three she had not been in any way equipped to be a mother.

Just before delivery it was discovered that Ms. T.'s baby was in a breech position and would need to be delivered by cesarean section. Ms. T. was disappointed, and again experienced thoughts and feelings about being defective, about being too old to have a child, and about having tampered with nature. She wondered if the breech position was additional evidence that she was not "meant" to carry a child. These notions, and their accompanying feelings, were short-lived. She was able to acknowledge them and put them to rest much more quickly than she had done previously.

At the end of her full-term pregnancy, Ms. T. delivered a son. He is now a healthy and thriving nine month old. Ms. T. states that she and her husband delight in their son, growing increasingly attached to him as time goes on. Both are relieved that Ms. T.'s fears about bonding have not materialized.

Although we cannot generalize from one woman's experience of pregnancy after anonymous ovum donation to all women, three themes that emerged during Ms. T.'s pregnancy may prove to be common in ovum donation pregnancies. They are themes that we discussed earlier in this section: feeling defective, feeling the child is a stranger, and feeling unauthentic. Through therapy, Ms. T. was able to understand these feelings as well as to gain a handle on them so that she could get on with and enjoy her life as a new mother.

We have seen in this chapter that although ovum donation is the female counterpart of donor insemination, in practice it is both medically and psychologically very different. Donor insemination has historically been surrounded by an aura of secrecy and shame leading to a denial of its occurance as well as prevalence. There has been little psychological counseling offered to DI couples, and virtually no psychological counseling offered to sperm donors. By contrast, ovum donation, though only a few years old, seems to be happening in an atmosphere of far greater openness. Most importantly, there is recognition among professionals in the field that ovum donation (as well as all third party options) are family building methods that have life long implications. If this attitude is conveyed to patients it is likely that they too will approach ovum donation seriously, thoughtfully and respectfully.

Surrogacy

Although it has a prominent place in this book on the new reproductive options, surrogacy is not new, nor is it an outgrowth of the recent advances in reproductive medicine. Rather, surrogacy, the first-known form of third-party reproduction, dates back to biblical times. Then, as now, it raised complex social and emotional issues.

Surrogacy history begins with Abraham and Sarah, the first known infertile couple:

> Now Sarah, Abraham's wife, bore him no children and she had a handmaid, an Egyptian, whose name was Hagar. And Sarah said unto Abraham, "Behold now, the Lord hath restrained me from bearing: I pray thee, go unto my maid: it may be that I may obtain children by her." And Abraham hearkened to the voice of Sarah. (Genesis 16:1–2)

Abraham's decision to follow his wife's advice and to have her handmaiden bear his child provided a solution to their childlessness. Hagar, history's first-known surrogate mother, conceived and gave birth to Abraham's first son, Ishmael. This event, however, did not resolve the pain of infertility for Abraham and Sarah. Instead, Sarah reacted with unexpected bitterness toward Hagar's pregnancy, saying to her husband, "The wrong done me is your fault!"

The Bible goes on to chronicle the problems that continued between Sarah and Hagar. These extended to Sarah's relationship with Abraham and continued even after Sarah gave birth to a long-awaited child, Isaac. Thus, even after Sarah's own prayers had been answered, she remained bitter and said to her husband, "Cast out that slavewoman and her son, for the son of that slave shall not share in the inheritance with my son Isaac."

Fortunately, the vast majority of couples who have turned to another woman to bear a child for them have not experienced the emotional pain that burdened the family of Abraham and Sarah. Nonetheless, their story is prophetic in that it introduces the idea that surrogacy is a complicated process. Sarah was the first, but by no means the last, woman to find that she had unanticipated reactions of jealousy and resentment to the pregnancy and childbirth experience of another woman, even one who was bearing a child for her.

This chapter presents a picture of surrogacy today. Although we recognize, as the story of Sarah demonstrates, that surrogacy is not a solution to female infertility; it is an alternative path to parenthood. However, many families have successfully been built through surrogacy. These families, now numbering over five thousand, are testimony to the fact that surrogacy, practiced with care, is a legitimate family-building option.[1]

In order to understand the status of surrogacy today, an option cherished by some and villified by others, we must look to its history. What becomes evident, in reviewing this history, is that several events conspired to keep surrogacy in a controversial place among reproductive options.

The Development of Contractual Surrogacy

Throughout history, there have been informal surrogacy arrangements between couples and women who were friends, acquaintances, or family members. However, it was not until the mid-1970s that contractual surrogacy became available to infertile couples. In 1977, Noel Keane, a Michigan attorney, made public the fact that he had advertised in college newspapers and found a woman who agreed to carry a baby for a childless couple. His announcement met with extensive publicity, including television and media appearances and magazine features. It was also followed by announcements, from other lawyers, as well as physicians and small business people, that they, too, could assist couples to become parents through surrogacy.[2]

The arrival of contractual surrogacy generated controversy, curiosity, and interest. The controversy, which has continued and intensified in some ways, focused in large measure on the question of the contract: can a woman make and then be held to a preconception and prebirth agreement to place a child?

On one side of this controversy are those who feel that surrogacy contracts represent a reproductive freedom—that surrogacy, like abortion, should be a matter of choice. They argue that it is insulting to suggest that women are incapable of making an agreement and holding to it. Fay Johnson, of the Organization of Parents Through Surrogacy (OPTS), states:

> In order for a woman to become a surrogate she most often goes through a rigorous application process, including psychological tests and physical examinations. Often she must travel, take time off of work, and attend meetings with lawyers and psychologists. Some women will have to go through several months of inseminations before conceiving. When I think of all that's involved, I have a hard time believing that this is a woman who doesn't know what she is doing! I have an even harder time with people who think that they know what is best for her and who imply that she is incapable of making informed decisions for herself![3]

William Handel, founder and director of the Center for Surrogate Parenting in Beverly Hills, California, also objects to the notion that a woman entering into a surrogacy contract is being exploited. Handel emphasizes that surrogacy contracts, which he has worked hard to develop, go to considerable lengths to protect the rights of all women participating in surrogacy. Today's contracts, unlike earlier ones which placed emphasis on producing a baby, compensate women for their time and energy and clearly stipulate that consent to relinquishment is not a precondition for payment.[4]

Despite these changes in the contracts, critics of surrogacy still argue that it is unreasonable to expect a woman to know how she will feel about placing a child whom she carries before she is even pregnant. They point to the experiences of women who intend to place their babies for adoption and then change their minds late in pregnancy or after birth. These critics fail to acknowledge, however, that surrogates, like birth mothers in adoption, can change their minds. A child born to a surrogate can be relinquished only with her consent and with the state social worker's approval.

Michelle Harrison, assistant professor of psychiatry at the University of Pittsburgh School of Medicine, is an outspoken critic of surrogacy:

> The last time in the history of the United States that human beings were bred for transfer of ownership was during slavery. Slave women bore babies, some of who were fathered by the slave owners themselves. Not since slavery have we attempted to institutionalize the forced removal of infants from their mothers—except in cases of abuse or clear lack of fitness.[5]

But Harrison fails to acknowledge that surrogacy does not involve forced removal of infants from their mothers. A more balanced approach to contractual surrogacy comes from the American College of Obstetricians and Gynecologists (ACOG), which supports a woman's right to enter a surrogacy agreement but stresses that certain measures must be taken to protect her reproductive freedoms during and after pregnancy:

1. She should have the right to make decisions during the pregnancy.
2. She should be the source of consent with respect to clinical intervention and management of the pregnancy.
3. The contract should include provisions for such contingencies as: the pre-natal diagnosis of a genetic or chromosomal abnormality, the inability or unwillingness of the surrogate to carry the pregnancy to term, the death of a member of the commissioning couple or the dissolution of their marriage during pregnancy, the birth of a handicapped infant AND the decision of the surrogate to retain custody of the infant.[6]

Frank Chervenak, director of ultrasound and ethics at New York Hospital, and Laurence McCullough, of Baylor College of Medicine, also support a woman's right to participate in surrogacy as long as she is protected during her pregnancy. They regard the fetus as a patient and oppose any provisions in the surrogacy agreement that would require or forbid diagnostic or obstetrical management during the course of the pregnancy. They write:

> Thus, any provisions in a surrogacy contract calling for antenatal diagnosis or abortion before viability or restricting either are ethically unfounded. That is, the commissioning couple is under an ethical obligation to the pregnant woman to respect her autonomy, based on her right to control her pregnancy before viability.[7]

The Introduction of Paid Surrogacy

Noel Keane's 1977 arrangement introduced both the idea of a surrogacy contract and the concept of payment for surrogacy. This payment, intended to serve as compensation to the surrogate for her expenses and inconveniences before, during, and immediately following pregnancy, became a source of tremendous controversy.

Critics of surrogacy have a twofold—and somewhat contradictory—argument regarding payment. On the one hand, they charge that fees for surrogacy are so large that poor women will be exploited by being induced to sell their bodies or their babies. At the same time, these critics acknowledge that the fee, when seen in terms of an hourly wage, is insultingly small. Gena Corea, a feminist writer, is a harsh critic of surrogacy. She calls surrogates "breeders" and suggests that surrogacy will lead to an "international traffic in women" in which poor women will be coerced, by financial need, to bear children for wealthy women. (Her prediction, made nearly nine years ago, has not come to pass.) Corea expands her argument that poor women will be exploited by pointing out all the physical and emotional risks that a woman undertakes to receive a mere $10,000 (the standard fee at the time *The Mother Machine* was published).[8]

Surrogacy supporters remind others that some of the first women to become involved in surrogacy did so without any thought of payment. They point out also that the fee—currently about $12,000—is not a sizable amount considering all that is involved. If a woman's primary interest was financial gain, she could surely find an easier way to make $12,000 than to serve as a surrogate. They add that it is sexist to expect women to do so much for no payment and wonder what the fee would be to a man were the situation reversed.

In an effort to address the issue of coercion and to avoid the risk of exploitation, some have suggested that there be minimum income guidelines for surrogates. However, many supporters of surrogacy object to this idea, saying that it would discriminate against poor women, and it implies that they are incapable of making reproductive decisions for themselves. Each of these arguments finds itself on a slippery slope supporting one side of the payment debate while inadvertently supporting the other.

Surrogacy in Court

The controversy that surrounds surrogacy was heavily fueled by two widely publicized legal cases that arose following surrogacy arrangements. It is important to note that only eleven of the over 5,000 surrogacy births to date have resulted in litigation. Nevertheless, the cases raise disturbing issues that must be examined and resolved in order for surrogacy to remain a viable family-building option.

The first case to put surrogacy in the public eye was the Malahoff-Stiver case in 1983, a surrogacy arrangement by attorney Noel Keane.[9] It had several troublesome features; perhaps the most damaging of these was that the disputing parties, Alexander Malahoff and Judy and Ray Stiver, chose to take their personal conflicts public and to air them on national television.

The Malahoff-Stiver surrogacy arrangement first went awry when Mr. and Mrs. Malahoff, the contracting couple, separated during their surrogate's pregnancy. This fact prompted questions about the stability of couples who enter into surrogacy arrangements, as well as the potential stress that such arrangements may place on marriages.

The second problematic aspect was that Mrs. Stiver, the surrogate mother, gave birth to a baby with microcephaly, a condition that is often associated with retardation. Mr. Malahoff refused to accept the baby, claiming that he was not the genetic father. Then he and the Stivers decided to settle this very personal question on national television. Hence, it was on the "Phil Donohue Show" that Mr. Malahoff and the Stivers learned that Mr. Malahoff was correct: Ray Stiver was found to be the genetic father of the baby. The Stivers reacted to this news by agreeing to take the baby home and raise him.

The case remained in litigation for several years. In September 1992, a federal appeals court in Cincinnati ruled that Mrs. Stiver could sue Noel Keane for negligence. She charged that he should not have allowed her to be artificially inseminated with Mr. Malahoff's semen without having Mr. Malahoff go through a thorough medical screening. Mrs. Stiver contended that her child's handicap may have been the result of the transmittal of cytomegalovirus through Mr. Malahoff's semen.

The Malahoff-Stiver case prompted charges that couples turn to surrogacy in pursuit of "a perfect baby." Surrogacy practitioners refute these charges, emphasizing that the couples they work with are reasonable people, with reasonable expectations. Like all other couples, they hope to have healthy children, but as veterans of years of frustration and loss, they also understand that the world is not perfect and that no pregnancy comes with the guarantee of a healthy child.

Steven Litz, director of Surrogate Mothers, an agency providing surrogacy services in Indianapolis, states that he occasionally encounters couples who are looking for what he terms genetic manipulation (a surrogate with 'perfect' genes). He notes that such couples are easy to identify and stresses that any responsible surrogacy practitioner would exclude them from participation in surrogacy.[10]

The Malahoff-Stiver case also prompted charges that couples seeking surrogacy do not have stable marriages (or do not have marriages that can withstand the stresses of the surrogacy process). Again, surrogacy practitioners take issue with this charge. Hilary Hanafin, clinical psychologist at the Center for Surrogate Parenting, stresses that most of the couples she sees demonstrate strong, resilient relationships that have been tested—and retested—by years of infertility. Gerry Tarlow, a clinical psychologist and director of Solutions, a surrogacy program in Los Angeles, agrees and emphasizes that he and other practitioners have a responsibility to accept only couples who are likely to remain married and committed to parenting together.[11]

The second case to put surrogacy in the national spotlight—again in its worst form—was the famous Baby M case in 1985, which generated even more attention than the Malahoff-Stiver case. This was a very different dispute: both sets of parents wanted the baby.[12]

The Baby M case pitted Mary Beth Whitehead, a married, working-class mother of two and a surrogate mother, against her contracting couple, Bill Stern, a research scientist, and his wife, Betsy, a pediatrician. Betsy, who suffered from multiple sclerosis, turned to surrogacy because pregnancy can exacerbate the symptoms of this chronic illness.

The Sterns and Whiteheads entered into a surrogacy agreement through Noel Keane's program. In preparation for the program, Mrs. Whitehead underwent a psychological evaluation with Joan Einwohner. Dr. Einwohner's report, which was never shared with either the Sterns or Mrs. Whitehead, expressed concerns about accepting Mrs. Whitehead in the program. Dr. Einwohner was specifically troubled by the fact that Mary Beth indicated that she wanted to have more children.

Unaware that the psychological evaluation had raised serious questions, the Sterns and Mrs. Whitehead went ahead with their surrogacy plan. The pregnancy was healthy and uneventful, but by the third trimester, it became clear that Mrs. Whitehead was having difficulty emotionally with the process. This difficulty intensified when she gave birth to a baby girl, whom she named Sara (the Sterns had named her Melissa).

Although Mary Beth Whitehead initially placed the baby with the Sterns, she changed her mind within weeks and began efforts to gain custody. These efforts took the case into the courtroom, where it drew tremendous media attention. Some of that attention focused on the obvious class differences between the Sterns and the Whiteheads, with some criticizing Betsy Stern for being a career woman and others scorning Mary Beth Whitehead for the choices she made.

In addition to court-appointed psychologists and psychiatrists, who were called in to make a determination about what was in the best interest of the child, the Baby M case attracted several self-appointed experts. These included a group of feminists and the Combined United Birthparents, an advocacy group for birthmothers. Both groups, as well as others critical of surrogacy, defended Mrs. Whitehead's right to change her mind after birth and to parent the child born to her. They were opposed by equally passionate adoptive parents' groups and others who sought to defend Mr. Stern's right to parent his child, as well as Betsy Stern's rights as an adoptive mother.

The Baby M case was initially tried by Judge Sorkow, who decided the case on the basis of what he found to be in the child's best interest. He terminated Mrs. Whitehead's parental rights and awarded custody to the Sterns stating, "The Sterns and Whiteheads have different life styles, social values and standards. The rancor is too great. This court doubts that they can isolate their personal animosity and 'all of a sudden' cooperate for the child's benefit."[13]

The Baby M case did not end with Judge Sorkow's decision. Mrs. Whitehead took her appeal to the New Jersey Supreme Court. Once there, the case put surrogacy on trial. No longer a private tragedy between two sets of parents, it now became a debate about the meaning of pregnancy and motherhood. Once again, groups with opposing points of view argued about women's rights, reproductive freedom, and the validity of contracts.

Although it raised many difficult issues, the one that was of most concern to everyone interested in the Baby M case was that of the best interests of the child. Critics of surrogacy argued that it is never in a child's best interest to know that he or she was the product of a contract. They charged that surrogacy is a form of baby selling and stressed that knowledge of the contractual arrangement would be detrimental to the surrogate's other children, as well as to the child born through surrogacy.

Supporters of surrogacy challenged these criticisms by saying that surrogacy produces children who are very much wanted and loved and who would not have an opportunity to live if it were not for the surrogacy arrangement. Surely this was in their best interest. They added that experience had shown that children of other surrogates did not perceive the baby born of surrogacy as their sibling but rather they saw it—from the start—as the child of another couple.

In 1986, a group of former surrogates formed the National Association of Surrogate Mothers. As advocates for surrogacy, they explained their reasons for participating in surrogacy, described the positive experiences that they had had, and addressed the ethical issues of reproductive freedom. They explained that they saw surrogacy, like abortion, as an issue of choice and that they objected to being characterized as "breeder" women.

The New Jersey Supreme Court reached its ruling on the Baby M case in February 1988. It reversed Judge Sorkow's opinion and stated that existing adoption laws applied to surrogacy arrangements. Consequently, the birthmother—in this case, Mary Beth Whitehead—could not receive payment and could not be held to a prebirth decision to surrender her parental rights. The court then designated her the baby's legal mother but awarded custody to the Sterns.

The Need for Legislation

The Baby M case had a dramatic and continuing impact on the practice of surrogacy. Even now, nearly ten years later, the mention of surrogacy prompts comments about the case. The general public remembers it well and has been left with the impression that surrogacy is a risky and highly problematic venture.

Although it is unfortunate that the Stern-Whitehead dispute left such an indelible negative mark on surrogacy, the case did present compelling evidence of the need for legislation. Efforts to draft effective laws that preserve reproductive freedoms, protect women from coercion, and, above all else, serve the best interests of children, have met with limited success.

Several states have enacted laws concerning surrogacy. Much of this legislation focuses on the contract, with twelve states (Arizona, Florida, Indiana, Kentucky, Louisiana, Michigan, Nebraska, North Dakota, New York, Utah, Virginia, and Washington) voiding paid surrogacy contracts and some voiding unpaid contracts as well. Couples remain free to enter into surrogacy contracts but must be aware that their agreements will not be upheld if contested. Other surrogacy legislation addresses payment to surrogacy practitioners (with several states prohibiting compensation for facilitating surrogacy arrangements); the question of who are the legal parents of the child (with some states assuming that the contracting couple are the legal parents of the child and others assuming that the surrogate and her husband are the child's legal parents); and providing for medical and psychological screening of surrogates and couples and requiring that contracts be submitted to a judge prior to any attempt at pregnancy.

Clearly there is need for further legislation, especially addressing four essential issues.

Who Should Practice Surrogacy?

The original surrogacy practitioners were primarily lawyers and physicians who entered the field without backgrounds in psychology or child welfare. Although their intentions may have been honorable—a desire to help infertile couples create families—they were probably naive about the emotional and social complications that might arise. The Malahoff-Stiver and the Stern-Whitehead disputes illustrated the need for a practice that is carefully regulated and adheres to predetermined guidelines.

In its policy statement on surrogacy, ACOG recommends that "surrogate parenting arrangements be overseen by private, non-profit agencies with credentials similar to those of adoption agencies."[14] ACOG is referring here to the fact that adoption agencies must abide by clearly delineated state laws in determining who can adopt a child and in providing counseling and other services to birthparents. Hagar Associates, in Topeka, Kansas, for example, is a fully licensed adoption agency, and it applies the guidelines of adoption practice to all of its surrogacy placements. Nancy Hughes, program director, states:

> Our being a licensed child placement agency gives us some standards and connects us, in several important ways, to the tradition of adoption practice. We find that both couples and surrogates are comforted by this and that it gives us additional credibility in the community, as well as in the legal system. For example, because we do a home study on all prospective parents, and because we are required to keep permanent records, there is some assurance that we are doing all that we can to act in the best interest of children.[15]

Who Participates in Surrogacy?

Closely related to the question of whether rich women (or men) will exploit poor women through surrogacy is the question of who pursues surrogacy and why. Although some critics have charged that there are couples who will employ surrogates for convenience—in order to avoid the discomforts of pregnancy—surrogacy practitioners report that virtually all couples who apply demonstrate clear medical need for surrogacy. The women are either infertile or have medical or genetic conditions that make pregnancy inadvisable. In fact, the current standard of practice in surrogacy is to make medical need a criterion for acceptance into a program. Beyond medical need, most surrogacy practitioners limit this arrangement to heterosexual couples who appear to be in stable relationships.

What If the Surrogate Wants to Keep the Child?

It is extremely rare for a surrogate to change her mind. William Handel, director of the Center for Surrogate Parenting, notes that the Baby M case is testimony to how unusual it is: "If there were a lot of surrogates changing their minds then Mary Beth Whitehead's decision would not have received such attention. The fact is that surrogates very rarely change their minds."[16] Others agree, saying that it is much more common for the surrogate to worry that the couple will change their minds and leave her with the baby.

The Center for Surrogate Parenting had 269 births (as of May, 1993), and no surrogate changed her mind. Nevertheless, it can happen, so legal provisions must be made for this possibility. A few states have passed legislation that attempts to address the question of who are assumed to be the legal parents.

Of special significance to this question was the California Supreme Court's May 20, 1993, ruling in the case of *Anna Johnson v. Calvert*, in which a gestational carrier, Anna Johnson, attempted to gain custody of the child whom she carried for Mark and Crispina Calvert. The Supreme court, like the lower courts, ruled in favor of the Calverts. What was noteworthy about the ruling was that the court went much further in supporting the rights of couples involved in surrogacy. It made few distinctions between traditional and gestational surrogacy (gestational care), stating that it is the intent of the parties involved in surrogacy that will determine parental rights. In a statement that had implications for surrogacy as well as gestational care, Justice Edward Panelli recognized payment to the surrogate as "compensation for her services in gestating the fetus and undergoing labor, rather than giving up 'parental rights.' "[17]

Who Can Be a Surrogate?

In an effort to protect women from being hurt or victimized by surrogacy, legislation should clearly spell out criteria for participation in a surrogacy program. In addition to certain objective criteria, most professionals involved in surrogacy believe that an extensive psychological evaluation should be required for all prospective surrogates.

Fay Johnson of OPTS emphasizes that very few women are suited to be surrogates, and it is realistic, rather than demeaning, to identify those people who are unsuited. She notes that there are criteria for the practice of law, medicine, accounting, etc. Similarly, according to Johnson, there should be criteria for becoming a surrogate.

The Development of IVF: Its Impact on Surrogacy

When surrogacy became available in the mid-1970s, a substantial number of infertile couples were interested in this option. Many found that the increased accessibility of abortion and the acceptance of single parenthood had vastly reduced the number of healthy white infants who were available for adoption. Couples who sought to parent a white infant welcomed surrogacy as a potential pathway to their goal. They felt that it had several advantages over adoption: they would know the birthmother, be relatively certain that she had good prenatal care, and have the opportunity to be involved in her pregnancy.

Surrogacy also had the advantage of creating a child who was genetically connected to half the couple. Those interested viewed surrogacy as the long-awaited equivalent of donor insemination. They argued that since couples who suffered from male infertility could have a child that was half biologically theirs, then infertile women with fertile husbands should also have this option. Welcoming the opportunity for some genetic continuity, as well as the chance to know and select their child's birthmother, couples turned to surrogacy with interest and cautious enthusiasm.

The arrival of IVF in 1978, just two years after contractual surrogacy began, altered the history of surrogacy. Many couples who might otherwise have pursued surrogacy instead turned to IVF, which offered them the possibility of experiencing a pregnancy and having a child genetically connected to both of them. IVF was costly and difficult to accomplish medically, but many preferred it to surrogacy. In addition to offering the couple a full genetic and gestational connection to their child, it also eliminated any of the legal questions associated with surrogacy.

IVF led to the development of two other advances in reproductive medicine that had special appeal to certain couples who might otherwise consider surrogacy. Once eggs could be fertilized outside the body, there was no reason that genetic and gestational motherhood could not be separated in those instances in which a woman had lost part of her reproductive function. In other words, IVF made it possible for a woman who could not produce eggs to become pregnant with an egg that was retrieved from another woman and fertilized in vitro (with the intended mother's partner's sperm). Similarly, it was now possible for a woman who could produce eggs but could not carry a pregnancy to have her eggs retrieved, fertilized in vitro (again, with her partner's sperm), and then transferred to the uterus of a gestational mother.

Ovum donation, the transfer of eggs from one woman to another, first became available in 1984. Couples who would otherwise have pursued surrogacy but were now candidates for ovum donation saw this new option as having several advantages over traditional surrogacy: the couple could share a pregnancy together, make all the decisions regarding prenatal and obstetrical care, and avoid the legal questions involved with surrogacy. The child born to them would not have to be adopted. Futhermore, they saw it as a family-building option that offered them more privacy than they were likely to feel with surrogacy. Finally, the financial costs were less.

Gestational care, commonly referred to as gestational surrogacy or host-uterus surrogacy, first became available in 1986. (Gestational care is the subject of chapter 8.) This option, which some opponents of traditional surrogacy tend to view as a minor variation of surrogacy, represented a significant opportunity for infertile couples. Unlike other alternative reproductive options—donor insemination, ovum donation, and traditional surrogacy—which all involve the donation of gametes, gestational care offered infertile couples the chance to have a full biogenetic child. Many recognized it as raising far fewer ethical questions than other alternative paths to parenthood and welcomed it as a much-needed medical treatment.

Had the ARTs, including ovum donation and gestational care, not come along on the heels of surrogacy, undoubtedly more attention would have been paid to establishing laws and guidelines for surrogacy practice. However, these new options diverted people's attention; they saw clear advantages to choosing IVF and some advantages, depending on their medical condition, to choosing either ovum donation or gestational care. The result was that relatively few couples pursued surrogacy.

Changes in the Field of Adoption: The Impact on Surrogacy

The decrease in the number of infants available for adoption was another change that affected surrogacy. This decrease was caused by the increased availability of birth control, by the 1973 U.S. Supreme Court decision of *Roe* v. *Wade* in which abortion was legalized, and by the gradual lifting of the social stigma regarding single motherhood.

The late 1970s and the 1980s brought increased awareness of and sensitivity to the experiences of adoptees and birthparents. The old myth that birthparents were able to place their children in the hands of adoption agencies and then move on in their lives without looking back, and the accompanying myth that adoptees had no need to know about their birthparents, were discarded. A new appreciation for the significance of genetic ties and for the emotional investment of birthparents replaced these myths.

This new appreciation increased the awareness of professionals in the field of adoption to the profound losses shared by all members of the adoption triad: the birthparents, the adoptee, and the adoptive parents. The increased understanding of these losses prompted many people to look more cautiously at surrogacy and to view the surrogacy triad as very similar to the adoption triad. Michael Grodin, professor of medicine and ethics at Boston University School of Medicine, has drawn several comparisons between adoption and surrogacy. He raises concerns about couples and surrogates entering into an agreement regarding the placement of the child prior to that child's conception. Agreements of this nature have the potential, Grodin cautions, to complicate a child's identity formation. Adoption is always complicated, even when parenting arrangements are "resolved at birth," and the child's later concerns about lineage, as well as about biological and social parentage, can become paramount.[19]

Another way that changes in adoption affected surrogacy involved the use of language. Prior to the 1980s, the language surrounding adoption promoted negative feelings about the adoption process and about all members of the adoption triangle. Adoptees were labeled "adopted children" even as adults. Birthparents were referred to as "real parents" (suggesting that the adoptive parents were not real) or "natural parents" (implying that the adoptive parents were not natural). Children were said to have been "given up," "given away," "put up," or "surrendered" for adoption. Patricia Irwin Johnston, a nationally respected professional in the field of adoption, makes this point repeatedly. She attempts to raise people's consciousness by reframing the terminology into positive adoption language. For example, birthparents now make "an adoption plan" and families are "built" through adoption.[20]

Heightened appreciation for the power of language has caused people to question the language of surrogacy as well. Supporters and critics of surrogacy alike have challenged the use of the word *surrogate* to describe the role of the woman who conceives, carries, and delivers a child. Critics of the practice have asked why she is not simply termed "the mother" or pejoratively referred to as "the breeder."[21] Supporters of surrogacy have struggled to find more constructive language, such as *pre-birthmother* or *birthing mother*.

The language of surrogacy is complicated by the fact that there are now two very different reproductive options—both frequently identified as surrogacy—one in which the surrogate bears her genetic child and the other in which she bears the genetic child of another woman. These options are genetically very different, and because having a genetic link to one's offspring is a major part of parenthood for many would-be parents, we will refer to traditional surrogacy as *surrogacy* and the process by which one woman carries another couple's full genetic child as *gestational care*.

In addition to changes in language, the 1980s brought increased openness in adoption. The old practice in which the birthparents and the adoptive parents received little, if any, information about each other was replaced in most agencies by a greater willingness to share information among all parties. The practice of 'Open Adoption,' whereby the two sets of parents meet and may or may not be given identifying information about each other emerged.

The shift toward contact between birth and adoptive parents has extended to the practice of surrogacy. We need only compare "Elizabeth Kane's" account of her experience as a surrogate in *Birthmother* with a recent cover story from People magazine. As an early surrogate, Kane was given a pseudonym and allowed to have only minimal contact with the contracting couple. By contrast, the *People* story celebrates the close relationship that developed between a television star and her look-alike surrogate. As this story implies, contact between contracting couples and surrogates has come to be supported, encouraged, and facilitated by many programs.[22]

Who Seeks Surrogacy?

The availability of the ARTs coupled with the fears provoked by surrogacy's troubled history and its continued state of legal ambiguity have limited the number of couples who choose to become parents through surrogacy. Nevertheless, there remain a significant number of couples who give careful consideration to this option.

Most couples who consider traditional surrogacy begin with little understanding of the process, and many have no idea where to begin to gather information. Although years of infertility have taught them to act, to explore, and to persevere, surrogacy represents uncharted territory. And although repeated disappointments have prepared them for further bumps along their difficult road to parenthood, surrogacy may seem far more frightening.

OPTS can help couples begin their exploration. In addition to keeping an up-to-date list of professionals who are involved with both surrogacy and gestational care, OPTS members serve as telephone volunteers. They answer questions and provide explanations about different approaches to building families through surrogacy. Contact with OPTS members removes much of the mystery from the surrogacy process and reassures hesitant couples that surrogacy and gestational care, are indeed viable options.

Most people seeking surrogacy are married, childless couples. Many are veterans of years of unsuccessful infertility treatments or of repeated pregnancy losses. By and large, they come to surrogacy having exhausted all other available options for biological parenthood. Some have first tried gestational care.

Some couples prefer surrogacy to adoption because it offers them the chance to have a child who is the genetic offspring of the father. Critics of surrogacy view this motivation harshly, saying that it comes from a sense of machismo and reflects male egotism rather than the desire to become a father. What these critics fail to address, is that many people have deep feelings about genealogy. For some, there is pride, perhaps tied to feelings about particular relatives who are part of their lineage. For others, who have suffered the loss of a cherished family member, there is a strong need to carry on the family bloodline by adding another member to the next generation. Still others feel a need for genetic ties that is based on their religious or cultural background. Finally, there are those who experience feelings that are less specific: an existential longing to bring a new life into the world.

Other couples choose surrogacy because they want the opportunity to select their child's birthmother. Infertility has left them feeling powerless over their destiny, and they feel that adoption comes with too many unknowns (this is changing to some extent with the proliferation of open adoptions). Surrogacy offers them a way to gain some control over having a family. They look forward to contact with their surrogate throughout her pregnancy and anticipate being present at their child's birth. (According to Hilary Hanafin, psychologist for the Center for Surrogate Parenting, 85 percent of the couples working with her center are present at the delivery.)[23]

Finally, there are couples who pursue surrogacy because they view adoption as unavailable to them. Being over a certain age, being married less than a certain number of years, or a recent history of serious illness are all criteria that can disqualify some people for adoption.

Who Becomes a Surrogate?

Although payment is a factor in a woman's decision to become a surrogate, it is rarely the only motivation. Most women have other reasons as well for making the decision. In studying eighty-nine women who had participated in a surrogacy program, Hilary Hanafin found that the two most frequently stated reasons for wanting to become a surrogate are the enjoyment of being pregnant and the desire to help childless couples. Similarly, Philip Parker, a psychiatrist who studied the first 125 applicants to a surrogacy program, found that although many were motivated by financial compensation, most identified other personal and altruistic reasons for choosing surrogacy.[24]

Women seeking to become surrogates often speak positively of their personal experiences with pregnancy, labor, and delivery. They say that they felt "happy" and "fulfilled" during pregnancy and enjoyed uncomplicated deliveries. Many add that as much as they like being pregnant, they are not prepared to add another child to their families at this time.

Prospective surrogates also speak of their compassion for infertile couples. Often they have had a friend or relative who has gone through infertility or pregnancy losses. Having been exposed to the pain that a childless couple endures, these women feel inspired to help. They see bearing a child as a way that they can help and have personal satisfaction at the same time.

Dr. Hanafin found that many of the surrogates she studied said that they loved being mothers and that they decided to become surrogates because they could not imagine life without children. Others added that they felt they had not yet done anything remarkable or made an impact, and this was an opportunity to do something of major significance—something that would surely make a lifetime difference for someone else. Some said that they had been very young when they had experienced their first, and often unplanned, pregnancy. They looked forward now to the opportunity to plan a pregnancy and to undertake it with more understanding of the process, a greater degree of control, and a sense of wisdom and maturity.[25]

Dr. Hanafin and others have found that there are woman who have borne children yet were once told that they were infertile. Having lived with the fear, but having been spared the reality of infertility, some say that they feel a responsibility to help those who have not been so fortunate. Similarly, we have spoken with surrogates who did experience infertility or pregnancy loss before successfully building their families. These experiences had a lasting impact on them; they were drawn to surrogacy hoping to reduce the pain of a childless couple.

Finally, some women decide to become surrogates because they are attempting to make amends for past losses. This reparation may be either conscious or unconscious. For example, women may turn to surrogacy because of unresolved feelings about past abortions or having placed a baby for adoption. In Parker's 1983 study, 35 percent of the surrogates reported they had had an abortion or placed a child for adoption.[26]

Psychologists involved in evaluating women for surrogacy pay careful attention to evidence that a woman is trying to undo a past loss through surrogacy. They try to help such women to see that although the surrogacy experience might prove healing in some ways, there is also the risk that it will become yet another loss, intensifying previously unresolved problems. Although some women with histories of abortions, and even some who made adoption plans for other babies, will be accepted for surrogacy, those whose central motivation seems to revolve around this earlier loss will be discouraged from participating in surrogacy.

Reproductive losses are not the only losses that a woman may be trying to reconcile either subconsciously or unconsciously when she decides to be a surrogate. There are women who have experienced rape, incest, or some other trauma, who may be hoping to repair damaged self-esteem through surrogacy. And due to the insidious nature of sexual abuse, there are survivors of childhood abuse who may unconsciously allow themselves to be further exploited when they are adults. It is therefore important that the screening process include a careful assessment of this issue. Although those who support surrogacy are quick to point out that it is a woman's choice about what to do with her body, they are not suggesting that this choice extends to doing psychological harm to herself.

When asked how they can carry a child and then place it with another couple, many surrogates respond by saying that they do not regard the child as their own. Some refer to the bond they feel with their husbands and state that in order for a child to be theirs, he or she has to be a child that they have with their husband. Being inseminated with another man's sperm is a very different process, and they consider the resulting child to be his child and that of his infertile wife. Many add that the egg from which the child was conceived would have otherwise been wasted and they believe they are putting it to good use by using it to bring a child to an infertile couple. As one former surrogate said, "The child could only exist because of the union and love of the infertile couple. It was created in their spirit, dreams and hard work. It was always meant to be their baby."

Another question that is frequently posed to prospective surrogates involves bonding. Assuming that bonding, a strong, unbreakable connection between mother and child, begins in utero, people often ask how surrogates can place the infants they have carried. Dr. Hanafin has found that most surrogates say that a form of bonding does occur, but primarily with the expectant parents, not with the baby:

> It is hard for me to find words to describe the relationship that developed between us. It didn't happen all at once, but grew over time and with the pregnancy. And although it happened among the four of us, it was most powerful between us—the two women. The bonds forged over our many phone calls, our lunches out, and most of all, our visits to the doctor, are strong, solid, and lasting.[27]

Although this may be a coping strategy in that surrogates may consciously or unconsciously strive to heighten their connection with the couple in an effort to diminish their connection to the child, it appears to work.

Cristie Montgomery, a former surrogate and now the director of Surrogate Parenting Services in Laguna Niguel, Californa, focuses on the meaning of the word *expecting*. She observes that in surrogate pregnancies, it is not the surrogate who is expecting but the woman who intends to raise the child.[28]

There have been accusations that surrogacy represents a two-class system: poor women have babies for wealthy couples. In fact, financial differences usually do exist between the two groups, but they are rarely as pronounced as has been charged. Dr. Hanafin and others have found that surrogates tend to be middle- and working-class women who are married, employed, and have completed high school and some college. Dr. Hanafin has participated in a few surrogacy arrangements in which the surrogate and her husband had higher incomes than the couple with whom they were working.[29]

Another charge leveled against surrogacy is that women who become involved in it are unstable and therefore cannot appreciate the significance and possible consequences of their decision. Dr. Hanafin addressed this question by administering the Minnesota Multiphasic Personality Inventory (MMPI) to a group of women following their surrogacy experience. The MMPI is a frequently used and empirically validated psychological test that provides measures of certain personality variables and screens for psychopathology. The results confirmed Dr. Hanafin's clinical impressions that the vast majority (98 percent) of the women were psychologically healthy individuals without significant psychopathology.[30]

Dr. Hanafin takes issue with the fact that surrogates have been described as breeder women who allow themselves to be exploited. This has not been her experience; the women whom she has known are strong, bright, clear-thinking, empathic, responsible individuals who have initiative. Most have established a clear sense of self by the time they are in their mid to late twenties and combine this sense of self with an ability to be other-centered. Dr. Hanafin adds, "Where I walk the fine line is when I fear a woman is too other centered—I need her to have a strong inner core so that she can make good decisions for herself."[31]

Dr. Hanafin also takes issue with the lack of attention and respect that is paid to the husbands of the surrogates, whom she identifies as the "unsung heros of surrogacy" and describes as "thoughtful, supportive, and non-possessive." Usually they love children, have a good sense of humor, and offer their wives tremendous support in this endeavor. "After all," she says, "there is self selection. What man will take a day off of work to talk about menstrual periods and cycles."[32]

Many women who initially express interest in surrogacy do not go on to carry a baby for another couple. Some drop out when they realize all that is involved or when they encounter serious opposition in their families. Others screen themselves out later in the process when they find that the experience is more stressful and demanding than they had imagined it to be. Finally, many are turned down from programs because something troublesome surfaces in their clinical interview, the psychological testing, or their medical exam. William Handel, director of the Center for Surrogate Parenting, reports that only one of every sixteen women who apply to his program goes on to be a surrogate.[33]

How Surrogacy Is Practiced

Couples who decide to pursue parenting through surrogacy find that there are many different ways to go about it. Nancy Hughes, of Hagar Associates, in Topeka, Kansas, observes that each program has its own personality, based, in large measure, on how and by whom it was founded. Hagar Associates, founded by social workers, continues to have strong ties to social work practice and this is reflected in several aspects of its program. Similarly, programs that were founded by lawyers tend to reflect this background in their practice.[34]

Interested couples can begin by contacting the Organization of Parents Through Surrogacy, an independent, volunteer-staffed organization that has no ties to a particular program or practitioner. Hence, it can provide couples a range of options, with objective information and observations about each. OPTS members serve as telephone counselors, providing couples with first-hand accounts of their experiences with surrogacy.

Couples who prefer predictability in terms of cost, time frame, and outcome will probably find that they are more comfortable working with a large, comprehensive surrogacy program. These programs offer a wide range of services, including locating and screening surrogates, psychological counseling for couples and surrogates, legal counsel, and medical expertise. Larger programs also have the benefit of experience; having worked with many other couples and surrogates, they know what they can do to make the process easier for all parties. An example of a large program is the Center for Surrogate Parenting. It offers gestational surrogacy and ovum donation as well as traditional surrogacy. It works with approximately seventy couples at a time, dividing them among its three professional counselors.

Some couples find that they are more comfortable working with a smaller program. Although there may be less history to inform them and probably fewer surrogates to work with, couples appreciate the personal connection they feel with a small staff that is involved with only a few surrogates and couples. An example of a smaller program is Solutions in Los Angeles, directed by Dr. Gerry Tarlow and Dr. Nan Tarlow, clinical psychologists who became involved in the practice of surrogacy after their own successful experience with a surrogate. The Tarlows work with only five couples at a time, so that they can be closely involved with each situation.

Finally, some couples prefer to undertake surrogacy individually. This may mean working with lawyers who are experienced with surrogacy but who do not offer a full-service program. These attorneys may help couples to locate surrogates and will have experience with surrogacy contracts but do not offer psychological, medical, and insurance services necessary to complete a surrogacy arrangement. Although many couples have successful outcomes when they undertake surrogacy in this way, this process does carry with it more risks than participation in an experienced program. These risks include the possibility of unexpected medical or legal expenses (an advantage of working with a program that provides all the services at a set fee is that costs can be predicted), the possibility of insurance problems (surrogacy programs are experienced in working with insurance companies and can help couples and surrogates avoid situations in which a surrogate pregnancy is excluded from medical coverage), and the chance that the surrogate or the couple will be insufficiently prepared for or supported through the psychological challenges of surrogacy (since there are very few mental health professionals who are experienced with surrogacy, a couple working independently might have difficulty locating a counselor who is skilled in this area).

Fay Johnson, director of National Headquarters for OPTS, cautions people about undertaking individual arrangements in an effort to save money. They may save the money that would otherwise go to administrative costs, but the legal, psychological, and medical costs in surrogacy add up rapidly, even when all is going smoothly.[35] Couples who enter a pay-as-you-go situation may be surprised by how many unanticipated costs they encounter.

For many couples financial considerations are a key factor in their decision making. Some want to compare surrogacy costs with those of adoption, since they are also investigating that option. Others are more concerned about the ethical issues associated with surrogacy and want to make sure that they will not become involved in a process that could be viewed as baby selling.

Although there are variations in the cost of surrogacy, the range is approximately $25,000 to $45,000. The surrogate generally receives a $10,000 to $15,000 fee for her time and effort; the remainder of the fee covers legal and psychological services to both the couple and the surrogate, medical insurance and clothing allowance for the surrogate, and the administrative costs of the surrogacy program. The surrogate also receives reimbursement for extra day-care costs, lost wages, and travel expenses. Additionally, the couple must figure in the amount of lost wages and travel expenses that they will incur.

Couples selecting a surrogacy program can be confused about expenses since some programs present itemized charges and others, such as the Center for Surrogate Parenting, are inclusive. Therefore, it is important that couples considering surrogacy take a careful look at what their total costs will be. For example, since medical complications can occur, it is critical that a couple understand the extent and limits of the surrogate's medical insurance policy (or work with a program that handles this for them).

In an effort to help couples avoid unnecessary costs and other potential pitfalls, the Center for Surrogate Parenting offers consultation to couples considering surrogacy, even if they are not planning to go through the center. During the four-hour consultation process, couples can meet with Handel, Dr. Hanafin, and the administrative staff and can learn a substantial amount about the legal, medical, and financial aspects of surrogacy.

Although there are many ways of approaching surrogacy, there are three steps that all couples must take prior to attempting conception:

1. Locating a surrogate.
2. Medical and psychological evaluation for themselves and their surrogate.
3. Legal consultation for themselves and their surrogate.

Locating a Surrogate

Couples who decide to locate prospective surrogates on their own do so by combining word of mouth with newspaper and magazine advertisements. Most find that if they are persistent, they are able to find a woman who seems suited to work with them as a surrogate. Many such women say that they had actually been considering surrogacy for a long time but had not known how to go about it until they came across the advertisement.

Couples going through established programs or working with lawyers who help to arrange surrogacy do not have to advertise on their own. Spared the stresses and strains of telephone calls or letters from strangers, they review profiles of women who have been accepted in their program. The information that contracting couples receive about the surrogates varies among practitioners, but all provide couples with some social, psychological, and medical background on the surrogate, as well as a physical description.

How couples and surrogates decide to work together varies considerably, depending on whether the couple is going through a program or working it out on their own. A couple working independently will probably select their first-choice surrogate before she has undergone medical or psychological evaluation. Therefore, it is possible that they will face a significant disappointment early in the process: they may choose a woman, feel enthusiastic about working with her, and then be advised against it for medical or psychological reasons.

By contrast, couples working with programs that locate surrogates usually consider only women who have already been cleared medically and psychologically. For example, at the Center for Surrogate Parenting, couples do not see a profile of the surrogate until she has completed 90 percent of the screening process. Hence, they are spared time and effort, as well as the potential frustration and disappointment that would arise if the surrogate they selected was not accepted into the program.

Although most couples and surrogates appreciate having the opportunity to pick each other, there is often a psychologist or other skilled person involved in the matching process. For example, Dr. Hanafin, who has brought together several hundred couples and surrogates, tries to introduce only couples and surrogates whom she feels are likely to work well together. She and her associates look for shared values, similar personalities and belief systems, and people who seem to approach situations in similar ways. They have found that surrogates, like couples, have highly individualized interests and needs, and the counselors try to be responsive to everyone's requests whenever possible.[36]

Cristie Montgomery, of Surrogate Parenting Services, expresses similar views. She feels that "there is someone for everyone" and cautions against trying to put people together who have little in common. Experience has taught her that even when a surrogate or a couple has a concern or request that seems highly unusual or even odd, there is usually someone who feels comfortable working with her or them.[37]

An important part of the matching process involves determining that surrogates and couples have shared expectations regarding the pregnancy, labor and delivery, and contact following birth. For example, couples who expect frequent communication with their surrogate during pregnancy need to work with a surrogate who has a similar expectation. Similarly, those who expect to stay in touch with their surrogate in years to come need to be matched with a woman who agrees that their relationship will not end with the birth of the child.

Special attention also needs to be paid to the possibility that there can be something wrong with the fetus. Before a couple and a surrogate can agree to work together, they must be in agreement about whether the surrogate will undergo an amniocentesis and if so, under what circumstances, if any, they would decide to abort the fetus. They must discuss the possibility that other medical or psychological situations could arise that might prompt the surrogate to seek an abortion. For example, she could develop a medical problem the treatment of which is complicated by pregnancy. Although not all such circumstances can be anticipated, it is important that the couple and the surrogate—together with their psychologist or social worker—review several "what ifs." This review will help them determine whether they are likely to respond to unexpected events in similar ways.

Evaluation of Surrogates

Surrogacy programs vary in the criteria that they use for acceptance into their programs. We are including criteria here that we feel represents a sound standard of practice.

Medical Criteria. Nonsmokers who are over the age of 21 and who have children are considered for surrogacy. Other criteria are that a woman be in good general and reproductive health, with no evidence of genetic or sexually transmitted diseases. Extensive family histories are taken in order to assess the risk of serious hereditary disorders.

Psychological Criteria. Psychological assessment of a prospective surrogate takes her determination into account. While determination is a positive factor, indicating that she is someone who knows what she wants to do, it may also prompt a surrogate to try to camouflage things about herself that she fears might cause her to be rejected. The clinician faces the challenge of developing an alliance with a prospective surrogate that will enable her to examine the process honestly and to carefully think through whether surrogacy is truly in her best interest.

Psychological assessment addresses two central questions:

Is she an emotionally stable individual?
Is she psychologically prepared to be a surrogate?

Since surrogacy involves complex and challenging physical and emotional tasks, some of which may extend years beyond the pregnancy, women who serve as surrogates should be emotionally stable and resilient. Being a surrogate is not a time-limited experience. It is an experience that she will never forget and that will remain part of her history regardless of whether she continues to have contact with the child and the family. A surrogate will always be the genetic and gestational mother of someone she did not parent, and that someone may want further contact with her for a variety of reasons.

The MMPI-2, a widely accepted psychological assessment tool, is often used to evaluate prospective surrogates. However, Donna Robertson of the Center for Surrogate Parenting in Beverly Hills, who uses the MMPI-2 in her practice, finds the Rorsharch, another widely respected psychological test, a more valuable tool in assessing surrogates. The Rorsharch, which is a projective test, gives a great deal of insight into an individual's personality, as well as their emotional and intellectual processes. In addition, it can predict the extent to which people respond objectively to their environment versus their own unconscious process. Robertson finds the Rorsharch especially helpful in evaluating prospective surrogates. She looks specifically at the way in which a woman responds to unexpected stresses and to crisis, hoping to include only women who can remain calm and clear thinking should unexpected difficulties arise.

In addition to testing, a psychologist will assess the extent and nature of the potential surrogate's coping skills. Discussions about her history, including mental health issues, sexual relationships, reproduction, drug and/or alcohol use, and social connections, can provide important information about her stability and about how she copes with the vicissitudes of life.

Preparation for Surrogacy. A woman may be a responsible and stable individual but unprepared to be a surrogate. Therefore, it is critical that time be spent exploring her understanding of surrogacy and her reasons for wanting to undertake this process. The psychologist must determine if surrogacy is something that she has thought carefully about and whether she has considered some of the ways in which the experience might prove difficult for her. If she has not thought about potential difficulties, it is important to understand why not and to get assurance that she is capable of exploring this issue in depth. Information as to whether she is naive, ill informed, or acting impulsively is essential, and a surrogate would be screened out if she were.

In determining preparedness, it is crucial that the psychologist try to understand why a woman wants to be a surrogate and how she feels it will affect her life. Other questions that must be explored are how much of her motivation is altruistic or conversely, financial and how much of her motivation may be an attempt to "undo" prior losses, especially reproductive ones. The psychologist needs to explore each of these areas so that the prospective surrogate does not act primarily on an unconscious motivation, which she may later regret.

Although there is no "good" or "bad" reason to become a surrogate, psychological exploration can help determine if a woman's reasons are likely to be good or bad for her. It is important that a woman try to anticipate how she will feel in years to come, after she has completed her surrogacy experience. In other words, it is crucial that her reasons for wanting to be a surrogate are later validated by her experience, rather than her experience as a surrogate making her more vulnerable to psychic injury.

Part of the psychologist's role is to try to talk a prospective surrogate out of surrogacy. As paradoxical as this sounds, hearing arguments about potential pitfalls can help her to decide whether surrogacy would be a mistake that could have long-term negative repercussions. Or she may conclude that she can live with (and accept) the difficulties that could ensue. In other words, while hoping for a positive outcome, she must be well prepared for potential pain. The clinician must be supportive of her right to change her mind, helping the prospective surrogate to see herself as acting responsibly and maturely should she decide not to go ahead with surrogacy.

Some of the questions that a psychologist should encourage a surrogate to examine include the following:

1. *In years to come, will I look back and feel that the child I birthed was mine? If so, will I have regrets? Will I feel guilty?* Although no one has a crystal ball with which to predict the future, it is crucial that a surrogate consider the extent to which she might bond with the baby during pregnancy, and therefore experience intense feelings of loss upon relinquishment. If she has had other children, it will be helpful to think about when and how she bonded with them—primarily in the gestational stage or during infancy. She must try to imagine herself as an older woman and think about whether she will wonder about the child or about grandchildren she may never know.

2. *Is there something that could happen in my life that might change the rightness of this decision?* Life is unpredictable. In order to help protect herself from later looking back with regret, the surrogate should try to think of circumstances that might prompt her to regret her decision, for example, how she would feel if one of her children became seriously ill or died. Would this sort of tragic event cause her to look back, reexamine her earlier decision, and feel she made a serious mistake?

3. *Am I prepared to handle the potential social consequences of my decision to become a surrogate?* Even the most informed surrogates may not have considered the complexity of the undertaking. Consequently, it is crucial that the psychologist assume an educational as well as an evaluative role, introducing a series of "what ifs" to the surrogate. For example, has she acknowledged the possi-

bility that: (1) she may not get pregnant, (2) she may conceive and then miscarry, (3) she may have an ectopic pregnancy (which could compromise her future fertility), (4) she may give birth to a handicapped child, (5) she may discover after amniocentesis that she is carrying a defective child? The surrogate must also consider that the pregnancy could place significant stress on her marriage, her relationships with her children, and her work and/or her relationships with colleagues and friends. Her responses to each of these possibilities can indicate the extent to which she has thought through this undertaking.

The psychologist must look specifically at the social context in which the prospective surrogate lives. Since surrogacy is stressful in some ways, it is essential that she have an active and reliable support network available to her. Although a large program, with a varied staff and several other surrogates, can provide some of that support, it helps for her to have people in her personal life who value what she is doing. This support is even more important for the surrogate working on her own or with a small program.

In her 1989 study, "Surrogate Mothers' Grief Experiences and Social Support Networks," Kathy Forest studied thirty-two surrogate mothers following their pregnancies. Her findings underscore the importance of social support, especially from husbands, during and after a surrogacy experience. The women she interviewed spoke of the importance of support from family and friends. This support was essential to them because there were times during their pregnancies when they felt ostracized.[38]

The psychological evaluation includes the surrogate's husband or partner in order to confirm that he not only understands why she wants to become a surrogate but is able to be supportive of her decision. He is asked whether he has considered the possible ramifications of the decision, in terms of their marriage and family life and in terms of possible health risks such as a bed-rest pregnancy, a multiple gestation, a pregnancy loss, or an obstetrical emergency. He is reminded that he will probably face questions and criticisms from others who will query him as to how or why he agreed to let his wife conceive and carry a baby for another couple. He is further alerted to the fact that some of these comments may involve negative insinuations about the insemination process and may make insulting references to the fact that his wife conceived with another man's sperm. Finally, he should be asked to consider how he might feel toward the baby, who will be the half-sibling of his children, as well as his wife's genetic offspring.

4. *How will my children understand my actions now and in the future?* A prospective surrogate should consider how her children understand her decision to have a baby for another couple. It is important that she remind herself that their reactions to the idea of a surrogate pregnancy may differ from their feelings when pregnancy has been established. Similarly, they may have unanticipated reactions following the birth of a child, as well as in years to come. Although they may see it now as an act of kindness and a way to help childless couples, they may also feel that their sibling was given away.

A prospective surrogate should consider her children's experience not only from the perspective of loss (the loss of a sibling) but also from the perspective of their security. Might this experience raise uncertainties for them about their own permanency in the family? It is essential that she consider how this decision may compromise or blur their sense of family boundaries.

The prospective surrogate needs to discuss whether she intends for her children to have any ongoing contact with their half-sibling, and, if so, it needs to be confirmed with the contracting couple. Dr. Hanafin has known couples who have felt strongly that their children should remain in touch with the surrogate's children, seeing this contact as an important part of their development. By contrast, other couples have wanted distance, feeling that the contact would be confusing to their child. It would be tragic if children wanted and expected to see their half-sibling and were refused the opportunity to do so.[39]

In helping the surrogate assess her children's needs, a psychologist should explore their social context. She should ask the surrogate and her partner if they will encourage their children to tell their friends, schoolmates, and teachers about their mother's pregnancy. If so, has the surrogate and her husband or partner considered how they will support and guide the children, should they encounter unkind or unsettling questions and comments? It is important that they not instruct their children to lie or to avoid others, since both reactions are likely to promote a sense of shame and dishonesty.

5. *How will I feel when the pregnancy is over, when I am no longer doing something so special?* Psychological preparation for surrogacy involves reminding a woman that a surrogate pregnancy is a time-limited event and that when it is over she will no longer be in a position of doing something that is so different and special. To the extent that attention and admiration have been part of her motivation for surrogacy, it is crucial that she be prepared for the letdown she may feel when the pregnancy is over. Careful discussion and consideration of what it means to be in the limelight and then out of it may help her to avoid feeling cheated by the experience, especially when she is also dealing with separation from the couple and the baby, as well as with postpartum hormonal changes.

The psychologist can help the surrogate to look at the larger context in which she lives. She must consider whether she lives in a community that is likely to be respectful of her decision and her privacy or whether her neighbors and community associates are likely to be judgmental and antagonistic. She must think about what it will be like for her to guide and support her family when they are confronted by negative attitudes and opinions about her decision.

In addition to in-depth interviews with a psychologist, prospective surrogates meet with other surrogates. At the Center for Surrogate Parenting, these meetings occur in support groups: all prospective surrogates are required to attend support group meetings before meeting a couple. These meetings provide women with firsthand knowledge of the surrogacy experience.

Evaluation of the Couple

Couples considering surrogacy generally undergo less evaluation and screening than do prospective surrogates. This discrepancy is by design: many practitioners do not wish to be gatekeepers. They feel that it is unfair to make infertile couples prove they will be fit parents when fertile couples are put to no such test.

Although it is true that fertile couples do not have to prove themselves in order to become parents, there is well-established precedent in adoption for the assessment of prospective parents.

The guiding principle in adoption, as it should be in surrogacy, is to act in the best interests of the child. Although critics of surrogacy would argue that it is never in the best interest to conceive and carry a child "for the explicit purpose of relinquishing the child to another at birth,"[40] supporters of surrogacy have a very different perspective. They believe that to bring a child into a home where he or she is wanted and will be loved is in the child's best interest.

Applying the "best interest" standard to surrogacy means determining that the prospective parents are likely to provide the child with a stable and loving home. Some surrogacy programs, such as Hagar Associates, are also licensed adoption agencies and conduct a formal home study with all couples who apply to them. In its policy statement on surrogacy, the American College of Obstetricians and Gynecologists firmly supports this approach:

> For the near future, surrogate parenting arrangements should be overseen by private nonprofit agencies with credentials similar to those of adoption agencies. Such agencies should seek to ensure that the interests of all involved parties are adequately protected. The agencies should conduct confidential counseling and screening of candidate surrogates and candidate commissioning parents. Their primary goal should be to promote the welfare of the future child, as well as the welfare of any existing children of the surrogate.[41]

Although many commissioning couples do not undergo a formal home study, there are criteria used for acceptance into a surrogacy program.

Medical Criteria. Since the surrogate will be artificially inseminated with the husband's semen, it is essential that he be screened for sexually transmitted diseases. The husband should also have a complete semen analysis since it is important to have a current assessment of his fertility.

Both members of the couple should have physical exams to confirm that they are in good health. Just as they have a right to know about the health of the surrogate, she has a right to know of any existing or suspected medical problems with the contracting couple. The risk in not providing her with pertinent medical information is that she may feel cheated or misled if she later learns of a medical problem.

Finally, couples participating in surrogacy programs are encouraged to have the husband undergo a genetics consultation to assess the potential for birth defects. This is recommended even when there is no known risk of congenital abnormalities.

Psychological Criteria. Psychological evaluation of commissioning couples attempts to identify people who should not become parents through surrogacy and those who are not prepared to undertake surrogacy. The former group includes people who exhibit serious psychopathology and those who have substance abuse problems. The latter group includes couples who remain unresolved about their infertility experience or have not clearly thought through their second-choice decision making. Although some of these couples may eventually be suited for surrogacy, the psychologist needs to help them understand that they are not yet ready to move ahead with this option. Some will be bringing medical efforts to a close; others will need to grieve their infertility more actively.

As with a prospective surrogate, the psychologist will try to determine whether a couple is prepared to do surrogacy and the extent to which they are in agreement about the process. Couples are seen together and separately. In the individual sessions, the psychologist can get a sense of how each partner feels about surrogacy; are they equally enthusiastic about pursuing this option, or has one member pushed the other to do something that he or she questions? For example, a woman feeling guilty about her infertility and fearing that her husband will want to leave her might urge him to try surrogacy, anticipating that this "solution" will assuage his disappointment, as well as her guilt.

The decisions surrounding surrogacy can try even the most stable marriages. Conjoint meetings can provide important information about the strength of a relationship. The psychologist can see how they communicate and resolve conflicts and can get a clearer sense of their shared history, especially concerning their infertility and how they have coped with this crisis. Some relationships are so conflict ridden that couples should be turned away from the surrogacy program; identifying them is but one goal of this exploration.

Equally important is to help essentially stable couples anticipate, understand, and prepare for their potential vulnerabilities in the surrogacy process.

As in the interviews with the prospective surrogates, the psychologist should review a long series of "what ifs." These unlikely but plausible outcomes remind couples that even the most carefully laid plans can go astray. Having experienced disappointment and frustration, it is important that they be reminded that this undertaking cannot promise to spare them further loss.

The couple, like the surrogate, is entering into uncharted waters. Therefore, they too need substantial support. An important part of the screening process is to help the couple assess their relationships with family and friends with regard to surrogacy. They need to discuss how important people in their lives view surrogacy and to consider how their decision may affect these relationships.

Finally, the psychologist should attempt to get a clear sense of the couple's expectations of the surrogacy process. It is important that they think through the kind of relationship they wish to have with their surrogate and the degree of involvement they want with her pregnancy. Dr. Hanafin has found, for example, that some couples are "hypervigilant" and have difficulty trusting as they go through the process. They tend to have so many questions and worries that they create tension in the relationship with the surrogate. Other couples tend to be more removed, preferring to let the surrogate manage her own pregnancy and wishing to remain more distant from her. Both groups can be challenging to work with, but Dr. Hanafin has found that it is usually the more distant couples who are the more difficult to work with. Their aloofness can be upsetting to their surrogate, leaving her feeling depleted and unappreciated. Given that a relationship with a surrogate lasts at least ten months, and more often fifteen months, couples need to be comfortable with some form of contact.[42]

Legal Counsel

Although most states do not have statutes that prevent couples and women from entering into surrogacy contracts together, there are ten states in which existing contracts will be considered void if the surrogate changes her mind (Arizona, Florida, Indiana, Kentucky,

Louisiana, Michigan, Nebraska, North Dakota, New York, and Utah). Furthermore, it is unlikely that a court of law in any of the other states will hold a contract binding if the surrogate changes her mind. This situation is similar to adoption in that a woman who agrees, prior to birth, to place her baby with a couple is free to change her mind after giving birth. In other words, prebirth placement contracts are not legally binding.

If this is the case—that a contract is good only as long as both parties are in agreement—one might wonder why so many people go to the trouble and expense of entering into surrogacy contracts. Susan Crockin, a Massachusetts lawyer specializing in reproductive law, sheds some light on why such contracts can be extremely helpful regardless of whether they will ultimately hold up in court. Crockin observes that the process of legal negotiation forces people to think through each aspect of their decision and helps them to determine the degree to which they are truly in agreement. Entering into a contract emphasizes the seriousness of the endeavor and alerts people to some of the disappointments that they may encounter.[43]

Most surrogacy practitioners work closely with lawyers or are lawyers themselves. In addition to the legal assistance provided by the program, most encourage their surrogates, and sometimes their couples, to secure independent counsel. Legal consulting offers them additional assurance that they are not being coerced or otherwise misled. Couples participating in a surrogacy program in another state may need to hire a lawyer in their home state to do the legal work to ensure that the wife will be the child's legal parent. In most instances, this involves a stepparent adoption shortly after the child's birth.

The Process of Pregnancy and Birth

Attempting Pregnancy

Once a surrogate and a couple have entered into an agreement and the surrogate has been tested to confirm that she is not already pregnant, inseminations begin. Depending on where the couple and the surrogate live, this can be a complicated process. In some instances, the couple delivers the semen to the surrogate, who inseminates herself. Other arrangements span long distances and involve freezing and shipping sperm (although the use of frozen semen lowered the pregnancy rate in the past, many programs are now using a special test yolk buffer for the transport of semen and report improved pregnancy rates).

Although husbands have been tested for HIV, the only way to be certain that the sperm is disease free at the time of insemination is to freeze it and retest the man several months later. This is not commonly done, since it will delay the process, but some surrogates insist upon it.

For an infertile couple who has gone through years of medical treatments, working with a surrogate means a shift in their expectations about pregnancy. Having come to assume failure, they are now in a position to expect success; the presumption is that the surrogate is fertile. Infertile couples, however, have a long history of being disappointed, so many approach surrogacy with only cautious optimism.

Some surrogates do become pregnant easily. When this happens, couples have a range of reactions. Some are startled, having been conditioned to failure. Others may experience a tinge of sadness, feeling that the wife's infertility now stands in stark contrast to the husband and the surrogate's fertility. None of these reactions is unusual, and overriding them are feelings of happiness and enthusiasm.

One of the advantages of having psychological support throughout the surrogacy process is that the psychologist can offer helpful advice to both couples and surrogate. For example, Carol Wolfe of the Center for Surrogate Parenting makes several suggestions to couples about how to structure their relationship with their surrogate. She recommends that they be in contact with her at least twice a month while she is attempting conception and at least three or four times monthly during early pregnancy. It is important for her to hear from both members of the couple and also important for her husband or partner to be included in many of the contacts. Dr. Hanafin encourages them to celebrate the news that she is pregnant, preferably in person, but with flowers and a card if they live at a distance.[44]

When the surrogate does not conceive after a reasonable length of time (six attempts), everyone is upset. They wonder whether the problem is in the insemination process itself (e.g., improper handling or preparation of semen or poor timing) or whether there is an undiagnosed male factor. They may begin to wonder about the possibility that the surrogate herself has impaired fertility. The couple then faces a dilemma: should they investigate possible problems in the surrogate or husband, or both, or seek out another surrogate? The latter decision is certain to bring with it some feelings of guilt on the part of the couple. The surrogate may share some of these feelings, particularly guilt over not having come through for them. According to Dr. Hanafin, 15 percent of the couples that she works with will have to meet a second surrogate because their surrogate did not conceive.

It is helpful to have an experienced person who can offer support and guidance to all parties. Efforts can be made to minimize the feelings of failure that are inevitable in both surrogate and couple. At a time of disappointment, they may need to be reminded that they did all that they could to make the process work.[45]

The Pregnancy

Most surrogates do become pregnant. Following conception, couples and surrogates enter into a new phase of their relationship. This time can be full of great excitement and satisfaction, but it also brings additional concerns. It is important that the couples, the surrogates, and their partners have psychological support available throughout the pregnancy.

The stresses that arise in a surrogate pregnancy vary and cannot be predicted. However, one inevitably is present, especially in the first trimester: the fear of pregnancy loss. The surrogate is not at increased risk for pregnancy loss, but miscarriage occurs in approximately one in five of all pregnancies. Since this pregnancy was a hard-earned one, fears of loss are heightened for all involved.

Cristie Montgomery has personally experienced miscarriage in her attempts to build her own family and in her experience as a surrogate. As director of a surrogacy program, she has also observed other surrogates and their couples deal with miscarriage. She reports that since it is the infertile couple who is "expecting" the baby, it is they who suffer the major loss. In her own experience, she recalls feeling very different emotions when she lost a baby whom she expected to parent, than when she lost the baby whom she expected to place with the infertile couple. In the latter instance, she remembers feeling sad but associates much of this sadness with her feelings for the couple and for their loss.[46]

Hilary Hanafin advises surrogates and couples to contact the program rather than each other if they have any concerns about the pregnancy. She encourages couples to try to keep their concerns about the health of the pregnancy to themselves and asks that they not speak frequently with their surrogate about their fears of loss. Extensive discussion about miscarriage might make the surrogate feel pressured and more vulnerable. Couples who need additional support regarding this issue can talk with a physician or a mental health professional.[47]

Although media attention has focused on the fear some couples have that their surrogate will change her mind and try to keep the baby, the surrogates too may be frightened that the opposite nightmare will occur: the couple could change their minds and leave her with a baby she is not prepared to parent. Hence, it is very important that couples not only be in frequent contact with their surrogates throughout the pregnancy but that they also let them know how much they look forward to the baby's arrival. For example, discussion about furnishing a nursery offers reassuring evidence that they are eager to provide a home for their new baby.

Like other expectant parents, couples may worry that something will go wrong. Although in all likelihood the baby will be born healthy, those who have experienced infertility are conditioned to disappointment and loss. Having worked so hard to achieve this pregnancy, they are vulnerable to further heartache. Once again it is important that couples not discuss these fears at length with their surrogate, who is already coping with the normal physical and emotional challenges of pregnancy.

In addition to the ongoing availability of an experienced clinician, some programs have organized peer support for surrogates. For example, Steven Litz, of Surrogate Mothers Inc., has established an informal "big sister" program within his agency, which he feels is of great support to the surrogates. He and his staff notify former surrogates about new pregnancies and ask that they be in touch with the current surrogates. The newly pregnant women are relieved to have their feelings and experiences validated by women who have gone through the process before them. Additionally, this arrangement offers women who have completed their surrogacy experience the opportunity to remain involved in the process. Those who were motivated primarily by altruism welcome the chance to support others who are helping infertile couples.[48]

The amount of contact that a couple and surrogate have during pregnancy varies from one couple-surrogate pair to another. There are also variations among programs; some programs promote contact, others discourage it, and still others allow the preferences of both parties to determine the amount of contact they will have. What is most important is that couples and surrogates have shared expectations and that all are comfortable with the level of contact that they maintain.

The Birth

Most couples want to be present at their child's birth. This event gives the couple the opportunity to bond from the beginning, and their surrogate the opportunity to participate in, and feel gratified by their joy. Although unexpected events, such as a very early or rapid labor or an unavoidable travel hindrance, sometimes conspire to prevent new parents from being in the delivery room, most make every effort to be there.

Couples and surrogates appreciate having practical help regarding their hospital stay, since this is a new and unfamiliar experience for each of them. They need information about stepparent adoption (in many states this is the requisite procedure so that the adoptive mother can assume parental rights), circumcision, birth certificates, pediatrician contacts, and car seats.

Many couples and their surrogates also welcome guidance regarding their evolving relationship, especially if something unexpected occurs, such as an obstetrical problem or a birth defect. However, since even couples and surrogates for whom all goes smoothly are in uncharted territory, it is helpful to have advice from their agency. The Center for Surrogate Parenting offers its couples a series of recommendations regarding the days and weeks following birth:

1. Couples should spend at least several hours at the hospital with their surrogate and baby. This time provides them with

an important opportunity to share their joy with their surrogate and allows her to see—first hand—how much the baby means to them.

2. New parents should introduce themselves to the hospital staff. Although there may be some people who are unfamiliar with surrogacy—or possibly even antagonistic to it—experience has demonstrated that many hospital staff members are eager to be helpful and inclusive.

3. Couples should stay in the town that the baby is born in for a minimum of two days. This helps the surrogate to have a chance to get some closure on the experience. During this time she needs not only to see them with the baby, but also to have her children see them with the baby.

4. Couples should give their surrogate a gift before leaving. This gift should be something that will last and which will provide her with an on-going reminder of their gratitude.

5. Couples and surrogates should make a specific plan about when they will next be in contact. This plan may include telephone calls or in person visits, depending on geography as well as personal styles and preferences.[49]

After Delivery

Psychologists working with surrogates and couples have observed changing relationships between them in the period following delivery. Although most agree that bonding has occurred between the surrogate and the couple—not between the surrogate and the baby—they see this bonding as taking different forms. Some couples and their surrogates have frequent telephone contact, especially in the first few weeks. Others need to establish some distance, possibly sending a note or some photographs regularly. Some new mothers turn to their surrogates (who are experienced mothers) for information and guidance; others need to be independent in order to establish their authenticity as mothers. What is most important during this time, as during the pregnancy, is that the couples and surrogates are in agreement regarding contact. When they are not, one or the other is likely to feel disappointed or even abandoned.

Although most couples and surrogates experience loss as they move away from the intense experience that they have shared, many also feel a mutual need to decrease their contact after the first year. At that point, the relationship usually takes the form of a correspondence, with letters and photos exchanged once or twice yearly. However, some couples and surrogates develop and maintain a much closer ongoing relationship.

Perhaps the most important determinant of whether the couple and surrogate maintain a relationship that includes visits and family get-togethers is the extent to which the surrogate and her children want to know the couple and their child. This issue must be discussed in advance, so that the couple, the surrogate, and the surrogate's husband have shared expectations about ongoing contact between the children. Some see contact as important for the well-being of their children; others feel that an ongoing relationship would be confusing.

Regardless of the degree of contact between them, most surrogates and couples following delivery move to a new phase in their lives. For the couples, there is the adjustment to parenthood; they are delighted to have a child to love and nurture. Some report that they proudly tell total strangers of their child's miraculous beginning. Others attempt to maintain more privacy by saying little or nothing about the circumstances of their baby's birth. Some even say that their baby is adopted, feeling that this half-truth is the best way to protect themselves and their child from intrusive questions.

For the surrogate, the months following delivery offer both opportunities and challenges. One opportunity is that she now has more time and energy to focus fully on her own family. Many report that the experience has given them increased self-confidence, and they are now able to pursue new ventures in their lives, such as schooling or a new career. But they also face the challenges of dealing with the loss of the special experience, the loss of the baby, the separation from the couple and the program, and the physical changes that are inevitable in the postpartum. Some must also deal with criticism for their participation in surrogacy. For the thirty-two former surrogates studied by Forest in 1989, social ostracism and negative media attention were the most difficult aspects of the surrogacy experience.[50]

Surrogates cope with feelings of loss following pregnancy in a variety of ways. Some become involved in another cause or project. Others volunteer or seek paid positions in their surrogacy program or become involved in surrogate parenting in some other way. For example, some are members of OPTS. Some surrogates begin to think about having another baby for the same couple or another couple.

Many couples also think about having a second child with their surrogate. When the relationship has been good, as it usually is, couples are eager to attempt another pregnancy. As Fay Johnson describes it, they see their surrogate as someone who "walks on water" and hope that she will agree to work with them again.[51]

For the surrogate, the decision about whether to have a second baby often depends on timing. Her life schedule and theirs may be in synchrony, making this something she can and would like to do. However, there are also instances in which the parents are eager to expand their family and their surrogate is not able or ready to undertake another pregnancy.

When a couple desiring a second child works with a new surrogate, or when a surrogate enters into an agreement with a second couple, each can experience some disappointment. Couples and surrogates report having such happy associations and memories of their first surrogate pregnancy that a second experience—with a new couple or surrogate—can be a letdown. However, Dr. Hanafin has also known surrogates who found their first experience somewhat mediocre and decide to have a second surrogacy pregnancy, hoping that it will be more satisfying.[52]

OPTS has surveyed its members regarding their ongoing contact with their surrogates. Although it was a small sample, many of their findings were interesting, including:

- 100 percent of their respondents remain in contact with their surrogates, the most frequent contact being photos and letters on birthdays and holidays.
- 83 percent of their respondents had seen their surrogate since the birth of their child, and all had included their children (and hers) in the visits.
- 67 percent said that contact was initiated equally between the surrogate and the couple.
- 42 percent rated that contact "very comfortable" (another 33 percent said it was "comfortable" and 25 percent said that they had some ambivalence about it).

- 67 percent reported that there was nothing that troubled them about having contact. Those who had some concerns cited: feeling awkward with their surrogate's family, viewing their surrogate as needy; and having to say good-bye again.[53]

Parenthood through surrogacy is a challenging experience that does not end with the birth of a child. In fact, many parents would say that the biggest challenges begin there.

First, there are the normal demands of parenthood. Much as they longed and toiled for the opportunity to raise a child, couples inevitably find that it is difficult. A cuddly baby soon becomes a curious toddler, who then turns into a demanding two year old. The years pass quickly. Before they know it, parents are on the daily roller coaster ride of adolescence, looking back upon the bygone days of the terrible twos as but a blissful dream.

Along with the normal demands of parenthood are the special challenges of parenting through surrogacy. Questions of privacy, of explaining the process to the child, and, most important, dealing with the child as he or she attempts to make some sense of these origins are continuous challenges that face couples who choose this option.

Finally, couples must grapple with issues of affiliation and advocacy. Some parents through surrogacy choose to maintain as much privacy as possible and do not openly identify themselves with surrogacy; some feel a need to affiliate with others who have taken the same road to parenthood; and some feel a responsibility to work to protect and preserve this option for other prospective parents. These couples become involved with OPTS, a growing organization that offers families through surrogacy an opportunity to know each other, to share their experiences, and to work together toward public acceptance and support of their chosen path to parenthood.

Conclusions

Negative media attention, especially following the Baby M case, caused many people to regard surrogacy with suspicion. Even now, several years after the courtroom drama put surrogacy on trial, this parenting option is regarded as risky, fraught with danger for both couples and surrogates. However, the experiences of both the couples and the surrogates, as seen in follow-up studies by Hanafin and Forest, paint a different picture.

The majority of those who have participated in surrogacy see it as a viable path to parenthood. However, they also acknowledge the need for information, support, and practical advice in every phase of the process. In the absence of public policy that guides and regulates surrogacy, it is the responsibility of professionals who are involved in the process—lawyers, mental health practitioners, and physicians—to ensure informed consent. Working together, they must help all those who enter into surrogacy arrangements to do so with a full understanding of the social, emotional, legal, and ethical challenges at hand.

8

Gestational Care

The development of in vitro fertilization brought a host of new possibilities for infertile couples. Once eggs could be fertilized outside a woman's body, there was a way to separate genetic and gestational parenthood. For that segment of infertile women who had lost part of their reproductive capacity, the separation of reproductive functions meant exciting new options. Now women who had no ovarian function could carry and deliver a baby who was conceived with a donated egg and their husband's sperm. Additionally, women with functioning ovaries who could not carry a pregnancy had the chance to have their embryo transferred to the uterus of another woman.

We begin examining the process by which one woman carries another couple's baby with a dilemma: how best to refer to it. Some people feel strongly that it should be identified as a form of surrogacy, since one woman is carrying a baby for another couple. (And in that sense, the word *surrogate*, which according to the *American Heritage Dictionary*, means "one that takes the place of another; a substitute," may be more appropriate here than it is in traditional surrogacy.). Those approaching it from this perspective commonly use the terms *gestational surrogacy* or, less commonly, *host-uterus* or *IVF surrogacy*. Others say this process is not surrogacy, as the public has come to know surrogacy, and therefore it should not be identified as such. Those who have this perspective stress its role as a medical treatment for infertility and view it as a medical treatment rather than an alternative to biogenetic parenting. Hence, they call the woman who carries the baby a *gestational carrier*, a term that emphasizes her physical contribution.

As clinicians, we have given a great deal of thought to each of these perspectives in order to determine what language to use. After considerable debate we decided to call the process *gestational care* and to refer to the woman who carries the pregnancy as the *gestational carrier*. We recognize that the term gestational care will be unfamiliar to most readers, but use it because it accurately describes the process. We also recognize that the term gestational carrier may trouble those practitioners who regard this option as a form of surrogacy. Therefore, when we quote practitioners who use the term *gestational surrogacy*, we will respectfully use the same language that they do.

The developments of in vitro fertilization and surrogacy coincided historically, and because of this historical coincidence, couples who might otherwise have turned to traditional surrogacy had other options. For many women who had been unable to conceive, particularly those with tubal disease, IVF was a miraculous treatment. When it worked, IVF enabled the women to become pregnant themselves, eliminating the need for a surrogate.

A second, and smaller, group of couples who initially considered or pursued traditional surrogacy were those in which the women had functioning ovaries and tubes, but were unable—because of medical illness, prior surgery, or congenital abnormality—to carry a pregnancy. For them, the concurrent arrivals of surrogacy and IVF represented a new and exciting possibility: they could have their eggs retrieved, fertilized in vitro with the husband's sperm, and transferred as embryos into the uterus of another woman. This possibility, which existed from the beginning of IVF, became a reality in the mid-1980s with the birth of the first baby through a gestational care pregnancy. From this point forward, gestational care offered a woman who was unable to go through pregnancy, labor, and delivery the opportunity to mother a child who was her genetic offspring.

Early in its development, gestational care was seen as a slight variation of traditional surrogacy, and, in the eyes of many, it still is. Because the process involves one woman carrying a baby for another, many practitioners involved in traditional surrogacy became involved in this new process. Although the medical complexities of the process required that they develop close working relationships with physicians and with IVF laboratories, many of the other essential aspects of a practice that involved legal, social and psychological services were already in place.

Although gestational care became closely associated with traditional surrogacy practice early in its history, reproductive endocrinologists, nurses, and mental health professionals who work with gestational care in a medical setting view them differently. One such group, Pennsylvania Reproductive Associates in Philadelphia, began a Gestational Carrier Program in 1988. By incorporating the necessary legal and psychological services into their medical team, they were able to offer IVF with embryo transfer to another woman's uterus as part of their medical treatment program.

The discussion that follows looks at the social, ethical, and legal questions associated with gestational care. As we examine these questions, it becomes clear that some of the controversy has arisen because gestational care inherited the complicated, sometimes troubled, legacy of traditional surrogacy. It is also clear that this process prompts some new and very different questions, focusing primarily on what it means for one woman to carry the genetic child of another couple.

A Social and Ethical Perspective

As we have noted throughout this book, people have different feelings about the importance of genetic versus gestational ties. There are those who believe that the most important link between parent and child is a genetic one: that genes are the bloodline connecting generations. Others emphasize the significance of the bond that develops between a woman and the child she is carrying; they see the gestational aspect of reproduction as equal to or even much greater than the role of genetics.

The identity of gestational care has been shaped not only by its origins in two fields but also by the complex and conflicting views concerning genetic and gestational bonds. Those who focus primarily on genetic ties tend to see gestational care as linked to the ARTs. They regard the use of a gestational carrier as an important treatment for certain reproductive problems that afflict women, in particular women who have a malfunctioning or absent uterus.

Representative of the view that gestational care is a medical treatment for infertile couples rather than a form of surrogacy is the group at Pennsylvania Reproductive Associates. They draw clear distinctions between their Gestational Carrier Program and the practice of traditional surrogacy:

> The importance of a genetic distinction has been reaffirmed through clinical experience. Women evaluated as potential gestational carriers report that they can accept carrying a child that is biologically unrelated to them, and they feel that they would have great emotional difficulty relinquishing a child that is, in part, biologically theirs. Being genetically inert, the carriers report that they are able to separate themselves emotionally from the baby and decrease the attachment process throughout the pregnancy.[1]

Others involved in programs that use traditional surrogates as well as gestational carriers do not share the views of these clinicians. Although they acknowledge the genetic differences between the two options, they emphasize the importance of what they have in common: one woman is carrying a baby for another. Cristie Montgomery, who has served as a traditional surrogate and directs Surrogate Parenting Services, stresses that in either situation, the women involved must separate pregnancy from motherhood. In both cases, it is the woman who intends to parent the baby, and her mate, rather than the woman who carries the baby, who sees herself as expecting.[2]

Practitioners involved with traditional surrogacy as well as gestational care report that some of the couples they work with focus on genetic ties, and others emphasize the importance of gestation. Gerry Tarlow, director of Solutions, a surrogacy program, notes that he has had several couples try one or two IVF cycles with a gestational surrogate. If pregnancy does not occur, many then request traditional surrogacy. Nancy Hughes, director of Hagar Associates, has a slightly different perspective. She agrees that this happens on occasion but reports that many of the couples she works with move directly on to adoption if they are not able to have a child through gestational surrogacy.[3]

However they feel about genetic and gestational ties, everyone involved with gestational care grapples with a complicated and potentially worrisome issue: a couple is entrusting their embryo/fetus/child in its prebirth care to another woman, often a stranger, and she is entrusting her body to nurture its growth and development. Embryos are very precious, especially when there is a finite number, as when a couple has undergone IVF in order to freeze embryos prior to the woman's cancer treatment. And since pregnancy is often a complicated process that can involve physical risks, there is also the possibility for conflict of interest between the couple and the gestational carrier. For example, a woman could develop serious medical problems during the pregnancy and require surgery that could harm the fetus. Less serious but also worrisome conflicts can arise if the couple, understandably anxious over the safety and well-being of their growing child, attempts to control the gestational carriers behavior and/or life-style during pregnancy. These are but a few of the situations that can arise when a woman agrees to carry another couple's baby.

Mental health providers, physicians, and ethicists involved in the new reproductive technologies have attempted to address the serious questions that surround gestational care. What are the rights during pregnancy and after of a woman who agrees to carry and deliver a baby for another couple? Is she a "mother" in any sense of the word, or is her role more akin to a prebirth caretaker or a nanny? What are the rights of the couple who agree to entrust her with their embryo? Do they have any jurisdiction over her body during pregnancy and, if so, what is it?

The American College of Obstetricians and Gynecologists (ACOG) has issued a policy statement emphasizing the significance of the woman who carries the child and affirming her rights as the mother:

> The woman who carries the child 1) Should be the sole source of consent for all questions regarding the prenatal care and delivery and 2) should have a specified time period after the birth of the infant during which she can decide whether or not to carry out her original intention to place the infant for adoption.[4]

George Annas, professor of health law at Boston University School of Medicine and Public Health and a respected expert in the field of reproductive law, makes this point even more emphatically.

In an article that clearly identifies the woman who carries and delivers the child as mother, he writes:

> The woman who gives birth to the child should irrebuttably be considered the child's legal mother. She could agree to give the child up for adoption, but only after its birth, and in accordance with the state's adoption laws.[5]

Nancy Reame, a professor in the School of Nursing and Reproductive Sciences at the University of Michigan, grapples with some of the complexities of a gestational care pregnancy. She acknowledges the ACOG guidelines and notes that they may help to protect a woman's rights regarding her own health care. However, she points out some of the pitfalls of allowing the gestational surrogate to be the decision maker:

> The autonomy of the gestational surrogate mother may compromise the rights and responsibilities of the genetic parents. . . . For example, the gestational surrogate would have the right to abort an unrelated fetus if she no longer wished to carry the pregnancy. Alternatively, she could be responsible for the custody of a child with birth defects rejected by its biological parents.[6]

The practitioners at Pennsylvania Reproductive Associates, as well as many others involved in gestational care feel that a gestational carrier's rights to make decisions related to her pregnancy can be protected and respected without having to designate her as mother. What they do, instead, is to prepare contracts that carefully delineate her rights: the right to make decisions about her obstetrical care and the right to make decisions regarding her body during pregnancy (nutrition, activity level, rest, travel). English Braverman and Corson take the following position: "Once the pregnancy is established, the carrier, in consultation with her physician, should be the sole source of consent for medical decisions and delivery."[7]

Similarly, Dr. Hilary Hanafin, of the Center for Surrogate Parenting, emphasizes that the woman who is pregnant and her physician have the right to make medical decisions during the pregnancy even if the fetus is not genetically related to her. However, every effort must be made in advance to anticipate potentially difficult obstetrical decisions and to confirm that couples and their gestational surrogates are in agreement about how these decisions should be handled.[8]

A Legal Perspective

Many people, including those in the field and those outside of it, associate gestational care with its precursor, surrogacy. From a legal standpoint, some of that association has promoted the development of this reproductive option while other aspects have interfered with the practice.

One positive contribution from the field of surrogacy has been the development and evolution of a surrogacy contract. The original surrogacy contracts focused on the baby who was to result from the agreement rather than on the services being provided by the surrogate. More recent contracts have emphasized the time, effort, and physical and emotional wear and tear involved in surrogate pregnancies and have compensated the women for their efforts rather than for the baby (baby selling is illegal in all states). This evolution is especially relevant to gestational carriers, who are providing a service rather than a product. Compensation for time and effort is also critical because of the low probability of success; chances are good that a woman will spend a great deal of time and effort simply trying to become pregnant.

Lawyers with traditional surrogacy practices bring crucial experience to gestational care. This family building option has also forced them to address some new issues, including the rights of the couple and the surrogate during the pregnancy and following delivery. Another question that arises with a gestational care pregnancy concerns identifying the legal parents at birth. Whereas traditional surrogacy usually requires stepparent adoption—the surrogate is initially the child's legal mother, having provided her ovum as well as her uterus—gestational care programs have developed some effective ways of establishing the parental rights and responsibilities of the biological parents.

William Handel, director of the Center for Surrogate Parenting, is reported to be the first person to have the genetic mother's name placed on the birth certificate in situations involving gestational surrogates. Handel accomplishes this task by filing maternity and paternity suits a few months prior to delivery. (Just as a father can file a paternity suit in instances in which he has not been recognized as his child's father, so also can genetic parents file prebirth maternity and paternity suits to "prove" that they are the child's parents.) Since the gestational surrogates are not seeking parental rights, the suits are uncontested, and they have proved to be an effective vehicle for enabling the genetic parents to be designated the unborn child's parents as early as the last trimester of pregnancy.[9]

Similarly, Steven Litz, of Surrogate Mothers Inc., petitions the court when the gestational surrogate is six months pregnant, seeking that a legal relationship be established between the genetic parents and their unborn child. Lawyers in other programs have developed similar mechanisms for ensuring that the biological parents are deemed the legal parents at the earliest point possible. This legal effort protects the couple and also protects the woman who is pregnant from any parenting obligations since she has never intended to parent the child she is carrying.[10]

Although various attorneys have been successful in establishing the parental rights of the genetic parents, this is not always the case. One New York court refused to acknowledge a "maternity action" filed in an attempt to establish that the genetic mother of twins born to a gestational carrier is the children's legal mother. This refusal occurred despite the fact that the genetic and gestational parents were in agreement. The court concluded that New York law did not allow an order establishing maternity; therefore the state legislature, not its courts, must be asked to expand the law to cover technological advances.[11]

Gestational care has also inherited some of the legal baggage that has burdened surrogacy arrangements. Effective legislation has been sorely lacking for both options, leaving practice largely unguided and unregulated. To the extent that laws have been passed, they are largely restrictive, and most fail to distinguish between the role of a gestational carrier and a traditional surrogate. A law that initially passed in the California legislature in September 1992, but was subsequently vetoed by the governor, was an important exception. It attempted to make some important distinctions between the two options by stating explicitly that a child born of a gestational care agreement is the legal child of the contracting couple.

For the most part, gestational care arrangements have been spared the dramatic court cases that have been so damaging to traditional surrogacy. There has, however, been one well-publicized case, *Johnson* v. *Calvert*. Anna Johnson, who carried a baby for Mark and Crispina Calvert, attempted to gain custody of the baby following delivery. The initial ruling, in October 1990, was that Ms. Johnson had no parental rights. On appeal, the California Supreme Court reached similar conclusions in February 1993. In May, the California Supreme Court made a second ruling and went much further in its support of the Calverts. It focused on the question of intent and said that the people who "intended" to raise the child should be designated as the parents.[12]

Although the Johnson v. Calvert case advanced the cause of gestational care by setting valuable precedent, it also had negative repercussions because it brought unwanted attention to it. The fact that Ms. Johnson sued for custody indicated that even a gestational carrier, who is not genetically related to the offspring, might change her mind.

Gestational Care Couples

Medical Indications

As with traditional surrogacy, couples who use established programs must go through extensive screening procedures before they are accepted into a gestational care program. First, they must demonstrate medical need, which can be established in a number of ways.

In the first category are women who have no uterus—either resulting from congenital absence of the uterus or removal because of cancer or other gynecological or obstetrical problems. Thus, they have suffered the loss of part of their reproductive capacity. If their ovaries are intact, the potential to have a genetic child remains. The prospect of gestational care may offer these women some hope.

Women with severe uterine scarring (often referred to as Asherman's syndrome) following a pregnancy loss, an elective abortion, or occasionally after a normal pregnancy fall in the second category. This scarring makes it difficult for an embryo to implant. Frequently minor surgery can correct the condition; when it cannot, a gestational care pregnancy may be the alternative of choice for these couples.

Couples in which the woman has uterine problems that preclude pregnancy and who choose gestational care usually do so after several unsuccessful attempts at pregnancy, perhaps including failed IVF cycles or early pregnancy losses, or both. These experiences provide probable justification for the theory that the couple's problem resides in the woman's uterus, not in the embryos. Faced with the irony of being able to create healthy embryos but lacking the ability to gestate them, some couples welcome gestational care as the solution for their infertility problem.

Women who have malformation of the uterus, often as a result of DES exposure, fall in the third category. They may be unable to carry a pregnancy safely to viability. Some of these women have experienced repeated pregnancy losses, which appear to have confirmed their inability to carry a pregnancy to term.

Other women who fall into a fourth category, have been advised not to attempt pregnancy for medical reasons. For example, heart problems or chronic illness, such as multiple sclerosis may contraindicate pregnancy. Usually such women are able to become pregnant, but pregnancy is likely to compromise their health. Gestational care offers them and their partners the opportunity to reproduce without undergoing the potential risks of pregnancy.

A growing number of women are surviving cancer, but at the expense of their fertility. They compose a fifth category. For some, this loss occurs as a result of surgery; they may have had a partial hysterectomy, leaving their ovaries available for egg retrieval. Women who have a partner and are about to undergo a chemotherapy regimen that will destroy or severely damage their ovarian function can elect, prior to chemotherapy, to undergo IVF for the purpose of obtaining embryos to cryopreserve for later use.

Many cancer survivors see gestational care as an important ingredient in their recovery. Having come face to face with death, they see having a child, and especially a child genetically related to them, as a link to their future. Many also see gestational care as a way of reducing the losses they have experienced; even in the face of significant losses, they have been able to salvage their ability to reproduce.

There is a sixth and final group of couples who are considered by some physicians to be candidates for gestational care pregnancies: those for whom several attempts at IVF have failed, despite the fact that the couple produces healthy embryos and the woman's uterus appears to be normal. When IVF repeatedly fails to result in pregnancy, some physicians conclude that the problem must reside in the uterus and that some unknown or untreatable factor is preventing implantation. They suggest that these couples might benefit from having their embryos transferred into another woman's uterus. Other physicians disagree with this rationale, believing it is unwarranted treatment and, furthermore, a long shot.

Social and Emotional Considerations

Many couples are introduced to the idea of gestational care when they are in crisis. Having endured an illness or surgery that resulted in the inability to become pregnant, many women receive offers from a close friend or family member who is willing to carry a child for them. Some of these offers, although made with sincerity, are later withdrawn when altruistic volunteers learn all that is involved in gestational care. Similarly, some couples who may initially respond to the offer with enthusiasm decide against pursuing the process because of its medical uncertainty, high costs, or psychological and legal complexities.

Couples and their volunteer gestational carriers may be advised against the process by physicians, psychologists, or family and friends. For example, prospective parents who are over age forty may be advised against it because their advanced age makes success very unlikely. Others may be dissuaded because it is not advisable that they undergo ovarian stimulation. Finally, there are couples, as well as gestational carriers, whom a psychologist or other mental health professional may feel are unprepared or ill suited for this unusual undertaking.

Not all couples with medical need for a gestational care pregnancy have a family member or friend who is willing or able to help them. Others may know a willing volunteer but conclude that the closeness of their relationship may in fact be detrimental to the process. Some couples decide that it is important enough to them to have a genetic child that they are willing to enter into an agreement with a stranger.

As we have noted, people feel differently about the importance of genetic ties. Hence, some couples might consider working with a gestational carrier but eventually decide against it, concluding that what is most important is for them to become parents. They then turn to adoption as a more expedient (and more certain) path to parenthood. For them, gestational care is appealing but too costly, too time-consuming, and, most important, too much of a long shot.

Other couples look at the challenges involved in gestational care and decide that the option is worth pursuing. Some base their decision on their feelings about bloodlines: they want a child who is genetically connected to them and to those who came before them. Others focus more on the idea of known versus unknown genes, fearing that adoption is too risky. Still others, especially cancer survivors, experience a powerful longing to have a genetic connection to their child as a way of reducing the pain associated with their illness or surgery. Having faced their mortality, they view genetic continuity as a way to live on.

Couples who have a genetic child and then suffer a subsequent reproductive loss are among those most drawn to gestational care. Having felt pleasure in genetic ties and having found that pregnancy is an experience that lasts nine months and then fades into the background, many of these couples regard gestational care as a perfect solution. They conclude that they can handle the high costs (probably $35,000 or more, assuming they do not have a volunteer carrier) and low odds for success if this is their only opportunity for another genetic child.

Gestational Carriers

Some women offer to undertake a gestational care pregnancy because they want to help a friend or family member in need. Some are women who never before imagined that they would carry a baby for someone else. Now, moved by a tragedy in the life of a loved one, they see an opportunity to help out in a most meaningful way.

Some women decide on their own, unrelated to any desire to help a loved one, that they want to carry a baby for a childless couple. Hilary Hanafin, psychologist at the Center for Surrogate Parenting, has worked with a large number of these women, some of whom were traditional surrogates and some gestational surrogates. In her experience, the motivation of traditional and gestational surrogates is similar: they want to give something meaningful to others and to do something that matters with their lives. Many have had friends or family members who were infertile and see no other contribution more important than helping a couple become parents.[13]

Surrogates and gestational carriers are women who enjoy pregnancy, labor, and delivery. Although their families are complete, they want to experience these pleasures again. For them, the prospect of carrying a child for another couple is a real opportunity: they can enjoy a pregnancy but be spared the parenting responsibilities that follow.

Although the longing to be pregnant and to reexperience labor and delivery may be similar for surrogates and gestational carriers, there are some women who wish to be gestational carriers but not surrogates. They want to carry a baby for someone else as long as it is not their baby. They are clear that if they provided the egg (the genetic material) in addition to the gestational environment, the child would feel like their own. Andrea Braverman, the psychologist at Pennsylvania Reproductive Associates, reports that the majority of women in her gestational carrier program feel this way. Only on rare occasion has a gestational carrier later served as a surrogate for a couple. In her experience, this has happened only after a couple and the carrier have gone through failed ART attempts together and have developed close bonds.[14]

Other practitioners report different experiences. Many women apply to Dr. Hanafin's program with an interest in either traditional or gestational surrogacy. Similarly, Cristie Montgomery, whose program offers both options, feels that most of the women she interviews to be surrogates have concluded that the baby they give birth to—whether conceived with their egg or the result of an embryo transfer—is not their child.[15]

Awareness of these different points of view—one that a genetic tie (or lack of one) makes all the difference in the world, and the other that it is almost irrelevant—helps us to understand why some potential surrogates/gestational carriers choose one option and not the other, while others do not draw a distinction between them. It also helps us understand why some women—those who would carry a child only if it was the other couple's embryo—apply to programs that are medically based and do not offer traditional surrogacy. Conversely, those who feel less strongly about their genetic material but more strongly about the gestational bond are more likely to become involved with surrogacy programs that offer both options and focus primarily on the shared aspects of the two experiences.

Beyond genetic considerations, there are additional reasons why some women who consider carrying a baby for another couple prefer gestational care and others prefer surrogacy. Those who are willing to carry a child only if it is the couple's genetic offspring may make this decision based on the perceived needs of their own children. They may feel that they minimize the risk of their children's feeling that a sister or brother is being given away (or, worse, sold) if the child they carry is biologically unrelated.

Some women choose to be gestational carriers because they feel that they are less likely to seen as baby sellers—exploited women who are giving up their children. Lori Capone, a former gestational surrogate and an articulate spokesperson, has addressed some of these issues:

> I did not receive compensation for selling my child—she was never mine—and her parents did not purchase her from me. I received monetary compensation for going through the physical and emotional trials of pregnancy. Certainly no one can begrudge me that. I had a difficult pregnancy and a complicated birth culminating in an emergency Caesarean section. Forgive my lack of altruism, but I feel I did deserve compensation for the physical labor involved. It's different when you bear your own child because having your own child is compensation enough.[16]

Not all women who draw a distinction between traditional surrogacy and gestational care prefer the latter option. Some conclude that surrogacy is medically easier and more likely to be successful. These women, also aware of the risks of multiple birth, feel that they would rather undergo a process that is more likely to result in a singleton pregnancy than one that carries with it a 20 to 30 percent chance of multiples. They do not want to undertake the rigors of a twin pregnancy and are concerned about the complex dilemmas they would face if the embryo transfer resulted in a triplet (or larger) pregnancy.

Another medical reason that some women prefer surrogacy relates to convenience and efficacy. With artificial insemination, a simple procedure that a woman can perform on her own, pregnancy is usually achieved within six normal menstrual cycles. By contrast, in vitro fertilization, with embryo transfer, is a complicated procedure, requiring carefully coordinated monitoring of both women's menstrual cycles. Even in the best medical centers, this process has only about a 30 percent chance per cycle of pregnancy, assuming the genetic mother is under age thirty-five and producing healthy eggs; otherwise, the chances for pregnancy are lower.

Women who do not draw distinctions between using their egg and someone else's will generally decide to become a traditional surrogate rather than a gestational carrier. Included also in this group are women who live far from medical centers and lack access to high-quality medical treatment. Rather than undertake the rigors of travel, which might require that they be away from their families for a few days, together with the increased risks of multiple gestation, these women choose traditional surrogacy.

The Process for Couples

Couples seeking a gestational care program typically go directly to a medical center that offers ART or to a surrogacy program. Both approaches can lead to the desired goal. Gestational care programs offering reproductive technology services have access to necessary legal and psychological services, and agencies specializing in surrogacy services are connected to medical centers that perform in vitro fertilization.

Fees for traditional surrogacy are high—around $35,000; gestational care may turn out to be even more expensive because of the complicated medical care that is involved each cycle and because it often takes more than one or two cycles to establish an ongoing pregnancy. Although there are some one-time costs, such as administrative, legal, and psychological fees, the medical costs of IVF are repeated each cycle. It is therefore essential that couples understand what they will be paying for and when. For example, they need to determine what their costs will be for subsequent cycles if the first does not work and for cryopreservation if they have extra embryos. Since IVF is covered by some health insurance carriers and only in certain states, (and many will not pay for IVF services if a carrier is involved) it is also critical that the gestational care program or practitioner be knowledgeable about what insurance companies, if any, are willing to pay medical expenses in a gestational care pregnancy.

Couples entering into gestational care arrangements need to take a careful look at the psychological services that will be available to them. Fay Johnson, of the Organization of Parenting Through Surrogacy, points out that couples working with a gestational surrogate may feel that they have even more at risk than couples undertaking traditional surrogacy because another woman will be carrying their full genetic child. Thus, couples working with a gestational surrogate may be even more fearful than those who are expecting through a traditional surrogate that she will change her mind and not want to relinquish the child. Contracting couples should have a good deal of trust in their gestational surrogate, as well as in the psychologist who is working with all of them.[17]

Assessment and Preparation of the Couple

Ethical Dilemmas. Some situations involving gestational carriers pose profound ethical dilemmas. One concerns women who have or have had cancer. It may not be in the best interest of a child to bring him or her into the world with a mother whose chance of raising him or her to adulthood is seriously compromised. On the other hand, there are no guarantees for anyone's future; thus, many professionals feel that it is unfair to exclude a couple from becoming parents on the basis of medical history, especially if the other parent is in good health.

One couple's story poignantly captures the dilemmas that can arise for caregivers and couples alike. The couple had contacted the IVF program in which they had embryos stored from a successful cycle that occurred three years ago. They told the staff that when their "IVF son" was a year old, the mother was diagnosed with a serious form of cancer and given a poor prognosis. The couple had a friend who was willing to be their gestational carrier and was determined to have their embryos transferred to her. Both the husband and wife said they hoped to witness the birth of their second child before the wife died. It was very important to them that she not die having left frozen embryos; she needed to attempt to give them life in order to die in peace. The medical team was in an ethical quandry: they felt tremendous empathy for the couple and wanted to grant them this last request. Yet they did not believe that it would be in the unborn child's best interest to do so.

This difficult and tragic situation illustrates a central dilemma that clinicians may face in the practice of gestational care—a dilemma that frequently revolves around the question of the best interest of children (born or unborn). If frozen embryos are transferred to a gestational carrier, a child (or children) may be born to a dying or recently deceased mother. The child's father, no matter how loving, caring, and capable, will be grieving, and may be unprepared for the challenges of single parenthood (which could mean parenting twins or triplets). These events will undoubtedly have psychological significance for the couple's child, especially if the mother dies shortly before or after the birth of a younger sibling. On the other hand, gestational care offers the embryos the opportunity for life that they would not otherwise have. Furthermore, the chance to try this option, whatever its outcome, might better fortify the father for the challenges of single parenthood that lie ahead.

Medical Assessment

The first question in assessing a couple for gestational care concerns medical necessity. Nearly all practitioners believe that it is unethical to undertake gestational care for reasons of preference or convenience and therefore require that a couple have a documented medical or surgical reason for pursuing this option. Only after a medical necessity has been established is a couple investigated further for medical appropriateness.

Physicians are not in agreement about whether couples who have had several failed IVF attempts but no documented uterine problems should be candidates for gestational care. Those who argue in favor feel that it is worth a try if several IVF attempts that resulted in healthy embryos failed to yield a pregnancy. They reason that there must be an undiagnosed uterine problem.

Those who argue against gestational care when a couple has had several failed IVF cycles see no reason to transfer one woman's embryos to another woman's uterus when the genetic mother has no known uterine abnormality (or any other medical reason that pregnancy is contraindicated). One such situation resulted in an interesting surprise. A couple had turned to gestational care after several failed IVF attempts that were eventually attributed to uterine problems. However, since they produced several embryos, they decided to maximize their efforts by having the better embryos transferred to the gestational carrier and the ones that appeared less optimal transferred to the mother. The unanticipated result was that both women became pregnant and delivered siblings two days apart. This story, although unusual, seems to support those who believe that gestational care should be reserved only for women with a known uterine problem. Nevertheless, it is important to remember that many explanations for infertility are undocumented; they are educated guesses at best. Thus, IVF may fail because of an unobservable uterine problem, or the uterus may have nothing to do with a failed cycle.

Couples who attempt pregnancy via gestational care must be able to produce healthy embryos or have cryopreserved embryos. Although fertilization is never guaranteed, a semen analysis provides helpful information about the quality of the sperm and whether they are likely to fertilize eggs. Similarly, hormonal studies on the prospective biological mother can help to identify potential problems in follicular development and in the quality of her eggs. These hormonal screenings can rule out couples for whom gestational care appears to be a very long shot, either because of a problem with the sperm or a problem with the egg quality that would impede fertilization.

Some couples interested in gestational care have good reason to believe it may be successful. For example, those who have had a child in the recent past know that they have a proved track record. Nevertheless, a history of pregnancy, especially if the intervening years put the woman in an older category, by no means guarantees future conception.

Finally, some couples turn to gestational care because they have frozen embryos and need someone to gestate them. They include those who have cryopreserved embryos from a previous IVF cycle (either successful or failed) and have subsequently encountered a medical or surgical problem that precludes pregnancy. This group may also include women who have been treated for cancer, who underwent IVF prior to surgery or chemotherapy in order to produce embryos.

When a couple has only a finite number of cryopreserved embryos, there is additional pressure on all involved. These couples have no additional opportunities for genetic parenthood; transfer of their existing embryos represents their last chance for a child who is genetically connected to each of them. Thus, they and their gestational carrier will approach the treatment cycle with keen awareness that the stakes are high.

Psychological Assessment

Mental health professionals recommend meetings with the couple together as well as individually. Conjoint meetings offer couples an opportunity to hear each other's perspective and to confirm that they are in agreement; individual sessions offer each of them a chance to speak in private with a counselor and to voice any concerns that they might be reluctant to share with their partner. In combination these meetings should answer several questions.

Are both partners in agreement regarding this choice? Arranging for gestational care is an expensive and difficult undertaking, with significant potential for disappointment. The psychologist must determine whether the couple has considered other parenting options and explore why they are pursuing gestational care rather than another alternative.

If the couple plans to use a family member as their gestational carrier, it is essential that they explore the full implications of this decision. Whatever the outcome, the process that they are embarking upon together will affect family relationships in years to come. They need to discuss with each other their feelings about the prospective gestational carrier and consider issues that might arise as a consequence of their decision.

Has the couple considered how stressful the process is likely to be? Are they prepared for possible disappointment? Choosing to try gestational care, like other alternative paths, means that couples must reembark on the emotional roller coaster that became all too familiar during their infertility treatments. The chances of ending up with a child through this option are less than they are for virtually all other options. Couples must acknowledge the series of obstacles that may lie ahead. There could be problems with egg retrieval, fertilization, transfer, implantation, or pregnancy loss. The most likely scenario is that everything will go smoothly but no pregnancy will occur. Each step along the way will be intensely stressful, with the threat of loss or disappointment always lurking.

Has the couple anticipated at least some of the challenging questions that could arise during a pregnancy involving a gestational carrier? No one can anticipate all the questions and issues that might surface during a pregnancy. Nonetheless, it is important that couples consider some of the issues that have arisen for other couples and think about what they would do if they found themselves in similar situations.

Psychologists stress the need for couples to discuss their feelings about amniocentesis, as well as about what they would want to do if the results indicated a problem. Accordingly, they need to be in agreement about the conditions under which they would want to terminate a pregnancy or engage in multifetal reduction. Only after they agree as a couple can the psychologist make sure that they are matched with a woman who shares their views on these key issues.

Has the couple grieved the loss of pregnancy and childbirth? It is essential that couples, in their eagerness to seize the possibility of having a biological child, not overlook all that they have been through. Since the need for a gestational care was often the result of a traumatic experience, such as a life-threatening illness or emergency surgery, it is important that couples take some time to grieve. Part of their grief process will involve acknowledging all that has been lost (see chapter 4). If they neglect this task, they are likely to be all the more vulnerable to the frustrations and disappointments that arise in the process.

Pregnancy is more important to some people than to others. In general, women experience a far greater loss than their partners when pregnancy is not possible, but some men do look forward to seeing their wife pregnant and to sharing the experience with her. His partner may not share that desire as intensely, viewing pregnancy solely as a means to an end and not as an experience to be treasured in itself. Consequently, the woman may feel less loss than her mate when she learns that she is unable to carry a pregnancy.

It is vital that couples talk together about what it means to each of them to lose the opportunity to share a pregnancy. Even if gestational care succeeds, there will be loss involved. The dimensions of that loss, including the process of conception itself, need to be identified and acknowledged.

Have they talked about their plans to family or friends? If so, what was their reaction? Couples trying gestational care will have to make some decisions about whom they tell and when and what they say. Those who are working with a friend or family member may have more difficulty maintaining privacy. Couples who decide to work with a stranger can more easily postpone telling others about their decision. Some wait to see if pregnancy is achieved, feeling that the wait spares them from having to give progress reports on their efforts. Others are open from the start; they do not want to be forced to hide their plans or account for the time lost at work from medical appointments.

Couples can try to anticipate how family and friends will act and react: with support or negative value judgments about their undertaking. They need to remind themselves that many people are misinformed about the process, and others feel negatively about one woman's carrying a baby for someone else. Prospective couples must consider whether they are emotionally equipped to embark on a family-building option that is so controversial.

In fact, couples who tell their families that they have decided to try gestational care are often surprised by the responses they receive. Some learn that their families are comfortable, perhaps even familiar, with this parenting option. Others are encouraged to pursue adoption, a more predictable and less costly path to parenthood.

Have they have decided to tell the child about his or her conception and birth? Thinking about how and when a child might understand and integrate information about his or her origins will help them focus on what is in the best interests of the child, i.e. whether they should tell or not tell that a gestational carrier brought him/her into the world. Talking with other couples undergoing this process or with parents who are part of the OPTS network can help them sort out the questions and decisions they will face. Chapter 5 includes a discussion of openness v. secrecy in using donor gametes. Although couples who turn to gestational care will parent their genetic child, much of the discussion involving secrecy pertains to all forms of third party reproduction and is thus applicable here.

Have they considered how many times they will try to conceive a child through gestational care and what alternatives they will pursue if pregnancy does not occur? In preparation for the likelihood of disappointment, couples may want to consider other parenting options. Some couples will move on to surrogacy, feeling that "half our genetic child is better than no genetic connection." Others will opt for adoption or for child-free living.

Some couples who do not initially consider surrogacy later develop an interest in this option after unsuccessful efforts with gestational care. Frequently this interest grows out of feeling connected to the woman with whom they are working; they have grown close to her and now feel comfortable having a child with her.

Have they explored the potential legal issues? Although there have been few legal disputes to date regarding gestational care, couples nevertheless need to work with a lawyer who is experienced in this process and can draw up a contract. The contract is unlikely to be upheld in court, since a woman cannot legally relinquish a child prior to birth; however, it may hold psychological, if not legal, weight. Furthermore, the process of entering into an agreement provides an important opportunity for couples and gestational carriers to discuss critical and potentially devastating issues, such as failed pregnancy attempts, amniocentesis, elective abortion, multifetal reduction, and birth anomalies.

Assessment and Preparation of Gestational Carriers

The assessment and screening of a gestational carrier is similar in many ways to that of a surrogate. However, there are some distinctions. (Chapter 7 contains a fuller account of the assessment process.) Here we discuss only those factors that are unique to gestational carriers.

Medical Assessment. Although the gestational carrier will not be passing on her genes to the child that she carries, she will be undergoing pregnancy, labor, and delivery, and so it is important that her general health, as well as her fertility, be assessed.

Medical evaluation looks for any evidence of a uterine problem that might interfere with implantation or with carrying a pregnancy. Since most programs require that a woman have at least one child before undertaking gestational care (this requirement is usually for psychological reasons—so she knows what it means to be pregnant and to bond with a child in utero), she has had a medical history that provides useful information about any prior pregnancy. For example, a program might decide not to work with a woman who has a history of recurrent miscarriages, premature delivery, or some other obstetrical problem that could compromise a future pregnancy. In all other respects, the medical screening is similar to that of traditional surrogates.

Psychological Assessment. The psychological evaluation includes a careful examination of her emotional stability and her readiness to become a carrier. In addition to most of the questions that are addressed in the evaluation of a prospective traditional surrogate (see chapter 7), a psychologist attempts to sort through a number of other issues.

Coercion. Some women volunteer to carry a baby for relatives or friends and then find that they have second thoughts. In this case, a woman may feel that she has no way out of the situation, especially if the couple is expressing a great deal of gratitude and enthusiasm.

Women who have volunteered to carry for their sisters or other relatives are likely to feel duty bound, especially if there is family support and encouragement. The notion of reneging probably seems unthinkable. This support may evolve to covert or even overt pressure, possibly involving gifts or financial rewards.

A psychologist working with prospective gestational carriers must give them every opportunity to change their minds. A woman who has serious doubts may need help figuring out how and when to tell the couple that she has decided against it. The psychologist can assist her with this task, possibly supplying a medical or psychological reason why she should not proceed. Having a 'valid' reason from a professional can reduce feelings of regret or guilt that burden the prospective gestational carrier.

Couples usually pay close attention to the feelings and reactions of their gestational carrier and may sense when the woman has had a change of heart or is confused about whether she should continue the process. Having a psychologist who will step in and clarify what is going on may be a relief to them; once told that she is not available, they can begin to grieve the loss of this particular woman and decide if they want to seek another.

Willingness to Gestate a Multiple Pregnancy. The superovulation that occurs in stimulated cycles carries with it a 25 to 30 percent chance of multiple gestation. Consequently, every prospective gestational carrier must consider how she might react to learning that she is carrying more than one fetus, and possibly more than two.

Psychologists working in reproductive medicine know that many women discount the possibility of a multiple pregnancy. Consequently, it is imperative that the psychological assessment and preparation of the carrier address multiple gestation. The woman and the contracting couple must agree on how such a pregnancy would be handled. Otherwise, potential gestational carriers may blind themselves to the realities of their undertaking and later find themselves unprepared to deal with the challenges of a multiple gestation.

A prospective gestational carrier needs to give special consideration to the prospect of multifetal reduction. Before she can present her thoughts on it to her couple and the program staff, she must decide whether she would be willing to undergo a reduction and if so—or if not—whether she is prepared to live with the outcome (e.g., guilt following the procedure or, alternatively, guilt and sorrow if she refuses it and the babies are born very prematurely). As in surrogacy programs, every effort is made to pair gestational carriers and couples who have the same views on this subject. A woman opposed to abortion under any circumstances would be matched only with a couple who has similar feelings.

Ability to Handle Failure. Even the most successful IVF programs have significant failure rates. Gestational carriers working with older couples and others who have a diminished chance of success need to be able to anticipate failure. A volunteer carrier needs to give special thought to whether she will feel that she has disappointed a loved one. She needs to consider also what she will do if the couple wants her to attempt additional cycles.

Attitudes Toward Bonding During the Gestational Period. Although she may feel clear that the child will belong to the biological parents, the gestational carrier needs to try to understand how she perceives her role and how she is likely to feel toward the baby she is carrying. She can reflect on her earlier pregnancies and the extent to which she bonded with her baby in utero. If she bonded deeply during pregnancy, she needs to consider whether this situation is likely to be different. For women who volunteer to carry for their sisters, the issue of bonding to the baby is all the more complex since they will be genetically connected to the baby they carry.

Relationship With the Couple. Although it is difficult to anticipate exactly how their relationship will evolve, it is essential for gestational carriers and couples to consider several aspects of their relationship before undertaking gestational care and attempt to determine to what degree they have shared expectations of the experience.

There is no single way for a couple and a gestational carrier to conduct their relationship, but there are ways of going about it that will be right or wrong for certain individuals. For example, it would be a mistake for a woman who prefers some privacy during the pregnancy to be teamed with a couple in which both members look forward to attending almost every doctor's visit. Similarly, problems would be likely to arise if a woman who expected to develop a close and long-term relationship with her couple was matched with people who felt that a Christmas card was sufficient contact.

Informed Consent. Nada L. Stotland, M.D. Associate Professor of Clinical Psychiatry and Obstetrics and Gynecology at the University of Chicago discusses some of the complexities of assuring that there is informed consent within an obstetrical-gynecological setting. She mentions that informed consent presents special challenges with the ARTs since little is known about their medical or psychological long-term effects. Women have powerful, often con-

flictual, feelings about their reproductive organs, and a woman's reaction to an event or procedure cannot always be predicted by the
patient or her physician. Hence, it is imperative that psychologists
working in the ARTs, and especially those dealing with alternatives
involving third parties, establish informed consent.[18]

A psychologist working with a woman who wants to carry a
baby for another couple must begin by assuming that she is not
fully informed. She may have given careful consideration to gestational care but have incomplete information about the medical and
psychological challenges of the process. The role and responsibility
of the psychologist is to educate her by providing medical, psychological, legal, and social information.

In their eagerness to be pregnant through gestational care, potential carriers may fail to hear all that is presented to them; thus,
in-person interviews are often followed (or accompanied) by
written information. For example, the Center for Surrogate Parenting gives prospective candidates detailed letters with information about all facets of the program. After each piece of information, there is a box for the woman to initial, indicating that she
has read the material and agrees to abide by the expectations of
the program.

The Gestational Care Experience

Like ovum donation in which one woman's fertilized eggs are
transferred to another woman's uterus, the medical aspects of gestational care are especially challenging due to the necessity of syn-
chronizing two women's cycles. Since embryos cannot be transferred into a uterus that is not receptive to them, gestational
carriers are prescribed hormones that enable their menstrual cycle
to synchronize with the embryos. In other words, the woman who
carries the pregnancy and the woman whose eggs are being used
must be in the same phase of their cycle or the embryos will be unable to implant and will need to be cryopreserved.

The period after embryo transfer is stressful in every ART attempt, and perhaps even more so when it involves a gestational carrier. The high costs of gestational care and the reluctance of insurance companies to pay for the treatment prevent most couples
from trying more than once or twice. For many couples, a negative

pregnancy test following embryo transfer may well represent their last chance at genetic parenthood.

If a pregnancy is achieved—and the odds per transfer cycle are at best 40 percent (based on statistics from Pennsylvania Reproductive Associates)—then new challenges arise for couples and their gestational carrier: the threat of miscarriage, the risk that the pregnancy will be ectopic, or the risk of abnormalities.

Confirmation of a gestational care pregnancy often means that couples must face the challenges of multiple gestation. This is complicated since most couples, eager to be parents, welcome the possibility of two babies "for the price of one." Having engaged in this costly process in which the stakes are very high and the odds are against them, many couples are drawn to the idea of instant family. Moreover, for couples with a finite number of embryos or limited straws of frozen semen, the arrival of two babies would be a special blessing. Nonetheless, news of a multiple pregnancy brings mixed feelings for all involved since any multiple pregnancy is high risk. This risk increases with each fetus.

Although every gestational carrier is informed about the possibility of a multiple gestation prior to undergoing embryo transfer, some are still unprepared for what it means. A multiple pregnancy is both risky and stressful. There is a heightened chance of miscarriage or prematurity, and the gestational carrier may be advised to stay in bed for prolonged periods of time, a difficult task for a woman with children. She is also likely to gain a substantial amount of weight, something that is uncomfortable and limiting. Finally, there will occasionally be a gestational carrier who faces the extraordinarily difficult question of multifetal reduction. Although she will have been prepared for this decision in advance, the reality of the decision may indeed be different from what she anticipated.

Emotional Support for Couples and Gestational Carriers

Some gestational care programs offer ongoing support for the pregnant women and for their couples. This support can take a variety of forms, depending, in part, on geography. Dr. Braverman of Pennsylvania Reproductive Associates notes that many people travel a great distance in order to participate in her program. With those who live far from her center, Dr. Braverman maintains regular telephone contact—at least once a month with the carriers and at least once each trimester with the couples.

Couples or gestational carriers who live close to their program can meet, as needed, with the staff counselor or attend support groups. Steve Litz, director of Surrogate Mothers Inc., which offers both traditional and gestational surrogacy, reports that both types of surrogates in his program find it helpful to talk with other women who have gone through the process and have already delivered.

The relationship between gestational carriers and the couples for whom they carry is highly individual and depends on a number of factors, including personality, geography, and pregnancy outcome. However, nearly all couples and their carriers are likely to feel the need for professional support at various times during the process. It is therefore critical that a program psychologist be available to them throughout their efforts to conceive, as well as during and after the pregnancy.

Women who carry a baby for a friend or relative already have an ongoing relationship but may benefit from some assistance in sorting out how this relationship will change as a result of their decision to try gestational care. Among the challenges they face together is deciding how to deal with other family members and friends. A program counselor can meet with them together and separately to help them identify and address potentially difficult situations.

Arrangements between strangers allow for a wider range of options, including the possibility, at least theoretically, of little or no contact. However, experienced practitioners stress the benefits of a close and mutually supportive relationship between couples and their gestational carriers. The relationship between the two women is especially important, and whenever possible, the mother-to-be should attend the doctor's appointment with her gestational carrier. When geography or other factors prevent regular visits, both parties usually rely on frequent telephone calls. Dr. Hanafin reports that the most problematic situations that she has seen—and ones in which her assistance has been called upon and needed—have occurred when women pregnant through gestational care have felt that their couples were disinterested. In such instances, a counselor may need to intervene and let the couple know how they might better communicate their interest and appreciation.

The Birth Experience

The arrival of a child through gestational care is a wonderous event—truly a miracle of modern science. Couples and gestational carriers who have undertaken a pregnancy together look forward to delivery as a time of shared celebration.

Most couples make every effort to attend the birth of their child. They must be prepared, however, for the possibility that something will not go as planned. The baby may come early or labor may progress very rapidly, causing the parents-to-be to miss the delivery. One woman we spoke with had traveled two hours each way, throughout her gestational care pregnancy, in order to attend all medical appointments. She and her husband were prepared to leave for the hospital, with plenty of time to spare, as soon as they got the call that their gestational carrier was in labor. Their plans failed them however, when a tractor trailer jackknifed on the highway, and they were stuck in a five-hour traffic jam.

Most couples and the woman who carried their baby spend some time together following delivery. They have forged a strong bond, and it is important to maintain it in the hours that follow the birth. Gestational carriers take great pride and delight in seeing the new parents with their baby. Moreover, the couples' expressions of joy and appreciation help the women who carry and give birth to their babies reaffirm the rightness of their decision.

Couples report few difficulties with hospital staff. Rather, they say that staff frequently go out of their way to be helpful, to accommodate the new parents, and to adjust to this new form of parenthood. However, not everyone in the hospital setting will be familiar with or supportive of gestational care. Personnel may say or do unkind things, and hospitals may have rules and regulations that prove restrictive to the new parents.

As we mentioned earlier, some lawyers experienced with gestational care have developed procedures for assigning parental rights to the biological parents. These procedures depend, in part, on the state in which the gestational carrier gives birth and sometimes on the hospital. Each couple must make sure that their lawyer is familiar with the laws that will apply in the hospital where their gestational carrier gives birth and that he or she has taken appropriate steps, well in advance if possible, to ensure proper preparation of the birth certificate.

After the baby has arrived, the new parents and the woman who made their parenthood possible generally spend at least a few days together. This begins in the hospital but should include some transition time outside the hospital in which the carrier sees the parents with their new baby. This is especially important if the couple lives at a distance and will be leaving the city in which the gestational carrier gave birth. But even in more local arrangements, it is useful for the celebration that began in the hospital to continue in another setting—a restaurant or hotel. Most couples and carriers view this as a special time, during which the bonds between the two women grow even stronger. They say that spending this time together helps them get closure on the pregnancy experience and helps prepare them for the next phase of their relationship.

The weeks and months following birth involve certain challenges. The separation can feel both awkward and uncomfortable to both carriers and couples. Some say that they were not sure when and how to contact each other. They describe trying to balance their fears of being intrusive with their need to stay connected. Each may wait and hope that the other will call. For this reason, Dr. Hanafin recommends that couples and their gestational surrogates make a plan for their next contact before they separate. Knowledge that they will speak by telephone or exchange letters within a week or two makes it easier for each to say good-bye.

Although there may be some sadness upon separation, everyone involved is also motivated to move on. The carrier has family to return to; the pregnancy, while satisfying, was distracting and required considerable time and energy. Now she can focus more attention on her own children. The couple, now parents, have the thrill of settling into their new life: an experience that they may feel only partially prepared for because they were so conditioned to expect disappointment.

Gestational care remains a new and relatively uncommon path to parenthood, reserved for those willing to take on uncharted waters. Both the women who volunteer for this process and the couples who enter into agreements with them are betting against the odds.

Those who do so should go with full awareness of the complex medical, ethical, social, and possibly legal challenges that lie ahead.

Our sense is that couples and gestational carriers who decide to work together are strengthened by their common goal of bringing life to a child who would not otherwise exist and bringing genetic parenthood to a couple who has suffered reproductive loss and now has an opportunity to diminish that loss. It is a goal that celebrates the advances in modern reproductive medicine. One gestational carrier described her experience in this way:

> I had the chance to help people become parents who should have had a child long ago. For me, that was a very wonderful thing to be able to do. Every time they send me a picture of her, I feel filled with pride. There are many things I haven't done in my life so far, but I have helped bring someone into the world who was trying very hard to be born.

Embryo Adoption

Embryo adoption is the process whereby an embryo, created from the egg of a woman and the sperm of a man, is gestated in the womb of another woman to be raised by her and her partner neither of whom provided the gametes. Although we refer to this process as adoption, we use that term strictly in a social sense rather than in a legal one. Like traditional adoption, the couple who raises the child has no genetic connections to him or her, but unlike traditional adoption, the couple does not have to go through a legal process in order to be declared the child's legal parents. Instead of legally adopting the child after birth, however, as is the case in all other adoptions, the couple biologically adopts during the early embryonic stage—at the point of embryo transfer.

Embryo adoption is an option for couples who want to share a pregnancy experience and have neither eggs nor sperm to contribute to that process. Candidates include couples in which both partners fall into one of the categories that we mentioned in chapters 5 and 6. Embryo adoption is also an option for single women desiring a pregnancy who do not have a designated sperm donor and are unable to use their own eggs.

From a medical-technical standpoint there are two ways to accomplish the process of embryo adoption. The first is for couples to receive a preexisting cryopreserved embryo(s) that has been donated by its genetic parents. The second is for an ART clinic to arrange a cycle of ovum donation for the couple and to inseminate the donated eggs with donor sperm. Although both methods result in an offspring who is not genetically connected to the parents, from an ethical, emotional, and social policy perspective, these two avenues to embryo adoption are decidedly different.

We call the first option, which results from the donation of an existing embryo, *embryo donation*, and the second option—the intentional creation of a child through donated eggs and donated sperm—*embryo creation*. In both cases, the offspring has no genetic connection to the parents; we thus decided to place both options under the general heading of *embryo adoption*. We do recognize, however, that in a sense the use of the word 'adoption' may be somewhat misleading, as traditional adoption has never involved the intentional creation of children for the purpose of being adopted. Thus only one of these new options—namely embryo donation, which 'finds' homes/wombs for existing embryos—bears any resemblance to adoption.

Embryo donation, like traditional adoption, began as a perceived solution to a problem. IVF programs and their patients were troubled by the prospect of having extra embryos cryopreserved after IVF treatment. This question was of particular concern to people who had moral or religious objections to discarding embryos. The idea of donating those embryos to other infertile couples was appealing; it offered a creative use for these surplus embryos and the opportunity for pregnancy and parenthood to childless couples. Embryo donation was attractive to ART programs from a legal perspective as well. ART programs using embryo donation could avoid violating laws in states that prohibited experimenting on or discarding embryos.

Embryo donation has not proved to be the popular option that physicians and programs anticipated. Surprisingly, there are fewer embryos available for donation than anticipated, for two reasons. First, most couples use their frozen embryos, either following an unsuccessful cycle or, later, after the birth of a child(ren) to expand their families. Second, many couples who once indicated they would willingly donate embryos later conclude they are not comfortable with this choice.

Because of the scarcity of embryos available for donation and the large number of couples needing of both donated eggs and sperm, some clinics are now offering IVF cycles in which male and female donor gametes are used. This process may be considered as a logical extension of single gamete donation. Another reason for creating embryos is that the pregnancy rates, and, more important, the birth rates, are slightly lower with fresh embryos—about 10 to 15 percent per cycle.

Although from a genetic and social standpoint, offspring of created embryos are the same as the offspring of donated embryos, (they are not genetically related to either parent) the ethical differences between their origins are substantial. In one instance, the couple gestates and raises a child that began as an embryo that the genetic parents intended to gestate and raise themselves. In the second instance, couples are intentionally taking gametes from two separate donors and creating an embryo for the sole purpose of "prebirth adoption."

Embryo adoptions are clearly new paths to parenthood, bringing with them complex psychological, social, emotional, and ethical considerations. We have neither experience nor psychosocial research to draw upon. Thus we must borrow insights from the fields of adoption and donor insemination, as well as from our growing understanding of ovum donation.

Reasons for Choosing Embryo Adoption

Many people, both outside and inside the field of infertility, wonder why a couple would choose embryo adoption rather than adopting a child who is already born. There are many reasons why this alternative is appealing, most of which apply to both forms of embryo adoption. There are also reasons unique to both embryo creation and embryo donation. First we discuss the reasons that they share in common.

For couples who have experienced long-term infertility, embryo adoption offers two out of the three major reproductive experiences they feared losing. Although they will still miss out on having a genetic connection to their offspring, they will have the opportunity to be pregnant and give birth, as well as the opportunity to parent. Furthermore, embryo adoption offers the couple a chance to bond with their child prior to birth. In addition, the woman has control over her child's prenatal environment, thereby eliminating potential problems caused by unhealthy gestational conditions.

For couples who have adjusted to infertility treatment and for whom the thought of additional treatment is tolerable, embryo adoption may be preferable to tackling what they perceive as a complicated and often daunting new world—that of adoption. Furthermore, depending on the clinic and on whether the couple's health insurance policy covers the procedure, embryo adoption may be much more affordable than adoption after birth. Embryo adoption also offers the couple the guarantee of known paternity (not always the case with traditional adoption), assuming the clinic shares medical, social, and psychological information about the father in the case of embryo donation and the sperm bank provides the same information about the sperm donor in the case of embryo creation. Embryo adoption also offers couples privacy. Traditional adoption, by definition, is always public, whereas embryo adoption can be private, allowing the couple to reveal it or not on their own time frame.

Embryo donation is appealing to couples who have problems with the idea of intentionally creating children/embryos to adopt. They prefer knowing that the embryo they adopt was conceived by a couple who longed to be parents and went to great lengths to make it happen. Embryo donation is also appealing to couples who believe that the genes of the donating couple, whom they may imagine to be a close, loving pair, are in some way preferable to the imagined genes of birthparents. Embryo creation, on the other hand, is preferable to couples who believe it can offer them greater genetic selection. Although they realize that ovum donors are scarce and that donor selection may be limited, they know they can carefully select the sperm donor. This process of combining their choice of gametes may give them a greater sense of control, as well as the illusion that they are creating an ideal child.

Ethical Issues in Embryo Adoption

Some in the field of reproductive technology believe that the ethical issues of embryo adoption are the same for both created and donated embryos. Others make a distinction between the two. Thus, some clinics offer embryo donation but refuse to create donor embryos; in other words, they will not use both donor sperm and donor eggs in an ART cycle. Other clinics combine donor eggs and donor sperm to create embryos for couples but do not have an embryo donation program.

The Creation of Additional Children

An important ethical issue that arises is whether it is morally right to create embryos when there are already children awaiting adoption. Those who feel it is not ethical to do so believe that the desires of infertile couples are taking priority over societal good, thereby ignoring the best interest of children. Because embryo adoption is genetically identical to adoption after birth, programs that will not create embryos for this purpose believe that the advantages that come with being able to gestate are not sufficient justification to create additional children. They also do not agree that adoption is difficult (especially the adoption of a healthy white child, the choice most couples prefer) and that embryo adoption may be an easier route to having a child. Those who question the ethics of creating embryos for prebirth adoption believe that families do not have to be either racially or ethnically similar—that the ties necessary for maintaining healthy, loving families transcend racial or ethnic lines.

Elizabeth Bartholet, an adoptive parent (after many failed IVF cycles), also questions these assumptions about families. She is an outspoken advocate of the rights of children and an outspoken critic of the new reproductive technologies. Bartholet, in writing about all reproductive technologies that involve the use of third parties, states:

> Taking children's interests seriously would require us to think about the children we are creating with these new arrangements and about the children who already exist in this world. It would require us to ask whether it is good for children to be deliberately created so they can be spun off from their biologic parents and raised by others. It would require us to ask whether encouraging adults who might provide adoptive homes to produce their own adoptees is good for the existing children in need of such homes.[1]

Those who question the morality of embryo adoption when so many children are in need of homes also have an objection to the way in which resources are being allocated. They cannot justify spending enormous sums of money to create nongenetic children for parents. They do not believe it is right for couples or insurance companies to invest tens of thousands of dollars in this process, especially when the odds are against them. Rather, they argue, the money would be far better spent on reforming the adoption system and helping couples who cannot afford to adopt but would like to do so find children.

The arguments that it is wrong to create children for adoption, when there are living children in need of adoption, and that spending vast amounts of money to do so only accentuates the injustice do not necessarily pertain to embryo donation. When an infertile couple donates surplus cryopreserved embryos to other infertile couples, the recipient couple is not receiving embryos that were created specifically for that purpose. Rather, the embryos were intended to be used by the genetic parents, but due to a change in circumstances—usually the births of their desired number of children—they no longer need them. Because the embryos already exist, the financial cost of adopting them (usually between $3,000 and $4,000, the same as a frozen embryo transfer cycle) is much less than it would be if the couple created their own embryos via ovum donation and donor insemination.

The Commercialization of Embryos

Those who question the ethics of embryo creation are particularly concerned about the potential for commercialization—that donated embryos, as well as gametes used to create additional embryos, will become subject to supply and demand. Infertile couples in their desperation to have children will be willing to pay a high price—whatever the market will bear—for embryos to adopt or for gametes with which to create them. Some fear that the creation of donor embryos will become big business, with entrepreneurs emerging who will serve as embryo brokers, matching couples who can produce embryos to infertile couples who need them.

Bartholet addresses the question of commercialization:

The IVF process is increasingly used to facilitate full adoptions, whereby one couple's embryos are donated or sold to another for implantation. The advent of embryo freezing can be expected to encourage such arrangements on a large scale. Tens of thousands of frozen embryos are now being stored for future reproductive use; most of them will probably not be used by the contributing couples.[2]

Although her concerns are understandable and the potential for commercialization of embryos exists, current practice does not suggest this is happening—nor that it is likely to happen in the future. Only a small fraction of couples undergoing IVF procedures are requesting to use both donor eggs and donor sperm. Furthermore, when they do so—and when programs accede to this request—they are using eggs and sperm for which donors have received only modest compensation.

There seems little evidence that existing cryopreserved embryos will be commercialized. Most of these embryos are used by their genetic parents, either following a failed IVF cycle or as a means of expanding their family following a successful pregnancy. In addition, most clinics will not allow couples to accumulate an indefinite amount of embryos. Once a couple has accumulated a certain number (approximately four), they must have them transferred before undergoing a fresh IVF cycle. (This limit does not apply if more than the designated number are obtained in a particular cycle.) Thus, although it is true that ART programs have some "unwanted" frozen embryos, they are only a small percentage of those that were originally frozen. Furthermore we are aware of no programs that allow couples to sell rather than donate them.

Bartholet's concerns are not completely irrational. The procurement of eggs and sperm and the "rental" of wombs do have price tags, which many ethicists, attorneys, and some feminists feel are coercively high, while others feel are insultingly low. Hence it must appear to Bartholet and others that embryos too have a price, despite the fact that states have laws against such transactions. It is important for this discussion, however, to underscore the distinction between existing embryos, which currently may only be donated, not sold (donated embryos), and embryos, which might be intentionally created from male and female donor gametes (created embryos). The former do not have a price tag; the latter, particularly because they require donated gametes, may have the potential for commodification and commercialization.

Unfairness to Genetically Related Siblings

Most couples who offer their embryos for donation have completed their families. Another argument by those who object to embryo donation is that the resulting children will have genetic siblings whom they will not know. This situation, they say, is unfair to both the children who were born to their genetic parents as a result of IVF and the children born as a result of embryo adoption. Many who agree in principle with this objection say that the solution is not to prohibit embryo donation but to allow it only if it is done openly, so the genetic parents and/or siblings can have access to each other should they choose to do so. Others counter this objection by arguing that genetic bonds mean very little in and of themselves—that the bonds formed by kinship and family are the significant ones.

Other ethical concerns that we discussed in chapters 6 and 7 apply to embryo adoption as well: the right to have a child, especially by couples who are older and may be past normal childbearing years; the separation of the gestational-social and genetic aspects of mother and father (whether it is in a child's best interest to do so); the changing nature of family (whether it is in a child's best interest to be born through such an alternative arrangement, to parents whose age and life-style may preclude them from providing an optimal environment for their child); and the potential medical risks to ovum donors in procuring eggs. (The issue of medical risk applies only to created embryos.) Because embryo donation is so recent, the long-term emotional and psychosocial effects on a couple who have donated their jointly created embryos to another couple, probably anonymously, are unknown.

Psychosocial Issues in Embryo Adoption

Traditional adoption has changed drastically in the past decade, and many of these changes can and should be applied to embryo adoption.

Genealogical Bewilderment: The Need for Information

In the past, most adoption agencies operated on the premise that it was in the best interest of all parties for the birthmother and the adoptive parents to have little or no knowledge of each other and for birthparents to have little or no contact at all with their baby. Adoption workers believed that birthmothers would not be able to "cut the emotional cord" if they were permitted to know or to connect in any way with their offspring and that they would have difficulty getting on with their lives if they were to learn information—even nonidentifying information—about the couple who was going to adopt their child. Similarly it was believed that adoptive parents would have trouble bonding with their child or claiming him or her as their own if they met or even had knowledge about the birthparents. The prevailing theory was that it was better not to know—to let genetics unfold in a mysterious fashion.

Mental health professionals who work with adoptive families have come to understand, from listening to many adoptees, the yearning they have to know their genetic roots. Clinicians describe this phenomenon as genealogical bewilderment—a sense of not knowing from where one came or to whom one belongs. This yearning appears to be of fundamental importance for some adoptees, and seeking their genetic origins may be instrumental in helping them solidify their identity. The information learned helps them feel complete. The need to know where one comes from in no way seems to be a statement about a lack of bonding with their adoptive parents. On the contrary, adoptees who search often have secure relationships with their families. It may be because of this security that they feel permission to search, without having to fear rejection from the family that raised them—to whom they truly belong.

It appears that all parties to adoption have been shortchanged in the past. Birthmothers as well as adoptees have stepped forward to describe the aftermath of having their babies ushered away into what felt like a black hole, having no knowledge of where they were going and who would be raising them. Adoptive parents too craved information, especially as the years unfolded and they had no guideposts, and no facts, to offer their children. As a result of this climate of separation and secrecy and an awareness of the potentially harmful effects of genealogical bewilderment, the open adoption movement emerged.

Open adoption, a process in which birthparents and adoptive parents share information about themselves through letters, telephone calls, and sometimes personal visits, has gained, increasing recognition and acceptance from many adoption professionals whose agencies currently practice open adoption to varying degrees. Current policy in the adoption world—even among agencies that practice closed adoption—is to gather as much information as possible from birthparents about their medical, social, and emotional history. This information is shared with adoptive parents while preserving the privacy and anonymity of all parties. As the children grow, their parents can share information with them about their genetic connections. This information can be extremely helpful in ensuring a feeling of being tied to the past, developing a strong sense of oneself in the present, and having a sense of continuity about the future.

Embryo adoption offers the experience of pregnancy and childbirth—an experience longed for by many women. As soon as a child is born as a result of embryo adoption, however, the family experience is identical to that of other adoptive families, except that the former allows the mother to nurse her baby if she chooses to. (While it is difficult, it is possible for adoptive mothers to nurse babies.) Hence it is important to apply what we have learned from traditional adoption in setting policy regarding embryo adoption, especially the sharing of information between the genetic and the adopting parents. In behalf of their potential child, it is crucial that all adoptive parents—whether the adoption takes place after birth or prior to it—have access to information about their child's genetic parents' physical, medical, social, psychological, and educational history, information that is likely to help the child's identity formation and self-esteem.

Secrecy versus Openness

As recently as a generation ago many adoptive parents kept adoption a secret from their child, having been advised that it was best for the child not to know the truth about his or her origins. To some extent this rationale was a result of the stigma attached to illegitimate children. According to the theory, if children did not know they were adopted, they would not be subjected to humiliation.

This advice was not only psychologically harmful but impractical; it is impossible to hide adoption unless a couple moves to another part of the country and severs ties with family and friends. As long as a secret is known to some people—and in the case of adoption many know—it can always be revealed. In addition, since adoptees often look and act very different from their parents, many guess the truth. Some who were lied to initially when they asked if they were adopted were told the truth later, only to feel intensely betrayed. Now it is recognized that adopted children must be told the truth, and they need information about their birthfamily as well.

Although there has been a movement toward openness in the use of donor sperm, most couples who build their families in this way keep the information a secret from their child. Their reasons vary, but the stigma attached to infertility—in particular, male infertility—is probably the underlying reason for secrecy, regardless of whether it is acknowledged as the reason. Because the mother's pregnancy camouflages the couple's method of reproduction, it is tempting not to tell.

In embryo adoption, it is also tempting not to tell; the secret is easily hidden. However, children who are adopted—regardless of whether the adoption took place at the embryo stage or after birth—deserve to know the truth about themselves. Furthermore they deserve to know facts about their genetic history, facts that will help in their development and maturation.

Chapter 5 contains an extensive discussion of the ethical and psychosocial issues involved in secrecy versus openness with donor gametes, and we refer readers to that discussion.

Availability and Practice of Embryo Donation

The American Fertility Society has no listing of ART programs that offer embryo donation. There are programs that offer this option, however, seemingly on an ad hoc basis, but how it is done, who is eligible, and how many embryo donation transfers are performed appear to be a mystery. Since many ART programs began in the last five years and many have only recently added cryopreservation services, it is probably too soon to know whether ART programs will have enough donated embryos to establish embryo donation as a special service. The recent experience at the IVF America Program-Boston is telling and may be predictive of what can be expected in the future regarding the availability of embryo donation.

Prior to undergoing an ART cycle at IVF America Program-Boston couples have an initial consultation. This three-hour process includes separate meetings with a physician, psychologist, financial coordinator, and nurse. Meetings with the physician, in addition to reviewing whether the couple is medically appropriate for ART, include the signing of consent forms, one of which refers to the future disposition of frozen embryos that they may not want. Although couples are free to change their mind in the future, almost all couples choose to donate their unwanted embryos—should any exist—to an infertile couple.

In April 1993, IVF America Program-Boston sent out letters to 107 couples who had had frozen embryos in storage for at least two years. The purpose of the letter was to remind them about their embryos and to inquire about what they wanted to do with them: (1) use their embryos in a cycle within the next six months to try to establish a pregnancy for themselves, (2) leave them in storage, (3) instruct IVF America to discard them, (4) donate them to an infertile couple, (5) remove them from the clinic, or (6) donate them to research. Shari Litch, director of laboratory services at IVF America Program-Boston, stated that eighty-five couples responded to the letter (and a subsequent follow up) as of Nov. 1993. The most popular response (48 percent) was to delay the decision, leaving them in storage; 19 percent chose to use them in a cycle; 13 percent indicated they wished to donate them to research; 12 percent opted to discard; 4 percent opted to move them to another clinic; and 5 percent—only four couples of eighty-five—wished to donate them to an infertile couple. Thus of the eighty-five couples who responded to the letter, sixty opted to keep the embryos (i.e. to delay the decision, cycle within six months, or move them to another clinic). And of the twenty-five couples who opted not to keep their embryos, only four couples—16 percent of them—chose to donate to another couple. What was surprising was not the low incidence of couples' opting for donation to another couple but rather the dramatic change of heart by almost all couples.

Why did so many couples prior to beginning ART treatment indicate that they want to donate embryos they cannot use and later have a change of heart? One explanation is that because most couples with frozen embryos that have been stored over two years have children (63 percent of those who responded to the IVF America Program-Boston survey), they have living examples of what an embryo can become and cannot imagine giving up a child like the one they see in front of them. Another related explanation involves siblings. Individuals who donate their gametes are aware that their own children will have half-siblings whom they will probably never know. Although this may be troublesome to some gamete donors, it is usually not an insurmountable obstacle to gamete donation. However, when the picture changes and couples realize that their children will have full genetic siblings they will not know, what was once viewed as an altruistic act may begin to feel emotionally impossible. Finally, couples who have no children but have had frozen embryos in storage for over two years may not be able to live with the possibility that another couple could raise their genetic child while they remained childless.

The initial decision to donate has several explanations as well. One reason may be that couples at this stage in their infertility are feeling extremely vulnerable, at the mercy of their physicians, and do not want to do or say anything they fear might jeopardize their care. They may believe that choosing to donate is the "right" response, the one that will enable them to receive the best care, despite the fact that physicians go 'out of their way' to assure them otherwise. Another is that many couples attempt ART not imagining that it will work, let alone produce the number of children they desire. They opt for donation because they believe they do not really have to take that option seriously; it will probably never come to pass.

Elaine Gordon, a psychologist in southern California who works with several ART programs, offers an observation that sheds light on the differences between how people regard their gametes versus their embryos. She perceives that far more people seem willing to donate their individual gametes than to donate their joint embryos. From screening numerous women for ovum donation, many of whom have children and are married, we agree with these conclusions. Frequently potential donors say that they do not feel an egg is in any way close to a person. Once it is fertilized with the recipient's husband's sperm, they feel it is a long way from being their child, adding that if it were fertilized with their husband's sperm it would be a very different story; then it would be their potential child, and they could not give it to someone else. These observations hint at why only a small percentage of couples appear to be willing to donate embryos they created jointly: it feels as if they are giving up their child.

Programs must determine how much information they will share with couples about the gamete donors. This is true regardless of whether the embryos were created for purposes of adoption or whether they were originally created for an ART couple who later decide to donate them. We have already stressed the need for adopting couples to have extensive medical, physical, intellectual, and psychosocial information.

A related and important issue for programs that do have embryos available for donation is whether they will mix embryos from more than one couple in a single ART cycle. Since many couples who might opt to donate their frozen embryos have only one available and because pregnancy rates are low when just one embryo is transferred, it may be tempting to transfer embryos from more than one donating couple, to maximize the couple's chances of becoming pregnant. From a psychological and ethical perspective, we feel this policy is not a good one because it fails to take into consideration the best interests of the potential children.

Even if clinics provided extensive information about each couple whose embryos were donated, the adoptive parents would never know—unless they agreed to have their child undergo genetic testing after birth—whose child they were carrying should a pregnancy occur. The confusion in their minds could interfere with the bonding process that normally develops during pregnancy. Couples carrying their own genetic child often wonder whether he or she will have the husband's blue eyes, the wife's dark hair, his musical talent, her athletic ability. Many characteristics unfold over time and are part of the intrigue of parenthood. However, if couples had embryos transferred from more than one donor couple, they would never know—assuming they receive information about each couple—whether couple A, couple B, or couple C were the genetic parents of their child. They might find themselves scrutinizing their child, overly preoccupied with signs that will indicate whether he is destined to become a professional athlete, a mathematical genius, or a jazz musician. Even if they were provided information about each donating couple, they would be likely to have preferences for one couple's embryo over another. Should genetic testing reveal the child came from a couple who was not their first-choice genetic parents, they could be disappointed and possibly convey, though unintentionally, their feelings to their child.

Knowledge about a child's genetic blueprint can help parents attach only to the child who is theirs. We all understand that genes are a random collection from our parents, that musical genius in one parent (or even two) does not guarantee that offspring will inherit the desired trait. Although much of the pleasure in parenthood involves the unfolding of a mystery, most parents can turn to genetic history for guidance. Couples who are able to conceive and bear their genetic children are in for fewer surprises and less bewilderment about how their children become who they are. Even more important than parental knowledge, however, is our obligation to the offspring, for children who have no knowledge of their genetic history must live with a sense of bafflement about how they came to be and bewilderment about who they are. Our current understanding about human nature and the psychological development of human beings indicates that a genetic void is not in the best psychological interest of a person.

Those who advocate mixing embryos—and they tend to be physicians—argue that because the chances for pregnancy are better when more embryos are placed into the uterus, that should be sufficient reason for mixing. They believe that couples should be informed about their options, including the possibility of transferring embryos from more than one donor couple. Furthermore, they argue, if couples desire to mix embryos, they should be allowed to do so, and to create a policy against such a practice would be not only discriminating but paternalistic. Mental health clinicians counter that argument by reminding physicians that infertility is a major crisis. Infertile couples are often so desperate to have children that they may turn to the most expedient alternative available without thinking through the medical or psychological ramifications of that choice. Whether this issue becomes one that is hotly debated in ART programs remains to be seen and will probably depend on whether the findings at IVF America Program-Boston are indicative of the feelings of most ART couples or a statistical anomaly. If they are typical, clearly there will be very few embryos available, and recipient couples will be fortunate to get any embryos, let alone, from more than one couple.

Embryo donation seems to be rare among ART programs, although it is being done occasionally, at selected clinics. However, there are clinics willing to procure both donor eggs and donor sperm, thereby creating donor embryos for couples who need (and want) both sources of gametes. Both methods of embryo adoption produce the same result: a child not genetically connected to the rearing parents but gestated by the mother. Embryo creation is a much more controversial means of obtaining embryos for adoption; however, because donor embryos are not readily available, it may ultimately prove to be the only option.

Conclusion

Infertile couples travel unexpected journeys. For some, the journey is long and arduous, but its course is clear. For others, there are a series of bumps in the road, points at which their hopes and dreams are tossed about, but eventually they reach their destination. Still others come to one or more forks in the road where they are forced to make difficult and unanticipated decisions.

Sooner or later, the journey through infertility ends, and a new journey, beyond infertility, begins. Most are accompanied on this new journey by young travelers, children who have come to them in unexpected ways. Some of these children were conceived through assisted reproductive technology; their lives began on the cutting edge of science. Others are born through third-party reproduction; someone who will not parent them was instrumental in giving them life.

As they move beyond infertility, people remember where they have been; no one endures the pain and struggle of infertility and then forgets it. Our hope, however, is that the next journey will be an easier one, filled with unexpected pleasures and satisfactions. Our experience with infertile couples who ultimately choose to be parents is that this is almost always the case. Parenthood, so long sought and hard earned, is treasured in unanticipated ways.

Although it is clear to us that people are drawn to the new technologies—and in some cases driven—out of profound and intense urges toward biogenetic parenthood, it is equally clear to us that couples do not have to give birth, or be a genetic parent, in order to experience the joys, challenges, and fulfillment of parenthood. Although this book has been about medical solutions and resolutions to infertility, many couples do move on to adoption, whether it is a second- or even a third-choice route for building a family. We do not wish to convey in any way that we feel adoption is a less desirable choice. Rather, it is an ideal way for children who need homes, and for adults who want to parent, to find each other.

Because we believe strongly that happy, healthy, families can be built in many ways, we conclude with a favorite passage about adoption written by Elizabeth Bartholet. Although she is not a fan of the new reproductive technologies, Bartholet is a true believer in adoption. After struggling long and hard with infertility, this veteran of several failed IVF cycles writes the following words about her two sons, whom she adopted in Peru:

> But I could not have expected these two particular magical children. I could not have predicted the ways in which they would crawl inside my heart and wrap themselves around my soul. I could not have known that I would be so entirely smitten, as a friend described me, so utterly possessed. And I could not have anticipated that this family formed across continents would seem so clearly the family that was meant to be, that these children thrown together with me and with each other, with no blood ties linking us together or to a common history, would seem so clearly the children meant for me.[1]

As people emerge from the painful journey of infertility, many discover unforeseen joys in unexpected families.

Resource List

American Fertility Society
1209 Montgomery Highway
Birmingham, Alabama 35216
(205) 978-5000

Center for Loss in Multiple
    Birth (CLIMB)
c/o Jean Kollantai
P.O. Box 1064
Palmer, Alaska 99645

Childfree Network
7777 Sunrise Blvd, Suite 1800
Citrus Heights, CA 95610
(916) 773-7178

Donor's Offspring
P.O. Box 37
Sarcoxie, MO 64862
(417) 548-3679

Organization of Parents
    Through Surrogacy (OPTS)
National Headquarters
750 North Fairview Street
Burbank, CA 91505
(818) 848-3761

RESOLVE INC.*
1310 Broadway
Somerville, MA 02144-1731
Helpline: (617) 623-0744

*RESOLVE is a national, nonprofit charitable organization which offers counseling, information, advocacy and support to people with problems of infertility and education to associated professionals. RESOLVE'S mission is: "to provide compassionate and informed help to people experiencing the infertility crisis, and to increase visibility about infertility issues via concerted advocacy and public education."

Glossary

ART assisted reproductive technology; high-tech procedures that usually include superovulation and the manipulation of eggs and sperm.

beta subunit See HCG.

biochemical pregnancy a pregnancy that barely begins and ends almost immediately; diagnosed slowly by a beta subunit test. Most women would not even know they were pregnant; probably the only sign would be a slightly late menstrual period.

cryopreservation the process of freezing for future use; can be used for sperm and embryos but not eggs.

DES diethylstilbesterol; synthetic estrogen, given primarily in the 1950s and 1960s, presumably to prevent miscarriage; Later proved to be ineffective and also determined to cause potentially serious side effects in the offspring of mothers who took it.

donor a person who donates eggs or sperm.

donor insemination (DI) the process of inseminating a woman with sperm obtained from a man who is not her partner.

ectopic pregnancy a pregnancy that occurs outside the uterus, most frequently in a fallopian tube.

egg retrieval the process of removing eggs from the ovaries, usually done under an ultrasound-guided needle aspiration procedure.

embryo a fertilized egg that has at least two cells; generally embryos are transferred into the uterus when they are between two and twelve cells.

embryo transfer the process of placing embryos back into the uterus, usually done transcervically with a small catheter. The process is similar to an intrauterine insemination.

fetus a stage of development after embryo, arbitrarily defined as when the eyelids fuse, at the end of organogenesis; approximately sixty days after conception.

follicle fluid-filled cystic structure in the ovary in which the egg matures.

FSH follicle-stimulating hormone; a hormone released by the pituitary, along with luteinizing hormone, that stimulates the ovary, leading to follicular growth and maturation.

gamete an egg or a sperm.

gestational care the process whereby a woman agrees to gestate an embryo/fetus/child for another couple who contributed the gametes.

gestational carrier the woman who gestates an embryo/fetus/child for another couple; also referred to as a gestational surrogate.

GIFT gamete intrafallopian transfer; a new reproductive technology whereby eggs and sperm are transferred into the fallopian tube via a catheter.

HCG human chorionic gonadotropin; the hormone produced by early pregnancy tissue and therefore measured to diagnose and monitor a pregnancy; also used to trigger ovulation in ART because it acts like LH.

hyperstimulation syndrome a usually mild but potentially serious condition resulting from ovaries that have overresponded to fertility drugs.

intracytoplasmic sperm injection (ICSI) a micromanipulation technique whereby a single sperm is injected directly into the center of the egg cell.

intrauterine insemination (IUI) the process of placing sperm directly into a woman's uterus.

IVF in vitro fertilization; the process whereby eggs are removed from a woman's body and fertilized with a man's sperm; usually involves superovulation.

laparoscopy an operation, usually done under general anesthesia, when the physician looks into a patient's abdomen with a thin telescope-like instrument. This can be done for diagnostic or operative procedures and is the procedure most frequently used for GIFT.

LH luteinizing hormone; a hormone released by the pituitary, along with FSH, that stimulates the ovary, leading to follicular growth and ovum maturation. A sharp increase or surge in LH triggers ovulation.

Lupron a drug, given by injection, that suppresses the ovaries by shutting down the body's normal production of LH and FSH.

Metrodin a fertility-enhancing drug that is composed of pure FSH; given by injection.

micromanipulation/microinsemination the use of sophisticated tools and equipment for the purpose of facilitating fertilization.

morphology appearance; one of the parameters used to indicate sperm function.

motility movement; one of the parameters used to indicate sperm function.

multifetal reduction the process of aborting one or more fetuses in a multiple gestation, thereby reducing the number of developing fetuses to a more manageable, and therefore less risky, number.

natural IVF cycle an IVF cycle in which superovulation is not induced.

oocyte an egg; also referred to as an ovum.

ovum an egg; also referred to as an oocyte.

partial zona dissection a micromanipulation technique that involves making a slit in the shell of the egg, allowing the sperm easier access.

pergonal fertility-enhancing drug that is composed of equal parts of LH and FSH; given by injection.

polyspermia the fertilization of an egg by more than one sperm. These embryos are not viable.

premature ovarian failure the premature cessation of ovarian function, usually defined as before thirty-five years old.

semen analysis   a diagnostic test assessing male fertility, measured by count, motility, and morphology of sperm.

subzonal injection (SZI)   a micromanipulation technique that involves injecting sperm directly into an egg, just beneath the shell (zona pellucida).

superovulation   the administration of medication for the purpose of producing multiple eggs.

surrogate   a woman who conceives and bears a child for another couple, using the sperm of the male partner of that couple.

third-party parenting   the process in which a third person is necessary in order to establish parenthood (sperm or ovum donation, surrogacy, or gestational care).

ultrasound technology   noninvasive technique of visualizing internal structures using high-frequency sound waves; in ART it is used to measure follicular growth and guide needle placement for egg retrieval; also used to monitor early pregnancy.

ZIFT   zygote intrafallopian transfer; a new reproductive technology in which zygotes are transferred into the fallopian tube via laparoscopy.

zona pellucida   the shell around the outer part of the egg.

zygote   a fertilized egg that has not begun dividing.

Notes

Chapter 1

1. C. Mazure and D. Greenfeld, "Psychological Studies of In Vitro Fertilization/Embryo Transfer Participants, "*Journal of In Vitro Fertilization and Embryo Transfer* 6, no. 4 (1989).

2. M. Seibel and J. McCarthy, "Infertility, Pregnancy and the Emotions," in Mind/Body Medicine, Editors, D. Goleman and J. Gurin, *Journal of Consumer Reports Book* NY (1993).

3. A. Domar et al., "The Mind/Body Program for Infertility: A New Behavioral Treatment Approach for Women with Infertility," *Fertility and Sterility* 53, no. 2 (February 1990), and "Psychological Improvement in Infertile Women after Behavioral Treatment: A Replication," *Fertility and Sterility* 58, no. 2 (July 1992).

4. B. Eck Menning, *Infertility: A Guide for the Childless Couple*, Prentice Hall, 1977 Englewood Cliffs, N.J.; E. Kübler-Ross, *Death: The Final Stage of Growth*, Prentice Hall, 1975

5. S. Cooper, "Female Infertility: Its Effect on Self-Esteem, Body Image, Locus of Control, and Behaviors" (Doctoral diss., Boston University, 1979).

6. M. Sandelowski, et al., "Mazing: Infertile Couples and the Quest for a Child," *Image: Journal of Nursing Scholarship* 21 (1989): 220–226.

7. E. W. Freeman et al., "Psychological Evaluation and Support in a Program of In Vitro Fertilization and Embryo Transfer," *Fertility and Sterility* 43 (1985).

8. P. Mahlstedt et al., "Emotional Factors and the In Vitro Fertilization and Embryo Transfer Procedure," *Journal of In Vitro Fertilization and Embryo Transfer* 4 (1987): 232–236.

9. A. Domar, The Psychological Impact of Infertility: A comparison to patients with other medical conditions. *J. of Psychosomatic Obstetrics and Gynaecology*, 12/93.

Chapter 2

1. Elaine Baruch, "A Womb of His Own," Women & Health, Binghampton, NY, Haworth Medical Press, 1987.
2. Elizabeth Bartholet, *Family Bonds* (Boston: Houghton Mifflin, 1993).
3. A. Whittemore et al., *American Journal of Epidemiology* (January 1993).
4. Vatican, *Instruction on Respect for Human Life in Its Origin and on the Dignity of Procreation*, Joseph Cardinal Rutzinger, Alberto Bovone approved by Pope John Paul II Rome, Feb. 22, 1987.
5. Ibid.
6. Ibid.
7. Ibid.
8. Ibid.
9. Committee of Inquiry into Human Fertilization and Embryology, *Report* HMSO, London (July 1984).
10. Davis V. Davis, Tennessee Supreme Court, 1/28/92.
11. John Robertson, Resolving Disputes over Frozen Embryos, Hasting's Center Report, Nov./Dec. 1989.
12. M. Sandelowski et al., "Pregnant Moments: The Process of Conception in Infertile Couples," *Research in Nursing and Health* 13(1990): 273–282.
13. A. C. Van Steirteghem et al. Intracytoplasmic Sperm Injection (ICSI). Scientific Program of the American Infertility Society, Vol. 49: 545, 1993, Abstract 0–096.

Chapter 3

1. Stefan Semchyshyn and Carol Colman, *How to Prevent Miscarriage* (New York: Collier, 1989).
2. Ecker, J.L. Laufer, M.R. & Hill, J.A., "Measurement of Embryo Toxic Factor is Predictive of Pregnancy Outcome in Women with a History of Recurrent Abortion." *Obstetrics & Gynecology* (1993) Vol. 81, p. 84–87.

3. Helene Deutsch, *The Psychology of Women II* (New York: Bantam Books, 1945).
4. Sandy Lee, Our Newsletter: A Multiple Birth Loss Support Network Vol. VI No. 1 p. 8–9.
5. Jean Kollantai, Center for Loss in Multiple Birth, Palmer, Alaska personal correspondence
6. Private Conversation, Anonymous.
7. Kollantai, personal correspondence.
8. *Insights into Infertility* (Spring 1992). Author anonymous "A Patients Dilemma: Pregnancy Reduction."
9. Anonymous patient interview

Chapter 5

1. David Berger et al., *Canadian Journal of Psychiatry* Vol. 31 (December 1986). Psychological Patterns in Donor Insemination Couples
2. Andrea Braverman, "Survey Results on the Current Practice of Ovum Donation," *Fertility and Sterility* (June 1993).
3. Sherman Elias and George Annas, "Social Policy Considerations in Noncoital Reproduction" (1986). The Journal of the American Medical Association Jan. 3, 1986; 255: 62–68
4. Susan Klock, "Psychological Aspects of Donor Insemination," *Infertility and Reproductive Clinics of North America* 4, no. 3 (July 1993).
5. Patricia Mahlstedt and Dorothy Greenfeld, "Assisted Reproductive Technology with Donor Gametes: The Need for Patient Preparation," *Fertility and Sterility* (December 1989).
6. Elizabeth Noble, *Having Your Baby by Donor Insemination* (1987). Houghton Mifflin, 1987.
7. Klock and Maier, Psychological factors related to Donor Insemination *Fertility and Sterility*, 56: 484–495, 1991
8. Mahlstedt and Greenfeld, "Assisted Reproductive Technology."
9. Annette Baran and Reuben Pannor, *Lethal Secrets* (1989). NY, Warner Books
10. Ibid.
11. Noble, *Having Your Baby By Donor Insemination*.
12. Turner, personal conversation.
13. George Annas, *Family Law Quarterly* 14, no. 1 (1980).

14. Mahlstedt and Greenfeld, "Assisted Reproductive Technology."
15. Baran and Pannor, *Lethal Secrets*.
16. Ibid.
17. Ibid.
18. Ibid.
19. New South Wales Infertility Social Workers Group, *How I Began: The Story of Donor Insemination* (Fertility Society of Australia, 1988).
20. Elaine Gordon, *Mommy Did I Grow in Your Tummy?* EM Greenberg Press, Inc. 1992
21. American Fertility Society, *Guidelines for Gamete Donation: 1993* (Birmingham, Alabama: American Fertility Society, 1993). These guidelines are not regulations; sperm banks are free to adhere to them or not. And although these guidelines were primarily written to ensure high-quality standards and practice for anonymous sperm banks, they also state that when a known donor is used, he too should be subject to the same standards as anonymous donors.
22. Baran and Pannor, *Lethal Secrets*.
23. Ken Daniels, "Psychosocial Issues Associated with Being a Semen Donor," *Clinical Reproduction and Fertility* (1986). 4, 341–351.
24. American Fertility Society, *Guidelines*.
25. Ken Daniels, "Semen Donors in New Zealand: Their Characteristics and Attitudes," *Clinical Reproductive Fertility* (August 1987). 5, 177–190.
26. Patricia Mahlstedt and Kris Probasco, Sperm Donors: Their attitudes toward providing medical and psychosocial information for recepient couples and donor offspring. Fertility and Sterility. Vol. 56 No. 4 Oct. 1991
27. Elias and Annas, "Social Policy Considerations in Non-Coital Reproduction."
28. Daniels, "Semen Donors in New Zealand."

Chapter 6

1. Lutjen et al. The establishment and maintenance of a pregnancy using in vitro fertilization and embryo donation in a patient with ovarian failure. *Nature 1984*; 207: 174–176
2. American Fertility Society, Guidelines for Gamete Donation: 1993 *Fertility and Sterility*, Supplement 1, February 1993, vol. 59, No. 2

3. A. Braverman, et al. "Survey Results on the Current Practice of Ovum Donation," *Fertility and Sterility* (June 1993).
4. Marcia Angell, "New Ways to Get Pregnant," *New England Journal of Medicine*, October 25, 1990.
5. Braverman, "Survey Results on the Current Practice of Ovum Donation."
6. Whittemore et al., *American Journal of Epidemiology* (January 1993).
7. Braverman, "Survey Results on the Current Practice of Ovum Donation."
8. Ibid.
9. Ibid.
10. Ibid.
11. Ibid.
12. Elaine Gordon, personal conversation.

Chapter 7

1. Center for Surrogate Parenting, Inc. Newsletter (May 1993).
2. *Between Strangers: Surrogate Mothers, Expectant Fathers, and Brave New Babies* (New York: Harper & Row, 1990).
3. Fay Johnson, Director of National Headquarters, OPTS, personal conversation
4. William Handel, Esq. Director, Center for Surrogate Parenting, Beverly Hills personal conversation.
5. Michelle Harrison, "Financial Incentives for Surrogacy," *Women's Health Institute Journal* 1, no. 3 (1991).
6. American College of Obstetricians and Gynecologists, Opinion 88 (November 1990). Reference in Women's Health Institute Journal Vol. No. 3 (Summer 1991: 133).
7. Frank Chervenak and Laurence McCullough, "Respect for the Autonomy of the Pregnant Woman in Surrogacy Agreements: An Elaboration of a Fundamental Ethical Concern," *Women's Health Institute Journal* 1 (1991).
8. Gena Corea, *The Baby Machine* (New York: Harper & Row, 1985).
9. Andrews, Lori *Between Strangers: Surrogate Mothers ...* pg 40–46

10. Steven Litz, Esq. Director of Surrogate Mothers, Indianapolis, In., personal conversation
11. Hilary Hanafin Phd; Gerry Tarlow Phd personal conversations
12. Lori Andrews, *Between Strangers*. Harper & Row, N.Y., 1989, pg. 127–38 pg 148–70 pg 171–88
13. Lori Andrews, *Between Strangers* Harper & Row, N.Y. 1989 pg. 167
14. ACOG, Opinion 88.
15. Nancy Hughes, personal conversation
16. William Handel, Esq personal conversation
17. Fagan, Ralph, Center for Surrogate Parenting, Letter, May, 1993
18. Fay Johnson, OPTS, personal correspondence
19. Michael Grodin, "Surrogate Motherhood and the Best Interests of the Child," Women's Health Institute Journal 1, no. 3 (1991).
20. Patricia Johnston, *Adopting After Infertility* (Perspectives Press, Indianapolis Indiana 1992).
21. Gena Corea, *The Mother Machine* New York: Harper & Row 1985
22. Elizabeth Kane, *Birthmother* (New York: Harcourt Brace Jovanovich, 1988); *People*, Sept. 28, 1992 pg. 69–75.
23. Hanafin, personal conversation.
24. Hanafin; P. J. Parker, "Motivation of Surrogate Mothers: Initial Findings," *American Journal of Psychiatry* 140 (1983): 117–18.
25. Hanafin, personal conversation
26. Parker, "Motivation of Surrogate Mothers."
27. Hilary Hanafin, "Surrogate Parenting: Reassessing Human Bonding (paper presented at the American Psychological Association Conference, New York, August 28, 1987).
28. Cristie Montgomery, personal conversation
29. Hanafin,
30. Ibid.
31. Ibid.
32. Ibid.
33. William Handel, personal conversation
34. Nancy Hughes Phd, Hagar Associates, Topeka, Kansas, personal conversation
35. Fay Johnson, personal conversation.
36. Hanafin, personal conversation.

37. Montgomery, personal conversation
38. Kathy Forest, "Surrogate Mothers' Experiences and Social Support Networks" (master's thesis, Colorado State University, 1989).
39. Hanafin, "Surrogate Parenting."
40. M. Grodin, "Surrogate Motherhood and the Best Interests of the Child," Women's Health Institute Journal 1, no. 3 (Summer 1991).
41. American College of Obstetricians and Gynecologists, Opinion No. 88 from the Committee on Ethics, *Women's Health Institute Journal* 1, no. 3 (Summer 1991): 133.
42. Hanafin, "Surrogate Parenting."
43. Susan Crockin, Esq, personal conversation
44. Carol Wolfe, personal conversation; Hanafin, "Surrogate Parenting."
45. Hanafin, "Surrogate Parenting."
46. Montgomery, personal conversation
47. Hanafin, personal conversation
48. Steven Litz, personal conversation
49. Center for Surrogate Parenting,
50. Forest, "Surrogate Mothers' Experiences."
51. Johnson, personal conversation
52. Hanafin, personal conversation
53. OPTS The Organization of Parents Through Surrogacy, News (Winter–Spring 1990).

Chapter 8

1. Mary English, Andrea Mechanick-Braverman, and Stephen Corson, "Semantics and Science: The Distinction Between Gestational Carrier and Traditional Surrogacy Options," *Women's Health Institute Journal* 1, no. 3 (Summer 1991).
2. Cristie Montgomery, personal conversation
3. Gerry Tarlow; Nancy Hughes. personal conversations
4. American College of Obstetricians and Gynecologists, Opinion 88 (November 1990).
5. George Annas, "Determining the Fate of Gestational Mothers," *Women's Health Institute Journal* 1, no. 3 (Summer 1991).

6. Nancy Reame, "The Surrogate Mother as a High-Risk Obstetric Patient," *Women's Health Institute Journal*
7. Mary English, Andrea Mechanick-Braverman, and Stephen Corson, "Semantics and Science: The Distinction Between Gestational Carrier and Traditional Surrogacy Options," *Women's Health Institute Journal* 1, no. 3 (Summer 1991).
8. Hilary Hanafin, personal conversation
9. William Handel, personal conversation
10. Steven Litz, personal conversation
11. *Fertility News* (June 1993).
12. Johnson v. Calvert, Daily Appelate Report, California Supreme Court, May 27, 1993. Case #S023721
13. Hanafin, personal conversation
14. Braverman, personal conversation
15. Hanafin; Montgomery personal conversations
16. Lori Capone, letter to the editor, Sacramento Bee, March 11, 1992
17. Fay Johnson, personal conversation
18. Nada Stotland, "Ethical Dimensions of Informed Consent: A Psychiatric Perspective," *Women's Health Institute Journal* 3, no. 1 (Spring 1993).

Chapter 9

1. Elizabeth Bartholet, *Family Bonds: Adoption and the Politics of Parenting* (Boston: Houghton Mifflin, 1993).
2. Ibid.

Conclusion

1. Elizabeth Bartholet, *Family Bonds: Adoption and the Politics of Parenting* (Boston: Houghton Mifflin, 1993).

Index